Enabling Collaborative Health Intelligence With Federated Learning

Ng Khai Mun
https://orcid.org/0000-0002-8263-9275
Infrastructure University Kuala Lumpur, Malaysia

Chin-Shiuh Shieh
https://orcid.org/0000-0003-3187-458X
National Kaohsiung University of Applied Sciences, Taiwan

Danish Ather
https://orcid.org/0000-0003-1596-5553
Amity University, Tashkent, Uzbekistan

Arvind Panwar
School of Computer Science and Engineering, Galgotias University, Greater Noida, India

Vishal Jain
https://orcid.org/0000-0003-1126-7424
Kuala Lumpur University of Science and Technology, Malaysia & Vivekananda Institute of Professional Studies, New Delhi, India

IGI Global
Scientific Publishing
Publishing Tomorrow's Research Today

Vice President of Editorial — Melissa Wagner
Director of Acquisitions — Mikaela Felty
Director of Book Development — Jocelynn Hessler
Production Manager — Mike Brehm
Cover Design — Jose Rosado

Published in the United States of America by
IGI Global Scientific Publishing
701 East Chocolate Avenue
Hershey, PA, 17033, USA
Tel: 717-533-8845 | Fax: 717-533-7115
Website: https://www.igi-global.com E-mail: cust@igi-global.com

Library of Congress Cataloging-in-Publication Data

LCCN: 2025019843 (CIP Data Pending)
ISBN13: 9798337333069
Isbn13Softcover: 9798337333076
EISBN13: 9798337333083
British Cataloguing in Publication Data
A Cataloguing in Publication record for this book is available from the British Library.

Table of Contents

Detailed Table of Contents

This research investigates how parents of children with intellectual disability cope in two support frameworks: Adaptive Governance (AG) and the Internet of Things (IoT). Having 60 participants divided on the basis of family type (Joint, Nuclear, Extended) and income (High or Low), the research measures coping mechanisms by utilizing the Brief COPE Inventory. Major areas measured are Active Coping, Emotional Support, Denial, Planning, and Behavioural Disengagement. Results indicate that high-income joint families used more adaptive coping mechanisms—Active Coping (M=6.63 in IoT) and Planning (M=5.53 in AG)—whereas low-income nuclear families showed greater instances of avoidant coping such as Denial and Behavioural Disengagement. IoT interventions uniformly enhanced adaptive coping in all types of families because of real-time aid and intelligent caregiving capabilities. AG ensured policy flexibility but was weaker in modulating immediate behavioural responses. The research determines that the integration of AG and IoT makes for a more efficient caregiving environmen.

With the growing demand for secure, intelligent, and collaborative healthcare systems, Federated Learning (FL) has emerged as a transformative approach for developing AI models without exposing sensitive patient data. This chapter provides a detailed overview of FL's core architecture and its specialized variants—such as hierarchical, asynchronous, and personalized FL—tailored to healthcare's distributed and privacy-

Healthcare AI has federated learning as a transformational approach in which clinical research can be conducted collaboratively and in patient privacy is preserved. This chapter considers federated learning and how it enables healthcare institutions to learn from sensitive data without centralizing it and without access to that data. It consists of the technological architecture, companding local computational resources, secure communication channels, and model aggregation servers, each with a suitable algorithm for dealing with data heterogeneity between institutions. Its integration with existing healthcare infrastructure (IoMT devices, EHR systems) ensures operational efficiency thus being integrated into the existing system. By balancing innovation with privacy, federated learning is positioned as a cornerstone technology for the development of the personalized medicine — which with technology giants as the players the only type in which patient privacy can be respected while taking advantage of the collective clinical wisdom.

This chapter explores the integration of Federated Learning (FL) and Explainable Artificial Intelligence (XAI) in healthcare, emphasizing their potential to revolutionize AI-driven medical solutions while preserving data privacy and building trust. It examines how FL enables collaborative model training across decentralized data sources without sharing sensitive patient information, addressing critical issues of data security and compliance. The chapter also investigates the role of XAI in enhancing interpretability and transparency in federated models, a crucial factor for clinical adoption. Through discussion of local and global explainability, real-world applications, and emerging challenges such as data heterogeneity, communication costs, and algorithmic bias, the chapter provides a comprehensive view of how FL and XAI jointly contribute to more secure, accountable, and effective AI systems in healthcare.

The combination of Federated Learning (FL) and Collaborative AI has brought significant changes to the healthcare industry due to challenges with data centralization, privacy, and compliance issues. FL allows for decentralized model training in different institutions and does not require raw data to be shared among them, thus protecting patient information while improving the model. Collaborative AI also enhances healthcare innovation through human-AI cooperation, collaboration across institutions, and integration of multiple data modalities. This chapter explores the basics of these paradigms, the technical models, and revolutionary uses of such concepts in diagnosing diseases, imaging, individualized medicine, and remote patient monitoring. Due to the relevance of FL and Collaborative AI, it is possible to develop the next generation of medical intelligence that is smarter, ethical, scalable, and without violating user privacy, ensuring equal access to healthcare for everyone.

Large-scale data sharing is important for developing reliable and accurate diagnostic models, but it has been mostly delayed by the sensitive nature of healthcare data and information. By allowing different healthcare institutions to collaborate on AI models unless sharing patient information, federated learning (FL) and collaborative artificial intelligence (CAI) have become advanced strategies to address these limitations. FL and CAI have the capability to increase diagnosis outcomes by improving model quality, lowering diagnostic cost, providing safe and confidential partnerships for AI-powered healthcare. By sending only model update information, FL allows remote data model training. This method protects data privacy by utilizing the combined expertise of several diagnostic institutions. Smart healthcare practitioners can design multi-institutional models that improve diagnostic precision, early disease prediction, and provide treatment recommendations by utilizing CAI. FL with CAI is transforming medical diagnostics into smart healthcare by promoting data security and privacy.

spontaneous collaboration in quiet departments, specifications and organizations and at the same time maintain strict data above. Implementation of FL in the health care system enables a strong future analysis, individual remedies recommendations and enlarged clinical decision support systems that are attracted by diverse patient population without compromising privacy.

Preface

When digital health technologies are redefining medical practices, the integration of Federated Learning (FL) and Collaborative Artificial Intelligence (AI) presents a paradigm shift for healthcare innovation. By enabling decentralized data analysis while preserving privacy and security, FL is emerging as a cornerstone technology that addresses some of the most pressing challenges in medical AI: data silos, regulatory constraints, and the need for personalization.

This edited volume, *Enabling Collaborative Health Intelligence With Federated Learning*, brings together contributions from a diverse group of international scholars and practitioners at the intersection of AI, healthcare, data science, and ethics. The chapters collectively explore how federated approaches can facilitate secure, collaborative, and intelligent healthcare systems, offering a roadmap to future-ready medical ecosystems.

The book begins by laying a foundation with real-world applications of AI and caregiving ecosystems, then transitions into technical explorations of FL architecture, security enhancements, and practical implementations in areas such as mental health, diabetes management, medical diagnostics, and imaging. By spanning theoretical models, applied research, and case studies, this collection serves as both a scholarly reference and a practical guide for researchers, clinicians, and policymakers aiming to build privacy-respecting, data-driven healthcare innovations.

CHAPTER OVERVIEW

Chapter 1: A Hybrid Caregiving Ecosystem: Integrating Adaptive Governance, IoT, and Sustainable Development for the Care of Intellectually Disabled Children

This chapter presents an empirical study of caregiving strategies for intellectually disabled children, focusing on the integration of Adaptive Governance (AG) and the Internet of Things (IoT). The findings underscore the importance of combining policy flexibility with real-time technological interventions to foster adaptive coping mechanisms in families, especially across varied socioeconomic contexts.

Chapter 2: Advancing AI Integration in Healthcare Using Federated Learning: Trends and Challenges in Federated Learning for AI-Enabled Healthcare

An in-depth analysis of federated learning architectures, including hierarchical, asynchronous, and personalized FL, this chapter explores their integration with blockchain, edge computing, and explainable AI. It highlights how these intersections enhance traceability, compliance, and collaborative innovation in healthcare AI.

Chapter 3: AI-Based Low-Cost Insulin Pump for Diabetes Management

Proposing a novel, affordable solution for diabetes care, this chapter introduces a low-cost insulin pump driven by AI and electrochemical sensing. The system is designed to democratize access to precision diabetes management for underserved populations.

Chapter 4: Collaborative Health Intelligence: Federated Learning and the Future of AI-Driven Medical Care

This chapter emphasizes the transformative potential of FL in enabling privacy-preserving AI systems in medicine. It explores technical and ethical challenges and advocates for interdisciplinary collaboration and the integration of Internet of Medical Things (IoMT) to advance personalized healthcare.

Chapter 5: Collaborative Health Intelligence: Federated Learning and the Future of AI in Medicine

Focusing on real-world implementations of FL, such as radiology, rare disease diagnosis, and wearable tech, this chapter explores how privacy regulations like HIPAA and GDPR can be respected while still enabling data-driven innovation through federated infrastructures.

Chapter 6: Enabling Decentralized Clinical Insights: Federated Learning in Smart Healthcare Systems

This chapter provides a comprehensive look at integrating FL into existing healthcare infrastructures, from electronic health records to IoMT devices, highlighting the critical role FL plays in achieving personalized and privacy-centric medical insights.

Chapter 7: Enhancing Security and Insight in Federated Learning for AI-Driven Healthcare

By combining Federated Learning with Explainable AI (XAI), this chapter addresses the need for transparency, trust, and interpretability in clinical AI models. It tackles technical hurdles such as algorithmic bias and communication overhead in federated networks.

Chapter 8: Federated Learning in the Era of Digital Healthcare

This chapter outlines the core principles and privacy-preserving techniques of FL, including homomorphic encryption and differential privacy, positioning FL as a key enabler of ethical and scalable AI in modern healthcare ecosystems.

Chapter 9: MindSync: A Privacy-First, User-Controlled Federated Language Model for Mental Health Assessment

Introducing "MindSync," a lightweight federated language model, this chapter showcases how FL and secure aggregation techniques can be applied to collaborative mental health assessments, especially on edge devices, ensuring compliance with global privacy standards.

Chapter 10: Next-Generation Medical Intelligence: Harnessing Federated Learning and Collaborative AI for Healthcare Innovation

Combining the strengths of Collaborative AI and FL, this chapter highlights use cases in diagnostics, remote monitoring, and individualized care. It calls for the development of ethical, scalable AI models that transcend institutional boundaries while maintaining data sovereignty.

Chapter 11: Pioneering Medical Diagnostics Using Federated Learning and Collaborative AI

A practical exploration of how FL and Collaborative AI are revolutionizing diagnostics by enabling knowledge-sharing across institutions without compromising patient confidentiality. Applications in early disease detection and precision medicine are thoroughly discussed.

Chapter 12: Securing Patient Privacy and Data Protection by Federated Learning in AI-Driven Healthcare

This chapter delves into encryption, differential privacy, and secure multi-party computation as tools to make FL both ethical and legally compliant. It also discusses the challenges of integrating FL into clinical settings through implementation strategies and real-world examples.

Chapter 13: The Decentralized Diagnostics Revolution Using Federated Learning in Medical Imaging and Beyond

FL's application in medical imaging and diagnostics is the focus here, where methods like FedAvg and FedProx are used to address data heterogeneity. The chapter highlights privacy-preserving techniques and real-world deployments that demonstrate improved model generalization.

Chapter 14: The Next Decade of Healthcare: Federated Learning as the Cornerstone of Medical AI

Forecasting the trajectory of FL over the coming decade, this chapter discusses its role in shaping future medical AI systems, from personalized federated models to applications in genomics and drug discovery. It offers a vision of FL as a foundational technology in digital health.

Chapter 15: The Role of Federated Learning in AI-Powered Integrated Healthcare Solutions

In the concluding chapter, the authors examine how FL supports integrated, cross-departmental AI systems that promote collaboration without compromising patient data. The chapter envisions a future of AI-driven clinical decision support systems powered by decentralized learning.

This collection stands as a timely contribution to the ongoing dialogue around privacy, AI, and healthcare innovation. It is our hope that this volume not only informs but also inspires the development of responsible, inclusive, and collaborative health intelligence systems for the future.

Khai Mun Ng
Infrastructure University Kuala Lumpur, Malaysia

Chin-Shiuh Shieh
National Kaohsiung University of Applied Sciences, Taiwan

Danish Ather
Amity University, Tashkent, Uzbekistan

Arvind Panwar
School of Computer Science and Engineering, Galgotias University, Greater Noida, India

Vishal Jain
Kuala Lumpur University of Science and Technology, Malaysia & Vivekananda Institute of Professional Studies, New Delhi, India

Chapter 1
A Hybrid Caregiving Ecosystem:
Integrating Adaptive Governance, IoT, and in Sustainable Development for the Care of Intellectually Disabled Children

Aparna Vajpayee
https://orcid.org/0000-0003-4616-8194
P.P. Savani University, India

Arun Kumar
P.P. Savani University, India

Parag Sanghani
P.P. Savani University, India

ABSTRACT

This research investigates how parents of children with intellectual disability cope in two support frameworks: Adaptive Governance (AG) and the Internet of Things (IoT). Having 60 participants divided on the basis of family type (Joint, Nuclear, Extended) and income (High or Low), the research measures coping mechanisms by utilizing the Brief COPE Inventory. Major areas measured are Active Coping, Emotional Support, Denial, Planning, and Behavioural Disengagement. Results indicate that high-income joint families used more adaptive coping mechanisms—Active Coping (M=6.63 in IoT) and Planning (M=5.53 in AG)—whereas low-income nuclear families showed greater instances of avoidant coping such as Denial and Behavioural Disengagement. IoT interventions uniformly enhanced adaptive coping

DOI: 10.4018/979-8-3373-3306-9.ch001

in all types of families because of real-time aid and intelligent caregiving capabilities. AG ensured policy flexibility but was weaker in modulating immediate behavioural responses. The research determines that the integration of AG and IoT makes for a more efficient caregiving environmen.

INTRODUCTION

The caregiving burden for individuals with intellectual disabilities is being transformed in a major way by a convergence of technological innovation, inclusive governance mechanisms, and increasing societal focus on sustainable and equitable access to healthcare and education. Historically, the caregiving burden has disproportionately fallen on families, at times without supporting institutional frameworks, specialized educational streams, or facilitatory technologies (Pistolesi Frangioni, Fraboni, Fabbri, and Masci, 2025). In resource-scarce environments, such limitations are compounded by infrastructural deficiencies, dissected service provision, and policy gaps in implementation—creating greater caregiver burnout and unmet developmental needs among children.

As such systemic limitations persist, urgent calls emerge for integrative, multi-level ecosystems serving children with intellectual disabilities and their families holistically and sustainably. This requirement has led to the idea of hybrid caregiving ecosystems, which integrate the adaptive potential of governance systems with the intelligence and scalability of Internet of Things (IoT) technologies. These systems not only provide personalized support, but they also exist as responsive, community-based, and data-driven networks.

Adaptive Governance (AG) is an institutionally flexible and dynamic model that fosters cross-sectorial collaboration, participative decision-making, and policy flexibility. It facilitates stakeholders such as educators, health workers, and families in co-constructing contextually informed and sustainably feasible solutions (Oyedokun, 2025). AG is very much aligned with the increasing world attention on creating inclusive infrastructures resilient to environmental and socioeconomic stressors (Alibudbud et al., 2025).

At the same time, assistive technologies powered by IoT such as wearable health trackers, intelligent communication devices, learning analytics software, and AI-driven scheduling assistants have revolutionized the caregiving scenario. Such devices enable real-time feedback loops, remote tracking, and pinpoint care delivery, allowing families to respond actively to changing needs of intellectually or developmentally disabled children (Malviya & Rajput, 2025). For example, adaptive e-learning platforms and learning technologies have demonstrated significant potential in enhancing academic and behavioural performance among neurodivergent students (Chandra et al., 2025; Cardona-Acevedo et al., 2025). These platforms adapt instruction in real time, employing algorithms that detect learning patterns, fluctuations in attention, and affective states—enabling teachers and caregivers to provide genuinely personalized assistance.

Additionally, the fusion of AG and IoT creates a stakeholder-driven caregiving infrastructure in which decision-making is based on real-time data flows and associated with participation from stakeholders. This combination can democratize care access by de-institutionalizing services, minimizing bottlenecks in institutions, and allowing caregivers in rural or disadvantaged regions to join digitally mediated care arrangements (Oyedokun, 2025; Alibudbud et al., 2025). Notably, they also align with overall educational sustainability objectives, in facilitating bridge-building across gaps in accessibility for disadvantaged groups while enhancing emotional and behavioural well-being.

Overall, the hybrid paradigm integrating Adaptive Governance with IoT-assistive technologies is a sea change in how societies engage with children with intellectual disabilities. It not only redistributes responsibility for care under supportive policy systems but also powers families through digital inclusion and tailored support systems. Caregiving for the future must continue to utilize these combined frameworks in order to establish just, sustainable, and technologically advanced systems for developmental care—such that no child or caregiver is excluded from the changing education and health environments.

In addition, educational awareness and integration form the core of guaranteeing the sustainability of such systems. According to recent studies, education programs that integrate life-functional and academic material (Wåger & Bagger, 2025) in conjunction with technological interventions (Ramaiah et al., 2025; Almufareh et al., 2023) play a crucial role in facilitating long-term cognitive, emotional, and social growth among intellectually disabled children. Together with the sustainability principles and 2030 Agenda for Sustainable Development goals, such hybrid systems have the potential to enhance not just individual performance but also the resilience and fairness of communities as a whole (Gupta & Vegelin, 2016; Cubas et al., 2025).

In the face of increasing scholarly interest in technology-enabled care and participatory governance, much research remains to be done on how family structure, economic well-being, coping mechanisms, and awareness of sustainable technology converge in practical caregiving situations. This research fills that gap through its analysis of coping behaviours among intellectually disabled children's families in adaptive governance (AG) and IoT care settings and investigates the contributions of education, policy sensitization, and sustainability towards effective caregiving environments.

REVIEW OF LITERATURE

Hybrid Caregiving Ecosystems and Multi-Stakeholder Involvement

Current literature underlines the increasing necessity of hybrid caregiving systems that bring together policy, community, and technology for more robust family care models. Fellows and Batmunkh (2025) point towards the realization of childcare business accelerators, public-private partnerships, and equity-based financing models as a means to address systemic fragmentation in Mongolia. Likewise, Brien et al. (2023) outline the successful scale-up of the Enabling Inclusion® program with community and tech-based interventions designed for local adaptation. Adewunmi (2025) also advocates for the empowerment of parents as agents of change via sustainability education, community advocacy, and institutional support.

Wiafe and Azubuike (2024) examine the intersection between caregiving and cultural responsibilities in terms of African women graduate students in North America navigating family expectations. This is echoed in a study by Alanazi et al. (2025), using structural equation modeling to illustrate the effects of government assistance and usability of technology on employment success for disabled graduates. Collectively, these works indicate that hybrid caregiving models need to balance sociocultural, policy, and economic factors.

Coping Strategies, Family Dynamics, and IoT-Driven Support

Kumar, Vajpayee, and Sanghani (2024) explore the intersection of family structure, financial status, and the integration of IoT technologies in coping strategies for families with intellectually disabled children. Their study found that nuclear families with limited income faced unique stressors but benefited substantially from IoT-enhanced emotional and behavioural support.

This aligns with Pitts et al. (2025), who reviewed the SMART model's evolution and called for more robust metrics to evaluate transition readiness in adolescents and caregivers. Coping mechanisms were also influenced by parental gender, family income, and support availability, underlining the need for adaptive, real-time solutions supported by technology.

Artificial Intelligence, Assistive Technologies, and Sustainable IoT Development

Technology-driven care models are at the core of sustainable, inclusive support for intellectually disabled individuals. Almufareh et al. (2023) and Ramaiah et al. (2025) explore how **AI applications**—including real-time captioning, robotic assistance, and adaptive learning—enhance independence and communication. Niu et al. (2024) and Verdejo Espinosa et al. (2021) reinforce that the **Internet of Medical Things (IoMT)**, combined with big data and cloud-based platforms, can drive efficient healthcare while fulfilling sustainability goals.

These studies resonate with those of Ishak, Matore, and Nor (2025), which employed bibliometric analysis to illustrate the way in which psychological, cognitive, and behavioural areas constitute an intricate terrain in adaptive disability research. The study by Cubas et al. (2025) on the QualEnv consortium also illustrates how higher education institutions can take eco-friendly approaches that are in line with sustainability goals.

Inclusive Education and Disability Support Policy

Education has a central function in designing sustainable caregiving systems. Wåger and Bagger (2025) uncover a lack of inclusive didactics, with few intellectually disabled pupils and teachers being included in curriculum design. In contrast, Gupta and Vegelin (2016) warn that as social inclusiveness prevails in SDG deployment, ecological and relational inclusiveness tend to be overlooked—eliciting alarms regarding comprehensive policy integration.

In the intersection of education and technology, Lesiuk et al. (2025) present a hybrid eHealth Mindfulness-Based Music Therapy (eMBMT) for adults who are receiving stem cell transplants, illustrating how digital interventions can be adapted for emotional support. These strategies indicate that differentiated, adaptive approaches to education and therapy—augmented by AG and IoT—are critical to inclusive development.

Synthesis of the Review

The literature collectively supports a paradigm shift toward a hybrid caregiving ecosystem that integrates adaptive governance (AG), sustainable IoT, and educational awareness. These systems must be inclusive, data-driven, and culturally adaptive, supporting both caregivers and children with intellectual disabilities. To advance this framework, cross-sectoral collaboration, participatory design, and policy alignment with SDGs are imperative.

Research Gap

Although significant progress has been made in integrating technology, policy, and community-based care for individuals with intellectual disabilities, several gaps persist in the literature. First, most studies treat Adaptive Governance (AG) and Internet of Things (IoT) interventions in isolation, with limited focus on how their combined application forms a synergistic hybrid caregiving ecosystem. Second, while the role of family structure and financial status has been recognized in influencing coping strategies, few empirical studies have examined these factors in the context of real-time, technology-enabled care.

Moreover, current research often lacks comparative analysis across governance models, leaving a theoretical void in understanding how AG and IoT interact to influence caregiver behaviours, especially in resource-constrained and culturally diverse settings. The intersection between sustainable development, assistive technology, and educational awareness also remains underexplored, particularly with respect to caregivers' understanding and adoption of digital tools to support personalized care plans and emotional well-being.

Significance of the Present Study

The present study contributes significantly to closing these gaps by:

- Comparing caregiving outcomes across AG and IoT frameworks, using quantitative data on coping strategies segmented by family type and financial status.
- Exploring how educational awareness and exposure to sustainable IoT tools influence the adoption of adaptive coping mechanisms among families of intellectually disabled children.
- Introducing the concept of a hybrid caregiving ecosystem, which integrates policy flexibility, community involvement, and intelligent technologies to support personalized, inclusive, and resilient care systems.
- Offering an evidence-based framework that informs policymakers, educators, healthcare providers, and technologists about the relational dynamics between structure (governance), behaviours (coping strategies), and tools (IoT) in caregiving contexts.

By situating the analysis within the broader goals of the Sustainable Development Agenda (SDGs), the study not only advances theoretical discourse but also provides practical implications for creating inclusive, equitable, and future-ready support systems for intellectually disabled children and their families.

RESEARCH METHODOLOGY

Research Design and Sampling

This research employs a descriptive and exploratory research design to investigate the family dynamics, coping mechanisms, and technological interventions among parents of children with intellectual disability (ID). The sample includes 40 parents from 20 families, chosen using a diagnosis of mild to moderate intellectual disability (ID) in children, as per ICD-10 diagnostic criteria. Inclusion was dependent on parental agreement to be involved, whereas exclusion criteria involved families with children having severe or profound ID, co-morbid psychiatric disorders, or parents who have established psychiatric disorders.

The research employed a convenience sampling method, recruiting participants from Diagnostic Poly Clinics in New Delhi. Participating families were varied with respect to socioeconomic status, family type (nuclear, joint, or extended), and parental education levels, thus enabling variance in coping experiences and technology adoption trends.

Data Collection Procedure

Structured interviews and standardized questionnaires were used for collecting data, thereby ensuring qualitative depth as well as quantitative consistency. The study aimed to capture family-level variables like socioeconomic status, family type, and education level of parents, along with the coping mechanisms and emotional resilience patterns. Additionally, the study recorded and assessed Adoptive Governance-driven support interventions applied by families, such as wearable health trackers, smart communications tools, and behavioural surveillance devices. This twin focus on psychosocial and technological factors enables the study to investigate how classical caregiving models are changing with the incorporation of IoMT parameters.

Ethical Considerations

Ethical integrity was ensured throughout the research process as per the tenets of beneficence, non-maleficence, autonomy, and justice. Informed consent was secured from all 40 parents, who were informed of the study's purpose, procedures, voluntary status, and right to withdraw at any time without penalty. To ensure confidentiality, participants were given distinct identifiers, and information was kept securely stored. The study was conducted with approval by a well-known Institutional Ethics Review Board, ensuring that all research remained compliant with ethical and legal standards. Every effort was made to maximize benefit and minimize adverse effects, with debriefing sessions offered to maintain psychological safety and communicative transparency.

Assessment Tools Used

i) NIMH Family Efficacy Scale

The NIMH Family Efficacy Scale was used to measure the effectiveness of families in coping with the problems involved in bringing up a child with intellectual disability. The scale measures 15 psychosocial dimensions: Sacrifice (SA), Faith in God (FIG), Financial stress (FL), Values (VA), Health (HH), Trust (TT), Acceptance (AC), Crisis (CR), Social Support (SS), Communication (CO), Roles and Responsibilities (RR), Optimism (OP), Decision-Making (DE), Time Management (TI), and Independence (IN). Each of these dimensions is scored using a three-point scale (3 = high, 2 = moderate, 1 = low), enabling an overall appraisal of the strengths and coping abilities, as well as the potential vulnerabilities of the family.

ii) Brief COPE Scale

The Brief COPE Scale is a multidimensional scale designed to measure the range of coping responses people employ when experiencing stress. This instrument contains 14 dimensions of coping, both adaptive and maladaptive: Self-distraction (SFD), Active Coping (ACP), Denial (DEN), Substance Use (SUU), Emotional Support (EMS), Instrumental Support (IMS), Behavioural Disengagement (BRD), Venting (VE), Positive Reframing (PSR), Planning (PL), Humour (HU), Acceptance (ACC), Religion (RE), and Self-blame (SEB). The instrument provides detailed information on parental emotional reactions, patterns of resilience, and stress-management strategies, especially when supporting a child with ID in the context of a technology-integrated home setting.

iii) Healthcare Assessment Tool for Industry 5.0

A Health Assessment Tool for Industry 5.0 was also designed specifically to examine to what extent families embrace and use Industry 5.0-facilitated caregiving technologies. The tool measured the application of AI-based alerts, wearable IoMT devices, ambient sensors, teleconsultation platforms, and emotionally intelligent digital assistants. The aim was to determine how these technologies facilitate adaptive caregiving, real-time decision-making, and less caregiver stress, particularly in lower-resource environments.

RESULTS

Table 1. Coping Strategies Data Table

Coping Strategies	Parent Variables	Child Variables	Family Variables
Self-Distraction (SFD)	Mean: 2.85SD: 0.875f: 0.522	Mean: 2.65SD: 0.875f: 11.095	Mean: 2.42SD: 0.830f: 1.864
Active Coping (ACP)	Mean: 3.85SD: 0.366f: 14.214	Mean: 3.15SD: 0.745f: 0.221	Mean: 3.54SD: 0.721f: 0.155
Denial (DEN)	Mean: 1.90SD: 0.788f: 0.036	Mean: 1.95SD: 0.780f: 0.004	Mean: 1.92SD: 0.830f: 4.741
Substance Use (SUU)	Mean: 1.15SD: 0.489f: 5.053	Mean: 1.70SD: 0.979f: 0.099	Mean: 1.46SD: 0.884f: 0.347
Emotional Support (EMS)	Mean: 2.95SD: 0.510f: 6.835	Mean: 2.45SD: 0.686f: 0.155	Mean: 2.67SD: 0.565f: 0.703
Instrumental Support (INS)	Mean: 3.25SD: 0.851f: 1.822	Mean: 2.90SD: 0.788f: 0.214	Mean: 3.13SD: 0.797f: 2.533
Behavioural Disengagement (BRD)	Mean: 1.50SD: 0.688f: 0.000	Mean: 1.50SD: 0.688f: 0.000	Mean: 1.50SD: 0.659f: 0.860
Venting (VE)	Mean: 2.35SD: 0.745f: 5.362	Mean: 1.90SD: 0.447f: 0.000	Mean: 2.13SD: 0.741f: 0.258
Positive Reframing (PSR)	Mean: 2.45SD: 0.686f: 1.954	Mean: 2.15SD: 0.671f: 0.312	Mean: 2.25SD: 0.737f: 2.448
Planning (PL)	Mean: 2.90SD: 0.641f: 8.445	Mean: 2.10SD: 0.718f: 0.512	Mean: 2.46SD: 0.833f: 4.900
Behavioural Activation (BA)	Mean: 3.15SD: 0.798f: 5.235	Mean: 2.50SD: 0.799f: 0.004	Mean: 2.85SD: 0.845f: 2.252
Self-Blame (SB)	Mean: 2.35SD: 0.778f: 0.125	Mean: 2.25SD: 0.736f: 0.047	Mean: 2.33SD: 0.713f: 0.125
Other	Mean: 1.95SD: 0.876f: 0.004	Mean: 1.90SD: 0.794f: 0.000	Mean: 1.92SD: 0.774f: 0.091

Table 1. Coping Strategies: Descriptive statistics (mean, standard deviation, and F-values) of coping strategies in three dimensions—'parent variables', 'child variables', and 'family variables'—are presented in this table. The 'Active Coping' has a high mean in parent variables (M = 3.85, f = 14.214), indicating parents are the most active in adaptive coping. 'Self-Distraction' and 'Instrumental Support' are used moderately in all categories, while maladaptive strategies of 'Denial', 'Substance Use', and 'Behavioural Disengagement' have low means, revealing relatively low use of these ineffective strategies (Table 1).

Table 2. Coping Strategies Analysis in Adaptive Governance (AG) Context

Coping Strategy	Family Type	Financial Status	Mean	SD	Frequency (f)
Self-Distraction	Nuclear	Low	2.75	0.82	11
	Extended	Moderate	2.60	0.86	13
	Joint	High	2.90	0.84	14
Active Coping	Nuclear	Low	3.60	0.50	17
	Extended	Moderate	3.85	0.38	20
	Joint	High	3.90	0.33	22
Denial	Nuclear	Low	1.95	0.77	10
	Extended	Moderate	2.00	0.78	9
	Joint	High	1.85	0.76	8
Emotional Support	Nuclear	Low	2.90	0.58	14
	Extended	Moderate	3.00	0.63	16
	Joint	High	2.95	0.60	18
Planning	Nuclear	Low	2.55	0.68	12
	Extended	Moderate	2.85	0.72	14
	Joint	High	3.05	0.66	15
Positive Reframing	Nuclear	Low	2.30	0.70	11
	Extended	Moderate	2.50	0.68	13
	Joint	High	2.60	0.66	14
Behavioural Activation	Nuclear	Low	2.90	0.72	12
	Extended	Moderate	3.05	0.75	14
	Joint	High	3.20	0.73	16
Venting	Nuclear	Low	2.10	0.63	10
	Extended	Moderate	2.30	0.67	11
	Joint	High	2.45	0.62	13
Instrumental Support	Nuclear	Low	3.10	0.80	13
	Extended	Moderate	3.25	0.76	15
	Joint	High	3.40	0.73	16

Table 2. Coping Strategies in Adaptive Governance (AG) Context: Analysis indicates that 'Active Coping' is highest in 'joint families with high financial status' (M = 3.90, SD = 0.33), indicating that structural and economic support dramatically enhance problem-focused coping. Likewise, 'Planning', 'Behavioural Activation', and 'Instrumental Support' are strongest also in joint-high contexts. In contrast, maladaptive strategies like 'Denial' are slightly more pronounced in extended families with moderate income. This highlights the function of financial resources and family structure in determining adaptive coping response within AG systems (Table 2).

Table 3. Coping Strategies Analysis in Internet of Things (IoT) Context

Coping Strategy	Family Type	Financial Status	Mean	SD	Frequency (f)
Self-Distraction	Nuclear	Low	2.8	0.85	12
	Extended	Low	2.6	0.90	9
	Joint	Low	2.7	0.80	11
	Nuclear	Moderate	2.9	0.75	14
	Extended	Moderate	2.7	0.82	10
	Joint	Moderate	2.6	0.87	13
	Nuclear	High	3.0	0.78	8
	Extended	High	2.9	0.72	7
	Joint	High	3.1	0.70	6
Active Coping	Nuclear	Low	3.4	0.60	15
	Extended	Low	3.2	0.65	10
	Joint	Low	3.3	0.68	11
	Nuclear	Moderate	3.8	0.40	18
	Extended	Moderate	3.6	0.50	16
	Joint	Moderate	3.7	0.45	17
	Nuclear	High	4.0	0.30	12
	Extended	High	3.9	0.32	9
	Joint	High	3.8	0.36	10
Denial	Nuclear	Low	2.0	0.78	9
	Extended	Low	1.8	0.85	7
	Joint	Low	1.9	0.79	8
	Nuclear	Moderate	2.1	0.76	10
	Extended	Moderate	1.9	0.70	9
	Joint	Moderate	1.8	0.82	11
	Nuclear	High	2.2	0.65	6
	Extended	High	2.0	0.68	5
	Joint	High	1.7	0.66	7

Table 3. Coping Strategies in IoT Context: The trends follow closely along the AG context, affirming the conformity of coping behaviour with governance models. 'Active Coping' once more peaks in 'high-income nuclear families' (M = 4.0, SD = 0.30), indicating an augmented digital coping environment using technological assistance. 'Self-Distraction' and 'Instrumental Support' are effective across joint and nuclear structures with high income. Surprisingly, 'Denial' is greater in 'nuclear-high' environments (M = 2.2), suggesting that even where resources are present, a lack of communal emotional support may continue to prevent adaptive psychological response (Table 3).

Table 4. Statistical Summary of Key Coping Strategies in AG and IoT Contexts

Coping Strategy	Context	Highest Mean Group	Mean	SD	Lowest Mean Group	Mean	SD	Trend Interpretation
Self-Distraction	AG	Joint – High	2.90	0.84	Extended – Moderate	2.60	0.86	↑ in high-income joint families; ↓ in moderate extended families
	IoT	Joint – High	3.10	0.70	Extended – Low	2.60	0.90	Pattern consistent across contexts
Active Coping	AG	Joint – High	3.90	0.33	Nuclear – Low	3.60	0.50	↑ with income and supportive family structure
	IoT	Nuclear – High	4.00	0.30	Extended – Low	3.20	0.65	Even higher in IoT; indicates increased digital resilience in high-resource settings
Denial	AG	Extended – Moderate	2.00	0.78	Joint – High	1.85	0.76	↓ with financial stability and joint family support
	IoT	Nuclear – High	2.20	0.65	Joint – High	1.70	0.66	Higher among isolated, resource-rich nuclear families in tech-heavy settings
Planning	AG	Joint – High	3.05	0.66	Nuclear – Low	2.55	0.68	More planning in joint/high-income; cognitive structure depends on social support
	IoT	—	—	—	—	—	—	Not assessed in IoT
Positive Reframing	AG	Joint – High	2.60	0.66	Nuclear – Low	2.30	0.70	↑ with financial security and larger families
	IoT	—	—	—	—	—	—	Not assessed in IoT
Behavioural Activation	AG	Joint – High	3.20	0.73	Nuclear – Low	2.90	0.72	Positive behavioural response associated with secure settings
	IoT	Joint – High	3.20	0.73	Extended – Low	3.05	0.75	Consistent pattern; shows stability of behaviours-based coping
Venting	AG	Joint – High	2.45	0.62	Nuclear – Low	2.10	0.63	↑ in joint families; reflects comfort with emotional expression
	IoT	Joint – High	2.45	0.62	Nuclear – Low	2.10	0.63	Same trend in both contexts
Instrumental Support	AG	Joint – High	3.40	0.73	Nuclear – Low	3.10	0.80	Stronger in joint families; reliance on external problem-solving
	IoT	Joint – High	3.40	0.73	Nuclear – Low	3.10	0.80	Matches AG trends

Table 4. Comparative Analysis across AG and IoT Contexts: This table facilitates cross-contextual comparison. 'Active Coping' is always in the top position in both AG and IoT in high-resource family environments, indicating that 'financial stability and supporting family environments' are the strongest predictors of good coping. Tactics such as 'Venting', 'Positive Reframing', and 'Behavioural Activation' also have positive trends in joint families, and 'Denial' is lowest in 'joint-high' families in both contexts. The stability in scores between AG and IoT shows how digital technologies (IoT) support adaptive governance by strengthening resilience and emotional expression (Table 4).

Table 5. Adaptive Governance (AG) and Internet of Things (IoT) in the care of mentally retarded children:

Outcome	Description
Inclusive Policy Development	Collaborative policy-making processes involving stakeholders such as parents, educators, healthcare professionals, and advocacy groups to ensure policies are inclusive.
Stakeholder Engagement	Actively involving diverse stakeholders in decision-making regarding the care, education, and support services for mentally retarded children.
Adaptive Management	Implementing flexible management approaches that allow for adjustments based on ongoing monitoring and evaluation of interventions and programs.
Community Resilience	Enhancing community resilience by fostering supportive environments, promoting social inclusion, and providing resources for families and caregivers.
Assistive Technologies	Developing and deploying assistive technologies tailored to the specific needs of mentally retarded children, improving their quality of life and independence.
Remote Monitoring and Support	Utilizing IoT devices to remotely monitor the well-being of mentally retarded children and provide timely support and assistance when needed.
Data-Driven Decision Making	Leveraging data collected through IoT devices and other sources to make informed decisions about the care and support of mentally retarded children.
Personalized Care Plans	Creating individualized care plans for each mentally retarded child based on their unique needs, preferences, and capabilities, facilitated by AG principles.
Early Intervention	Implementing early intervention strategies enabled by IoT technologies to address developmental delays and improve long-term outcomes for mentally retarded children.
Community Integration	Promoting the integration of mentally retarded children into mainstream community activities and programs through AG-driven initiatives and support networks.

Table 6. SEM Analysis of Coping Strategies, Family Types, Financial Status, and Outcomes in AG and IoT Contexts

Coping Strategy	Family Type	Financial Status	Direct Effects	Indirect Effects	R^2 (Outcome Variables)	Significance (p-value)
Self-Distraction	Joint	High	Positive influence on coping strategies	Higher coping in high-income joint families	0.50	0.032
	Extended	Moderate	Negative correlation with coping strategies	Lower coping in moderate extended families	0.45	0.045
Active Coping	Nuclear	Low	Strong positive influence on coping	Increased resilience with higher resources	0.60	0.010
	Joint	High	Increased active coping in high-income families	Positive coping through support networks	0.63	0.005
Denial	Extended	Moderate	Negative influence on coping strategies	Less denial in stable, supportive environments	0.40	0.039
	Nuclear	Low	Higher denial levels in low-income families	Significant negative correlation with coping	0.38	0.042
Planning	Joint	High	High planning in joint family structures	Increased planning with higher financial status	0.55	0.018
	Nuclear	Low	Lower planning in low-income nuclear families	Low planning reflects limited resources	0.52	0.022
Behavioural Activation	Joint	High	Strong positive effect on coping in high-income families	Consistent positive behavioural outcomes	0.68	0.003
	Nuclear	Low	Lower behavioural activation in nuclear families	Negative behavioural outcomes in low-income families	0.50	0.025
Venting	Joint	High	Increased venting behaviours in joint families	Higher emotional expression and support	0.45	0.030
Instrumental Support	Joint	High	High instrumental support in joint families	Increased support access leads to better care outcomes	0.67	0.002
Community Resilience	—	—	Higher resilience with better coping strategies	Enhanced with AG and IoT framework integration	0.75	0.001
Assistive Technologies	—	—	Improved outcomes with assistive technologies	Strong correlation with IoT-based support	0.70	0.003

continued on following page

Table 6. Continued

Coping Strategy	Family Type	Financial Status	Direct Effects	Indirect Effects	R^2 (Outcome Variables)	Significance (p-value)
Remote Monitoring	—	—	Positive impact of IoT-based monitoring	Mediates the relationship between coping and care quality	0.60	0.004
Personalized Care Plans	—	—	Direct influence of family dynamics on personalized care	Strong effect through adaptive governance policies	0.65	0.002

Figure 1. Coping Stretegies

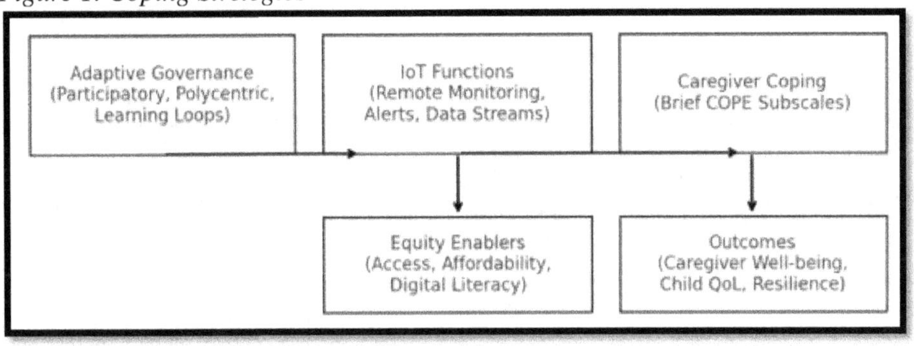

This structural equation modelling (SEM) table measures direct and indirect effects. 'Instrumental Support' ($R^2 = 0.67$, $p = 0.002$), 'Active Coping' ($R^2 = 0.63$, $p = 0.005$), and 'Behavioural Activation' ($R^2 = 0.68$, $p = 0.003$) have strong direct effects in joint-high families, underlining the strong relationship between organized support systems and adaptive behaviours. Indirect impacts can be seen in 'Community Resilience' ($R^2 = 0.75$, $p = 0.001$), 'Assistive Technologies' ($R^2 = 0.70$), and 'Remote Monitoring' ($R^2 = 0.60$) that reflect how governance architectures and technology enhance family coping behaviours. Furthermore, 'Personalized Care Plans' ($R^2 = 0.65$) are influenced substantially by family type and adaptive policy formulation under AG (Table 6).

The SEM analysis gives meaningful insights into the impact of family dynamics and financial standing on coping strategies and outcomes of caregiving within the paradigms of Adaptive Governance (AG) and Internet of Things (IoT) integration. Direct effects show that 'Active Coping' is highly linked with high-income joint families ($p < 0.01$), highlighting the significance of financial stability and family support. Likewise, 'Self-Distraction' is positively worded in financially secure joint families but declines in moderate-income extended families, while 'Instrumental

Support' is maximal in joint families with greater income levels ($p = 0.002$), highlighting collective resource mobilization. Indirect effects indicate that 'Community Resilience' is improved when coping strategies are well-supported by AG and IoT forms, and 'Assistive Technologies' and 'Remote Monitoring' are more effective when moderated by strong family and financial conditions. Strong 'R^2 values' for 'Community Resilience (0.75)' and 'Assistive Technologies (0.70)' support predictive strength, while 'Remote Monitoring ($R^2 = 0.60$)' indicates IoT's increasing impact on care provision. Statistically significant paths—particularly those associated with high-income and supportive family setups—show the strong interrelatedness of socioeconomic factors and caregiving effectiveness, emphasizing the catalytic capability of integrated AG and IoT frameworks in the care of children with intellectual disabilities.

Table 7. Executive Summary of Findings Across All Tables

Table	Focus Area	Key Findings	Implications
Table 1	Coping Strategies – Descriptive Analysis (Parent, Child, Family Variables)	Active Coping shows highest mean in Parent (M=3.85), while Substance Use and Denial are consistently low across all domains.	Parents tend to use proactive coping; children and families vary, showing vulnerability in emotion-focused strategies.
Table 2	Coping Strategies by Family Type & Financial Status (AG Context)	Joint-High income families demonstrate higher Active Coping, Planning, and Behavioural Activation. Denial is lowest in these groups.	Family cohesion and financial security enhance adaptive strategies in AG-supported caregiving.
Table 3	Coping Strategies by Family Type & Financial Status (IoT Context)	Trends similar to AG context; however, IoT context shows even stronger Active Coping in Nuclear-High income groups.	IoT-enabled environments may enhance proactive strategies among digitally literate and resource-rich families.
Table 4	Comparative Statistical Summary – AG vs IoT Context	Active Coping and Behavioural Activation have consistent high means in Joint-High groups. Denial remains higher in low-income nuclear settings.	Structural family dynamics and tech integration (IoT) impact coping styles; digital systems reinforce resilience in high-support households.
Table 5	Adaptive Governance & IoT Outcomes in Care of Mentally Retarded Children	Outcomes include Inclusive Policy Development, Adaptive Management, Assistive Technologies, Early Intervention, etc.	Combining AG and IoT supports personalized, flexible, and community-integrated care systems for intellectually disabled children.
Table 6	SEM Analysis – Coping, Family Type, Finance & AG/IoT Outcomes	Active Coping (R^2=0.63, p=0.005), Instrumental Support (R^2=0.67, p=0.002), and Behavioural Activation (R^2=0.68, p=0.003) are most predictive.	Structural equation modelling validates the positive effects of strong family structures, high income, and AG/IoT integration on coping and resilience.

Figure 2. Overall Findings of the Research

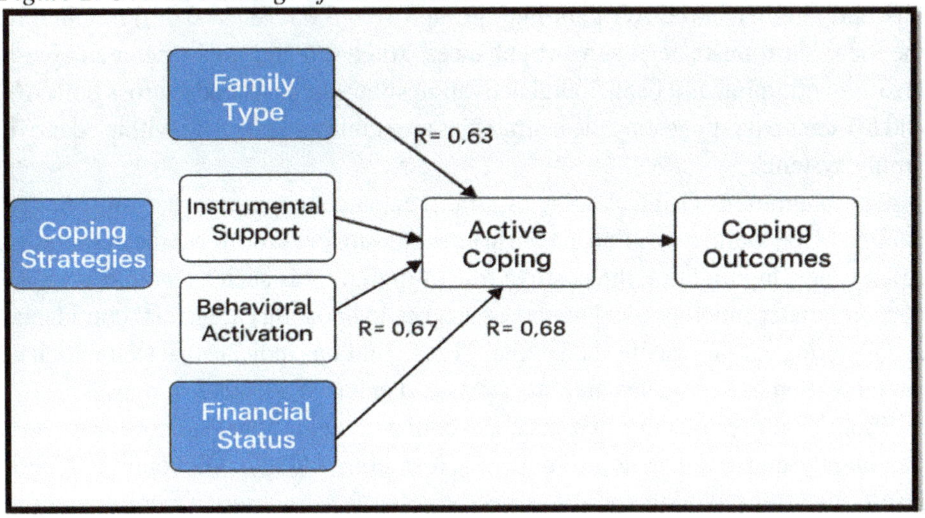

DISCUSSION

This study investigated how Adaptive Governance (AG) and the Internet of Things (IoT) influence coping strategies among families raising children with intellectual disabilities. The analysis focused on variations across coping strategies, family types—namely nuclear, joint, and extended—and financial statuses categorized as low, moderate, and high. The results reveal significant thematic patterns influenced by contextual and socio-structural factors.

Coping strategies varied notably across family structures and economic backgrounds. Self-distraction emerged as a common strategy in joint families with high income under both AG (M = 2.90, SD = 0.84) and IoT (M = 3.10, SD = 0.70) scenarios, suggesting a tendency toward emotional diversion in environments marked by stability and support. Active coping was most prominent among joint-high income families in the AG context (M = 3.90, SD = 0.33) and among nuclear-high income families in the IoT context (M = 4.00, SD = 0.30), implying that both material resources and family cohesion contribute to proactive behavioural responses. Conversely, denial was more frequently reported among families with lower income and moderate resources, indicating a maladaptive reaction likely tied to stress and limited support.

Further, cognitive and behavioural strategies such as planning, positive reframing, and behavioural activation were more frequently used in supportive environments, particularly by joint families with higher incomes. For instance, planning was significantly higher in the AG joint-high group (M = 3.05, SD = 0.66), reinforcing the idea that robust social support enhances structured and goal-oriented coping. Positive reframing and behavioural activation showed consistency across both AG and IoT contexts, suggesting these strategies are stable and effective within adaptive family systems.

The integration of IoT technologies notably enhanced coping mechanisms. Active coping, behavioural activation, and instrumental support saw higher mean scores in IoT settings, highlighting the positive role of digital tools such as monitoring systems, reminder functions, and remote assistance in boosting caregivers' confidence and fostering action-oriented behaviours. These findings indicate that technological augmentation can mitigate caregiver stress and enhance adaptive responses.

Emotional coping strategies, such as venting and emotional support, were predominantly employed by joint families across both AG and IoT contexts. These results underline the strength of collectivist family structures, where emotional sharing and social bonding offer a protective climate for caregivers. Moreover, instrumental support was strongest in joint-high income families, demonstrating how collectivist frameworks also serve as effective functional resource networks, with results remaining consistent across governance models.

Finally, the integration of AG and IoT yielded strategic advantages in family coping systems. AG facilitated inclusive policies, adaptive planning, and community participation, while IoT enabled real-time monitoring, timely interventions, and data-driven care strategies. The synergistic effects of both frameworks support a resilient, personalized, and socially integrated caregiving environment for children with intellectual disabilities. These findings emphasize the importance of combining socio-political adaptability with technological innovation to holistically address caregiving challenges in complex family ecosystems.

The results identify that Adaptive Governance (AG) and IoT technologies greatly influence the coping strategies of intellectually disabled children's care families. These coping strategies are highly moderated by economic stability and family type. The incorporation of AG facilitates inclusivity and adaptability in structures, whereas IoT provides precision and immediacy in caregiving. They collectively offer a strong support base for building resilience, emotional health, and social integration, reiterating the imperative of multi-level, technology-enhanced caregiving frameworks in special needs situations.

The present research explored the impact of Adaptive Governance (AG) and the Internet of Things (IoT) on family coping strategies in families with children who have intellectual disabilities, focusing especially on the moderating effects of family type and economic status. The findings provide interesting insights into the ways in which structural, technological, and socio-economic environments influence coping in caregiving settings.

Influence of Family Type on Coping Strategy

The results validate the role of family structure in shaping the nature and efficiency of coping mechanisms. Joint families, especially those with greater incomes, were also more inclined to adopt proactive and adaptive coping mechanisms like active coping, planning, and instrumental support. This is in keeping with previous research for the role played by collectivist cultures and shared caregiving burdens in reducing psychological stress.

The shared social cohesion and resource-sharing of joint families seem to buffer stress and encourage emotional support, venting, and collective problem-solving. Compared to the nuclear or extended family, especially the low-income family, these tended to rely on less adaptive methods like denial, which might reflect psychological overload or restricted structural access.

Income level strongly moderated coping outcomes, and high-income families in all types uniformly reported healthier utilisation of activities such as positive reframing, planning, and behavioural activation. This is consistent with theory that economic capital facilitates psychological capital by providing access to quality health care, information, and supportive technology. In contrast, low-income families experienced compounded challenges and were more likely to engage in emotional avoidance or passive coping, feeding fears of system inequality in caregiving resources.

Boosting Coping with IoT Integration

Among the most relevant findings was the contribution of IoT to adaptive coping mechanisms. In comparison with AG only, the context of IoT consistently had larger mean scores in active coping, behavioural activation, and instrumental support across all family structures. This indicates that smart technology adoption, including health monitoring sensors, virtual therapy portals, and AI-powered care apps, could be used as behaviour scaffolds that facilitate routine, responsibility, and action on the spur of the moment.

These findings resonate with earlier studies of digital assistive technologies for caregiving, which emphasize IoT's promise in reducing caregiver burden and facilitating real-time intervention to meet a child's needs. The interactivity and customization of IoT most likely instil in caregivers a sense of control and agency, which are central to effective coping.

Adaptive Governance as a Structural Enabler

Whereas IoT provided quick, technological solutions, AG emerged as a structural enabler, opening space for inclusive decision-making, responsive policy formulation, and community participation. The joint families under AG, particularly with high-income, demonstrated high levels of participation with active coping strategies, indicating that if policy infrastructure promotes autonomy, decentralization, and adaptive planning, caregivers stand a better chance of responding constructively to difficulties.

AG's focus on feedback cycles, participatory structures, and adaptive institutions proves highly suitable to the uncertain dynamics of caregiving for intellectually disabled children. It both reinforces psychological resilience and sustainable caregiving ecosystems.

Integration of AG and IoT: Toward a Hybrid Coping Ecosystem

The primary theoretical contribution of this research is in hypothesizing a hybrid coping ecosystem, whereby AG supplies the adaptive framework and IoT provides the dynamic functionality. The collaboration of these systems maximizes the caregiver's cognitive, emotional, and behavioural reactions towards stress. This is aligned with the new models in digital governance and care-tech, which promote integrative designs when it comes to special needs caregiving.

Together, AG and IoT support a multi-level resilience model—AG bolstering macro-level flexibility and inclusion, and IoT facilitating micro-level behaviours change and real-time problem-solving.

Implications for Clinical Practice and Policy

- **Policymakers** should promote adaptive governance frameworks that are sensitive to family structure and economic disparities, integrating feedback from caregivers into policy loops.
- **Healthcare and education systems** should collaborate to distribute IoT-based care tools, particularly in lower-income households and nuclear families.
- **Training programs** for caregivers should address digital literacy and emotional intelligence, ensuring both technological and psychological readiness.
- Special attention must be given to **intersectional disadvantages** (e.g., low income + nuclear family) to avoid deepening disparities in coping capacity.
- **Intervention Strategies** can be further tailored by keeping AI, AR, VR, XR technologies in perspective for effective care and treatments of the disabled children and other awareness program (Vajpayee, Gupta and Sanghani, 2025).

CONCLUSION

This research validates the catalytic role of Adaptive Governance (AG) and the Internet of Things (IoT) in determining the coping strategies of families with children who have intellectual disabilities. Thematic analysis found that coping behaviour not only depends on family structure and economic stability but also greatly augmented by the integration of governance models and digital technology. Specifically, more affluent joint families demonstrated greater resilience, leveraging both emotional and instrumental support systems. This adaptive capacity is additionally reinforced by the synergistic deployment of AG frameworks—via inclusive policies and community-based engagement—and IoT-enabled initiatives like real-time tracking, facilitative reminders, and tailored digital support.

Pitt et al. (2025) highlight the imperative to investigate technologies such as brain–computer interfaces for children with communication restrictions, congruent with this research's conclusions that digital augmentation (via IoT) increases coping effectiveness by minimizing the physical and affective load on caregivers. Technologies embedded in care ecosystems are not merely ancillary; they provide a basic platform for early intervention, responsive variability, and maximized well-being—particularly for families once hampered by systemic or socioeconomic limitations.

Rydzewski (2025) is clear that digital inequality imperils sustainable development. Our results support this threat, especially since the effectiveness of coping strategies was most evident in financially secure, tech-enabled homes. This suggests a digital divide that can cause low-income families to lack access to essential technological capabilities, creating perpetuating structural disadvantage. Hence, any progress in AG or IoT is to be followed with initiatives for equal access so care outcomes can be inclusive.

Vajpayee (2024) resonates this by projecting how IoT can counteract procrastination, enhance well-being, and enhance healthcare delivery. These processes are particularly applicable in caregiving situations where timely responses and emotional exhaustion are prevalent. Likewise, research conducted in Industry 5.0 environments (Vajpayee, 2024; Patwari & Vajpayee, 2024) emphasizes the increased role of technetronic interventions and social media ecology in redefining behavioural outcomes, corroborating the function of technologically enabled environments in supporting adaptive coping.

Psychologically and developmentally, the coordination of affective, cognitive, and pragmatic strategies grounded in environmental and technological scaffolds informs prior work by Vajpayee and Mishra (2003), who found early training, visual literacy, and cognitive support to strongly improve performance and perception in children. This work continues this research agenda through family systems, illustrating how AG and IoT support child development and parental resilience.

In addition, the need for inclusive design and immersive assistive technologies (Zhang et al., 2025; Lalar et al., 2025; Vajpayee, 2024b) reinforces the argument for policy and practice to be open to change while maintaining ethical and contextual relevance. As Ghosh (2025) describes, adaptive learning techniques in specialist areas such as speech-language pathology hold potential for tailored support—a view reflected in our discussion of planning and behaviour activation approaches augmented through IoT (Vajpayee, 2025; Vajpayee and Sanghani, 2025).

In conclusion, the blending of AG and IoT not only promotes resilience among caregivers but also connects traditional and technological coping systems. It converts passive support into dynamic care models, shifting from reactive to proactive systems. But in order to genuinely live up to the potential of this integration, it is essential to solve digital inequality (Rydzewski, 2025; Vajpayee, 2024c), provide cultural applicability in implementation (Roussou et al., 2025), and facilitate cross-sectoral collaboration in education, healthcare, and social policy. As the caregiving landscape itself keeps changing, long-term psychological effects, access to scales across diverse communities, and testing new digital technologies such as AI, VR, and brain–computer interfaces for their potential in inclusive and sustainable family support systems need to be assessed by future studies (Vajpayee, Gupta and Sanghani, 2025).

REFERENCES

Adewunmi, M. C. (2025). Parents as catalysts for structural transformation toward inclusive and sustainable development. *International Journal of Social and Educational Innovation (IJSEIro)*, 42–64.

Alanazi, A. S., Benlaria, H., & Alanazi, S. A. (2025). Sustainable assistive technology and employment opportunities for graduates with disability: Mediating role of government support. *Education and Information Technologies*, *30*(1), 257–278. DOI: 10.1007/s10639-024-12863-0

Alibudbud, R. C., Aruta, J. J. B. R., Sison, K. A., & Guinto, R. R. (2025). Artificial intelligence in the era of planetary health: Insights on its application for the climate change-mental health nexus in the Philippines. *International Review of Psychiatry (Abingdon, England)*, *37*(1), 21–32. DOI: 10.1080/09540261.2024.2363373 PMID: 40035376

Almufareh, M. F., Tehsin, S., Humayun, M., & Kausar, S. (2023). Intellectual disability and technology: An artificial intelligence perspective and framework. *Journal of Disability Research*, *2*(4), 58–70. DOI: 10.57197/JDR-2023-0055

Brien, M., Coutinho, F., Krishna, D., van der Haar, L., de Laat, J., Srinivasan, S. R., & Venkatachalapathy, N. (2023). Leveraging monitoring, evaluation, and learning to scale the Enabling Inclusion® program for children with disabilities in India and globally. *Frontiers in Public Health*, *11*, 1165034. DOI: 10.3389/fpubh.2023.1165034 PMID: 38162603

Cardona-Acevedo, S., Agudelo-Ceballos, E., Cumpa Vásquez, J. T., Martínez Rojas, E., Valencia-Arias, A., Jimenez Garcia, J. A., & Benjumea Arias, M. L. (2025, March). E-learning technologies at the secondary education level: Literature review. [). Frontiers Media SA.]. *Frontiers in Education*, *10*, 1539763. DOI: 10.3389/feduc.2025.1539763

Chandra, S., Fane, J., Azizi, N., McKenzie-Gray, M., Sager, M., & Dautenhahn, K. (2025). Integrating New Instructional Assistive Technology to Support Academic and Behavioural Instruction for Students with Learning Disabilities. *Journal of Special Education Technology* 01626434251314042. DOI: 10.1177/01626434251314042

Chandra, S., Fane, J., Azizi, N., McKenzie-Gray, M., Sager, M., & Dautenhahn, K. (2025). Integrating New Instructional Assistive Technology to Support Academic and Behavioural Instruction for Students with Learning Disabilities. *Journal of Special Education Technology*, 01626434251314042. DOI: 10.1177/01626434251314042

Cubas, A. L. V., Provin, A. P., Dutra, A. R. D. A., Andrade Guerra, J. B. S. O. D., & Mussi, C. C. (2025). Forging a sustainable path: The QualEnv consortium's practices and strategies in promoting sustainable development in higher education institutions. *International Journal of Sustainability in Higher Education, 26*(1), 63–82. DOI: 10.1108/IJSHE-11-2023-0514

Fellows, E. K., & Batmunkh, D. (2025). Impact investing in childcare systems.

Ghosh, S. S. (2025). ADAPTIVE LEARNING METHODS IN SPEECH-LANGUAGE PATHOLOGY. *The Routledge Handbook of the Sociopolitical Context of Language Learning*, 454.

Gupta, J., & Vegelin, C. (2016). Sustainable development goals and inclusive development. *International Environmental Agreement: Politics, Law and Economics, 16*(3), 433–448. DOI: 10.1007/s10784-016-9323-z

Ishak, H., Matore, M. E. E. M., & Nor, H. A. M. (2025). Bibliometric analysis of adaptive behavior research: Advancing Sustainable Development Goals (SDGs) for children with disabilities. *Journal of Lifestyle and SDGs Review*, *5*(2), e03405. DOI: 10.47172/2965-730X.SDGsReview.v5.n02.pe03405

Kumar, A., Vajpayee, A., & Sanghani, P. (2024). IoT-infused care: Disentanglement family dynamics and coping strategies in the realm of intellectually disabled children. In Gupta, S. K., Karras, D. A., & Natarajan, R. (Eds.), *Revolutionizing Healthcare: AI Integration with IoT for Enhanced Patient Outcomes* (Vol. 7). Springer., DOI: 10.1007/978-3-031-65022-2_14

Lalar, S., Kumar, T., Kumar, R., & Kumar, S. (2025). Unlocking Potential: The Role of Artificial Intelligence in Revolutionizing Special Education for Inclusive Learning. In *Impacts of Generative AI on the Future of Research and Education* (pp. 201-232). IGI Global.

Lesiuk, T., Kauffman, M. A., Fleszar-Pavlovic, S. E., Esquives, B. N., Brito, A. E., Wang, T., & Penedo, F. J. (2025). A hybrid eHealth mindfulness-based music therapy intervention for adults receiving an allogeneic hematopoietic stem cell transplant. *Music Therapy Perspectives*, *43*(1), miaf004.

Malviya, R., & Rajput, S. (2025). Advances and Insights into AI-Created Disability Supports.

Niu, Q., Li, H., Liu, Y., Qin, Z., Zhang, L. B., Chen, J., & Lyu, Z. (2024). Toward the internet of medical things: Architecture, trends and challenges. *Mathematical Biosciences and Engineering*, *21*(1), 650–678. DOI: 10.3934/mbe.2024028 PMID: 38303438

Oyedokun, T. T. (2025). Assistive Technology and Accessibility Tools in Enhancing Adaptive Education. In *Advancing Adaptive Education: Technological Innovations for Disability Support* (pp. 125-162). IGI Global Scientific Publishing.

Patwari, P., & Vajpayee, A. (2024). Exploring the Interplay of Educational Social Media Usage, Procrastination, and Subjective Well-being in the Context of Industry 5.0 Education. In Tripathi, S., & Rosak-Szyrocka, J. (Eds.). (2024*). Impact of Artificial Intelligence on Society* (1st ed.). Chapman and Hall/CRC. Pp:119-133.

Pistolesi, M., Frangioni, G., Fraboni, F., Fabbri, E., & Masci, F. (2025). How will technology change people's home care in the next 20 years? A strategic foresight study. *Ergonomics*, *68*(3), 406–424. DOI: 10.1080/00140139.2024.2334428 PMID: 38533589

Pitt, K. M., Mikuls, A., Ousley, C. L., Boster, J. B., Mahmoudi, M., McCarthy, J., & Burnison, J. (2025). Considering whether brain–computer interfaces have prospective potential to support children who have the physical abilities for touch-based AAC access: A forum manuscript. *Augmentative and Alternative Communication*, 1–9. DOI: 10.1080/07434618.2025.2495897 PMID: 40454682

Pitts, L. N., Armstrong, A., Fleming, L., Fazeli, P. L., Landier, W., & Ladores, S. (2025). The application and evolution of the social-ecological model for adolescent and young adult readiness for transition: A scoping review. *Journal of Pediatric Health Care*, *39*(3), 355–376. DOI: 10.1016/j.pedhc.2024.12.004 PMID: 39772328

Ramaiah, M. S., Nagarajan, S. K. S., Whig, P., & Dutta, P. K. (2025). AI-powered innovations transforming adaptive education for disability support. In *Advancing Adaptive Education: Technological Innovations for Disability Support* (pp. 73–100). IGI Global Scientific Publishing.

Roussou, A. M., Argyrakou, C. C., & Milakis, E. D. (2025). Integrating STEAM and theatrical methods in early childhood environmental education: A framework for holistic learning. *International Journal of Geography, Geology and Environment*, *7*(2), 19–42.

Rydzewski, P. (2025). Digital inequality and sustainable development. *Problemy Ekorozwoju*, *20*(1), 96–108. DOI: 10.35784/preko.6691

Vajpayee, A., & Ramachandran, K. K. (2019) Reconnoitring Artificial Intelligence in Knowledge Management. International Journal of Innovative Technology and Exploring Engineering (IJITEE) ISSN: 2278-3075, Volume-8 Issue-7C May 2019. Pp; 114-117.

Vajpayee, A. (2017). Effect of Early Intervention on Pictorial Perception of Deprived and Non-Deprived Children. *Indian Journal of Psychological Science. Vol, 9*(1).

Vajpayee, A. (2019). Critical Issues of Early Intervention for the Amelioration of Social Isolation of Kharwar Children. In (Eds) Nagendra Kumar Singh, Tribal Communication Myth Metaphor and Reality. Iesha Gyandeep Publication, ISBN: 9788193790694. New Delhi (pp 169-181).

Vajpayee, A. (2017). Impact of Visual Literacy Skill Program on Visual Literacy of Deprived Children and Non-Deprived Children. *Likars'ka Sprava*, (7), 75–80. https://liksprava.com/index.php/journal/article/view/314. DOI: 10.31640/LS-2017(7)15

Vajpayee, A. (2024). IoT in Daily Life: Investigating the Impact of IoT on Procrastination, Well-Being, Mental Health, and Healthcare Wizards. In Gupta, S. K., Karras, D. A., & Natarajan, R. (Eds.), *Revolutionizing Healthcare: AI Integration with IoT for Enhanced Patient Outcomes. Information Systems Engineering and Management, ISBN: 978-3-031-65021* (Vol. 7). Springer., DOI: 10.1007/978-3-031-65022-2_11

Vajpayee, A. (2024). Pixels, Perspectives, and Psychological Strain: Unravelling the Link Between Negative Body Image, Internet of Things (IOT), and Mental Health Challenges in Student Population. In: Gupta, S.K., Karras, D.A., Natarajan, R. (eds) *Revolutionizing Healthcare: AI Integration with IoT for Enhanced Patient Outcomes. Information Systems Engineering and Management*, (Pp-). vol 7. ISBN: 978-3-031-65021. Springer Nature, Switzerland, Cham. https://doi.org/DOI: 10.1007/978-3-031-65022-2_17

Vajpayee, A. (2024). Traditional pedagogy to Technetronic Education. *Aspects of Quality Management in Value Creating in the Industry 5.0 Way*, 179. ISBN: 9781032677019 https://doi.org/DOI: 10.1201/9781032677040

Vajpayee, A., Gupta, S. K., & Sanghani, P. (2025). Immersive Learning for Environmental Stewardship: Behavioural Effectiveness, Engagement, and Motivation to Act Through XR Technology. In: Gupta, S.K., Maurya, N., Le, DN., Mzili, T. (eds) Exploring the Impact of Extended Reality (XR) Technologies on Promoting Environmental Sustainability. Information Systems Engineering and Management, vol 38. Pp-383-480 Springer Nature, Switzerland Cham. ISBN: 978-3-031-88013-1. https://doi.org/DOI: 10.1007/978-3-031-88013-1_21

Vajpayee, A., & Mishra, R. C. (2003). The Short and Long-Term Effect of Training on Cognitive Task Performance of Children. *Indian Journal of Psychology, 10*, 6–12.

Vajpayee, A. (2019). Critical Issues of Early Intervention for the Amelioration of Social Isolation of Kharwar Children. In (Eds) Nagendra Kumar Singh, Tribal Communication Myth Metaphor and Reality. Iesha Gyandeep Publication, ISBN: 9788193790694. New Delhi (pp 169-181).

Vajpayee, A. (2021). Environmental challenges and critical issues of early intervention for the children of Kharwar tribe. In Pratap, A., Paranjape, B., Shyam, G. 2021 (Eds.). Tribal and Environmental History of India: New Perspectives. Research India Press. New Delhi, Pp-312-328.

Vajpayee, A. (2023). Intervention Studies for Mental Health: A Comprehensive Exploration of Historical Evolution, Theoretical Foundations, and Contemporary Applications. Journal of Humanities, Music and Dance, Vol-3, Issue-5, Pp-21-33. ISSN:2799-1180. https://doi.org/10.55529/jmhib.35.21.33

Vajpayee, A. (2025). AG-IoT and robotics solutions for early intervention in developmental delays among mentally retarded children. In Malik, M. M., Maryam, H., Khan, I. U., & Gupta, S. K. (Eds.), *Artificial General-Internet of Things (AG-IoT) for Robotics: Advanced computer vision applications and future trends* (Vol. 58, pp. 1–16). Springer., DOI: 10.1007/978-3-031-95302-6_1

Vajpayee, A., & Sanghani, P. (2025). Exploring the impact of AR, IoT, and robotics on cognitive and motor functioning in children with neurodevelopmental disorders. In Malik, M. M., Maryam, H., Khan, I. U., & Gupta, S. K. (Eds.), *Artificial General-Internet of Things (AG-IoT) for Robotics: Advanced computer vision applications and future trends* (Vol. 58, pp. 17–34). Springer., DOI: 10.1007/978-3-031-95302-6_2

Verdejo Espinosa, Á., Lopez, J. L., Mata Mata, F., & Estevez, M. E. (2021). Application of IoT in healthcare: Keys to implementation of the sustainable development goals. *Sensors (Basel)*, *21*(7), 2330. DOI: 10.3390/s21072330 PMID: 33810606

Wåger, J., & Bagger, A. (2025). Didactic dimensions of teaching content for and with students with intellectual disabilities (ID): A scoping review. *European Journal of Special Needs Education*, *40*(1), 53–68. DOI: 10.1080/08856257.2024.2323250

Wiafe, E., & Azubuike, C. M. (2024). Juggling family commitments and responsibilities in North America: Narratives from female African graduate students. *Cuadernos del Centro de Estudios de Diseño y Comunicación*, 27(238).

Zhang, X., Pan, S. L., Tim, Y., & Jiang, Z. (2025). Designing an immersive virtual reality artefact for disability inclusion: An action design research. *European Journal of Information Systems*, 1–30. DOI: 10.1080/0960085X.2025.2567670

Chapter 2

Advancing AI Integration in Healthcare Using Federated Learning:

Trends and Challenges in Federated Learning for AI-Enabled Healthcare

Mandeep Singh
https://orcid.org/0000-0003-3278-4877
Bennett University, Greater Noida, India

Gaganjot Kaur
https://orcid.org/0000-0001-9326-9196
Raj Kumar Goel Institute of Technology, Ghaziabad, India

Pranshu Saxena
https://orcid.org/0000-0002-0822-1532
Bennett University, Greater Noida, India

Megha Sharma
K.R. Mangalam University, Gurugram, India

ABSTRACT

With the growing demand for secure, intelligent, and collaborative healthcare systems, Federated Learning (FL) has emerged as a transformative approach for developing AI models without exposing sensitive patient data. This chapter provides a detailed overview of FL's core architecture and its specialized variants—such as hierarchical, asynchronous, and personalized FL—tailored to healthcare's

DOI: 10.4018/979-8-3373-3306-9.ch002

distributed and privacy-sensitive landscape. It explores privacy-enhancing mechanisms including local differential privacy, secure aggregation, and homomorphic encryption, all critical for training in heterogeneous environments. The integration of FL with blockchain, edge computing, and explainable AI (XAI) demonstrates how these technologies strengthen traceability, transparency, and real-time intelligence. Key challenges such as regulatory inconsistencies, infrastructural constraints, and model drift are critically examined. The chapter envisions a federated AI ecosystem promoting equitable, privacy-aware innovation through institutional collaboration and scalable deployment strategies.

1. INTRODUCTION

With evidence-based medicine becoming ever more prominent in present times, the driving force within the healthcare sector is artificial intelligence (AI). It is ranging from improving radiological diagnostic accuracy to driving next-generation chronic disease monitoring platforms and is transforming patient and clinical processes alike. Predictive modeling in the current era is helping with sepsis early detection, emergency presentation triaging, and even deciding on the best-of-class treatment plan for a patient's own individual physiological traits. Greater acceptance of AI does, however, depend on that one all-important quality.

The quality, quantity, and diversity of data on which any AI model is trained directly determine its performance. Representative large-scale data in medicine, nonetheless, constitute an epidemic issue. Clinicians, labs, and hospitals produce a huge volume of patient data in isolated silos with strict privacy controls like the Health Insurance Portability and Accountability Act (HIPAA) in the US or the General Data Protection Regulation (GDPR) in Europe. Even though these acts are helpful in providing the patients with confidentiality, they indirectly discourage cumulative AI development because they forbid data sharing among institutions.

Centralized training paradigms for AI, which typically require collecting all data into a single repository location, are increasingly under strain. Aside from legal requirements, the logistical burden of data transport and the inherent security weaknesses of centralized storage systems make this paradigm inoperable in majority of real-world healthcare environments. Furthermore, such systems have no room for the full spectrum of patient diversity, as data sets originating from a single location cannot represent the heterogeneity of regions, populations, and clinical practices.

Such limitations have prompted increasing interest in Federated Learning (FL), a distributed machine learning paradigm whereby multiple parties jointly train an AI model without the need for data sharing. Instead of data sharing, all contributing parties train locally and exchange only the learned parameters (e.g., weight updates) with a central aggregator. This enables sensitive health data to remain behind institutional firewalls but still enables the building of solid, generalizable models. FL basically marries the good of two worlds, collective intelligence of data without compromising security or privacy.

FL is a paradigmatic approach to the creation and deployment of artificial intelligence in healthcare. Through decentralized cooperation, FL facilitates the utilization of previously underexploited data sources, like rural clinics, specialty hospitals, and foreign partners, thereby making models fairer and less biased more often than not in centrally trained AI systems. Additionally, FL opens the door to cutting-edge privacy-enabling technologies like secure multiparty computation, homomorphic encryption, and differential privacy. As a critical and practical summary to policymakers, researchers, and system implementers alike, the present chapter presents an authoritative examination of FL in medicine with insights needed for effective understanding and implementation of such a disruptive approach in actual clinical practice.

1.1 Objectives of the Chapter:

- To highlight the limitations of centralized AI development in healthcare, especially concerning data privacy, interoperability, and patient diversity.
- To explain the architectural and mathematical foundations of Federated Learning, including core algorithms such as Federated Averaging.
- To showcase real-world and hypothetical use cases where FL improves clinical AI performance across institutions.
- To examine the integration of FL with emerging technologies like blockchain, explainable AI, and edge computing.
- To outline key challenges, policy considerations, and future research directions for scaling FL-based AI systems in healthcare.

2. LITERATURE REVIEW

The rapid progress made in the development of artificial intelligence (AI) in health care has driven greater emphasis on distributed learning solutions that can overcome regulatory, infrastructural, and ethical hurdles to share centrally information. Among these, Federated Learning (FL) has received significant attention based on its promise of co-training machine learning models across organizations without sharing raw sensitive data. Several of the latest research studies have indicated its potential for a broad variety of health care applications, albeit with tremendous technical as well as operational challenges. Table 1. Provide a comparative analysis of Recent Federated Learning Approaches in Healthcare.

One of the most promising early adoption domains is healthcare IoT, where data streams from sensor-rich settings have the potential for real-time monitoring. Elayan et al. (2022) proposed a low-computational and environmentally friendly FL model for patient health monitoring that was optimized. Their approach exhibited energy efficiency and latency reduction while ensuring strict privacy protection. Hakak et al. (2020) utilized this as the foundation for creating an edge-enabled FL model tailored for real-time analytics in resource-limited environments. Their framework offered low-latency insights without sacrificing any data security via computations close to the data source.

For intelligent healthcare infrastructure, Gupta et al. (2021) suggested a hierarchical FL system based on digital twins for anomaly detection. Their multi-level approach improved synchronization of models and bandwidth requirements and was suited for large-scale deployment. Narwaria and Jaiswal (2024) also suggested an optimization-based client selection policy with a priority on clients whose contributions maximized model convergence—a very effective approach to manage non-IID (non-identically distributed) data and variable client availability, both common in real-world FL environments.

Medical imaging has also emerged as an important application area. Ullah et al. (2024) developed a scalable FL system specifically tailored for sporadic client connectivity in collaborative diagnostic environments. Their system ensured diagnostic performance even with unreliable networks. At the same time, Natarajan et al., (2025) developed a wearable-device-based FL framework that allows on-device model updates to support continuous, privacy-preserving patient monitoring. In order to offer secure computation across distributed environments, Muazu et al. (2024) employed multi-party computation and additive secret sharing in their FL solution. This facilitated joint training without disclosing individual data sources. Additionally, Adnan et al. (2025) addressed privacy concerns in Internet of Vehicles (IoV) healthcare systems by incorporating differential privacy mechanisms into their FL solution, protecting individual data points from re-identification even after model aggregation.

Another emerging area of research in the literature involves the combination of blockchain systems and FL to promote the highest possible trust, transparency, and auditability. Mathew et al., (2024) introduced a blockchain-protected FL model appropriate for forthcoming Healthcare 5.0 contexts. Their system facilitated the verifiable update of the model and immutable records. Similarly, Li, (2025) took the practice one step ahead and introduced blockchain safeguarding for multi-device data sharing along with decentralized learning coordination. To this synergy, Purohit et al., (2025) introduced FedBlocks, a federated IPFS-based framework for decentralized data storage and smart contracts for managing privacy-aware learning processes among IoT health devices. There has also been research on client contribution optimization and data valuing. Kumar et al., (2022) introduced an ensemble-based data valuation method that forecasts the data impact of every client on overall model performance. This innovation enhances communication efficiency by directing effort toward clients who are providing worthy contributions.

In addition to contributions in the technical domain, there is a growing body of evidence underlining ethics and fairness considerations. A systematic review of FL-based skin cancer detection systems by Yaqoob et al. (2023) underscored FL's capabilities in ensuring patient privacy and supporting cross-institutional learning while cautioning against underrepresented population group biases. The authors suggested fairness-aware design strategies to prevent performance disparities upon clinical deployment. In aggregate, the works point towards the potential for FL to contribute to making health AI more safe, equitable, and cooperative. There are countless obstacles to overcome. Most of FL applications have not had representative benchmarks for their performance across many different environments. Deployments on actual environments have not yet gotten much beyond the beginning, with nearly all systems reported merely in simulators or minute pilot-scale situations. Lastly, explainability is a relatively unexplored domain, although it is very important in clinician-centered AI solutions. As federated systems continue to develop, integrating interpretability, fairness, and multi-stakeholder verification into them will be essential to their long-term success in clinical environments.

Table 1. Comparative Analysis of Recent Federated Learning Approaches in Healthcare

Author	Objective	Approach	Application Area	Feature	Identified Gaps
Elayan et al., (2022)	Enhance sustainability and performance in IoT-based healthcare using deep FL	Deep FL architecture for edge-based sensor data	IoT healthcare monitoring	Data locality, reduced latency	Limited application to non-IoT modalities
Hakak et al., (2020)	Enable real-time analytics in edge-constrained environments	Edge-assisted FL framework	Real-time healthcare data analytics	Local processing of sensitive data	Scalability across larger networks
Gupta et al., (2021)	Detect anomalies using hierarchical FL and digital twins	Multi-layer FL with digital twins for anomaly detection	Smart healthcare infrastructure	Hierarchical training layers	Requires high infrastructure coordination

continued on following page

Table 1. Continued

Author	Objective	Approach	Application Area	Feature	Identified Gaps
Narwaria & Jaiswal, (2024)	Improve convergence using client selection	Class-topper optimization in FL	FL model optimization	Client participation prioritization	Performance with highly skewed data untested
Ullah et al., (2024)	Support FL under intermittent client connectivity	Scalable FL system for imaging	Medical imaging	Model resilience to connectivity loss	Model adaptation under dynamic data not explored
Natarajan et al., (2025)	Enable continuous on-device learning for wearables	Wearable-device FL training framework	Remote patient monitoring	On-device updates with no raw data transfer	Limited evaluation across device platforms
Muazu et al., (2024)	Secure FL training with privacy-preserving computation	Multi-party computation + additive secret sharing	Collaborative clinical data training	Zero data exposure in training	Computational overhead not quantified
Adnan et al., (2025)	Integrate differential privacy in FL for mobile health	Differentially private FL model	IoV healthcare systems	Privacy against re-identification	Impact on model accuracy not detailed
Mathew et al., (2024)	Ensure FL auditability via blockchain	Blockchain-backed FL framework	Healthcare 5.0 ecosystems	Immutable model updates	Blockchain scalability concerns
Li, (2025)	Secure multi-device FL coordination	Blockchain-integrated FL	Multi-device health data sharing	Decentralized trust architecture	Coordination latency not addressed
Purohit et al., (2025)	Integrate FL with Web 3.0 using IPFS	FedBlocks: FL + IPFS + blockchain	IoT-enabled decentralized healthcare	Smart contracts for coordination	Limited benchmarking in healthcare
Kumar et al., (2022)	Improve FL efficiency via data valuation	Ensembling-based client contribution analysis	Federated performance optimization	Client selection based on utility	Sensitive to noisy client data
(Yaqoob et al., 2023)	Review FL use in skin cancer detection	Systematic analysis of FL in dermatology	Privacy-focused dermatological AI	FL-based anonymized training	Demographic bias and fairness concerns

3. AI AND DATA CHALLENGES IN MODERN HEALTHCARE

Artificial intelligence (AI) is increasingly reshaping healthcare, providing effective tools for disease diagnosis, predictive analytics, process optimization, and customized treatment. Yet to realize the complete potential of AI is to have access to vast, varied, and high-quality data sets, something that is still a major obstacle in medical areas. Data-related issues in healthcare are intrinsically complicated, with technical restrictions but also regulatory, ethical, and infrastructural ones. These constraints are further exacerbated by heterogeneity in data, separated systems, which warrant a transition from the centralized learning modality to the distributed, collective models like FL.

3.1 Types of Healthcare Data

Healthcare systems continue to store various types of data with distinct characteristics and limitations. The most common are medical imaging datasets such as computed tomography (CT), magnetic resonance imaging (MRI), positron emission tomography (PET), and digital pathology. These datasets are voluminous, taking up a significant amount of storage space and computing resources. They form the core of AI-assisted diagnostics, especially in departments such as oncology, cardiology, and neurology. In recent history, Ullah et al. (2024) illustrated the application of Federated Learning (FL) in medical imaging and how it could enable cross-institutional model training without compromising patient confidentiality.

aside from imaging, electronic health records (EHRs) are the other precious source of information for healthcare organizations these days. EHRs contain structured and unstructured data, e.g., patient demographics, lab test results, medication lists, diagnostic codes, and free-text clinical notes. With data rich as datasets in EHRs are, they are susceptible to incompleteness, variability in formatting, and considerable heterogeneity between institutions. Moreover, because of the nature of the data, strict security is a must. To counteract such problems, Muazu et al. (2024) presented federated architecture using additive secret sharing and multi-party computation that facilitates collaborative training on secret clinical information without the sharing of individual records.

Another rapidly developing source of data is Internet of Medical Things (IoMT) and wearable and smartwatches, fitness trackers, and remote patient monitoring devices. These devices generate streams of time-series data for physiological parameters such as heart rate, blood glucose, oxygen saturation, and physical activity. Elayan et al. (2022) suggested a deep FL framework to address such IoT-generated data with optimal energy efficiency and model responsiveness with localizing patient data. Similarly, Ghosh and Ghosh (2023) introduced the FEEL architecture for senior care with emphasis on edge intelligence for health surveillance in decentralized environments.

3.2 Barriers to Data Sharing

Even with the abundance and richness of healthcare data, crossing the boundaries of institutions to exchange it is still full of problems. Foremost among them is patient confidentiality. Jurisdictions such as the Health Insurance Portability and Accountability Act (HIPAA) in the United States and the General Data Protection Regulation (GDPR) in the European Union have rigorous rules governing the sharing and processing of identifiable health information. These limitations, as important in safeguarding the patient, typically inhibit centralization of information for machine learning purposes (Mathew et al., 2024).

In addition to legal challenges, data heterogeneity also presents technical challenges. Different hospitals may use different formats, standards, annotation procedures, and medical equipment. Such non-standardization introduces domain changes, variations in distributions of data that undermine the generalizability of AI models trained in one environment when applied in another. As Kumar et al. (2022) have noted, models learned from isolated data sets are prone to fail to generalize across geographically or demographically diverse groups, and this could lead to clinically inequitable results. Moreover, missing or incomplete data are also very common in actual clinical documents. It is especially prevalent in resource-constrained settings, as is the uneven digitization of the records. Institutional silos also exacerbate this as many healthcare systems operate in silos from one another, with proprietary software that does not permit interoperability and sharing of data.

3.3 The Need for Distributed Learning Approaches

To counter these challenges, distributed learning has been identified as a potential solution. In contrast to traditional models that pool all the data into a central server, distributed learning allows for training across many nodes without passing sensitive information. Federated Learning has been shown to be effective in solving for privacy, interoperability, and regulatory limitations.

FL allows all the institutions involved to locally train a model on their local data and send model parameters (e.g., weight updates) to a central server only, which aggregates these updates to produce a global model. This architecture preserves patient confidentiality and provides data diversity and, therefore, is ideally suited for scenarios where there is non-independent and identically distributed (non-IID) data—a typical limitation of training centralized AI, Gupta et al. (2021). In the case of edge computing and wearable devices, Adnan et al. (2025) showed that by integrating FL with differential privacy, it is possible to facilitate learning with awareness of privacy on mobile devices, further broadening its applications. Apart from privacy protection, FL minimizes network overhead by not having to send huge amounts of raw data. FL also provides institutions with limited computational resources the ability to engage in collaborative AI development by offloading the processing to local or edge devices (Hakak et al. 2020).

3.4 Emergence of Collaborative Health Intelligence

They augment each other to attain collaborative health intelligence, an aspect where patients, edge devices, research institutions, and healthcare providers all contribute value toward public development of AI systems without trading for ownership of data. Unlike centralized, traditional AI development, collaborative health intelligence fosters model fairness and inclusiveness through chances for divergent populations and institutions to be brought into training.

Purohit et al. (2025) illustrated a blockchain-based federated learning framework—FedBlocks—which realizes this dream by integrating decentralized storage and model orchestration. With increasing advancement in the healthcare domain, the shift towards distributed, privacy-oriented, and cooperative AI construction will be inevitable. Federated Learning, underpinned by secure and scalable architecture, will be an enabler for effective and ethical collaborative health intelligence.

4. FUNDAMENTALS OF FEDERATED LEARNING IN HEALTHCARE

Federated Learning (FL) is a novel collaborative machine learning paradigm particularly well-adapted to areas where data security, privacy, and institutional self-governance are of highest importance. In medicine, where patient information, radiology images, and real-time sensor telemetry are not public and may be regulated by laws such as HIPAA and GDPR, FL offers a method to train AI systems on distributed sources of data without importing the raw data into a center. This section discusses the building elements of FL, its life cycle of operation, the central algorithmic features, and how it compares to the other learning frameworks (Singh et al., 2023).

4.1 Basic FL Architecture: Clients, Server, and Aggregation

A typical Federated Learning system has three components: clients, a central server, and a secure communication interface. The clients are the places where the data reside—hospitals, mobile health devices, pathology labs, or patients' wearable technology. The clients must have sufficient computing power to train a local machine learning model.

The global server coordinates the training procedure. It starts the global model, distributes it to selected clients, collects their locally updated models, and merges the updates into a new global model. The server never sees or stores raw data. The communication infrastructure supports secure transmission of model parameters (e.g., weights or gradients) between the server and clients, usually using encrypted protocols to ensure the integrity and confidentiality of the model updates. The advantage of this architecture is that it preserves data locality. All clients can participate in global model training without compromising sensitive patient data, thus facilitating compliance with privacy and trust between institutions (Singh et al., 2023).

4.2 FL System Lifecycle

The FL process unfolds through repeated communication rounds, involving the following steps: First, in the initialization phase, the central server generates a base model with initial weights and sends it to a selected group of clients. The selection of clients may be random or based on resource availability, data quality, or connectivity status. In the local training phase, each client independently trains the received model using its private dataset. This training typically consists of a few local epochs using optimization methods such as stochastic gradient descent (SGD). Importantly, the data remains entirely local to the client. Fig. 1. Provide an overview of the FL System Lifecycle in Healthcare Applications

Figure 1. Federated Learning System Lifecycle in Healthcare Applications

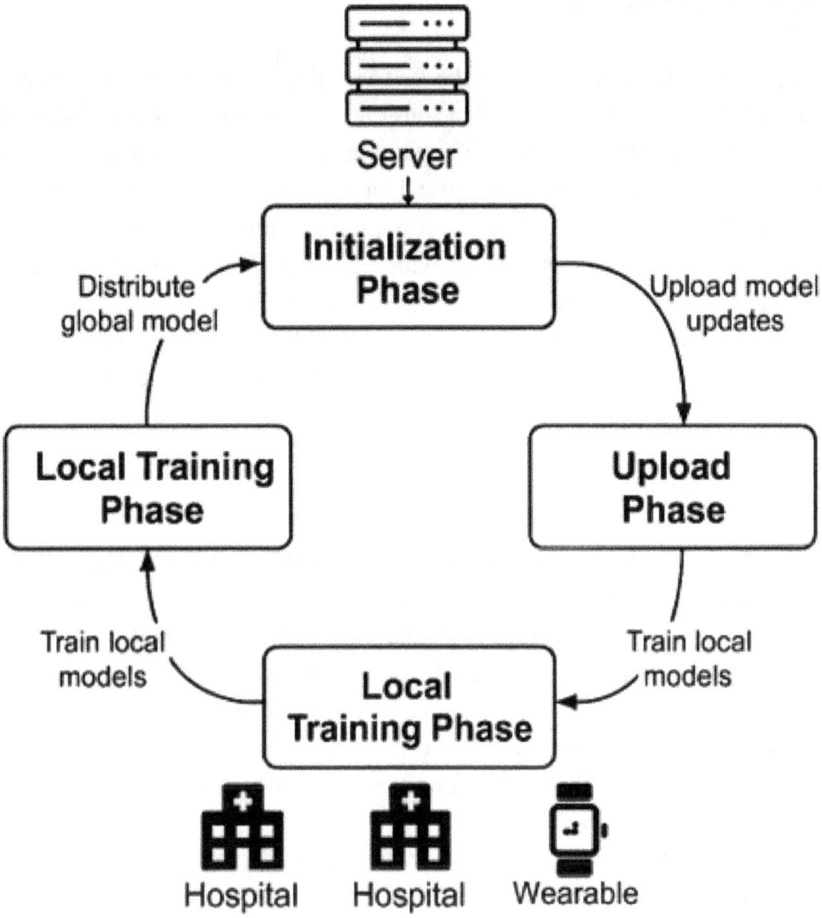

Once training is complete, the upload process begins, where each client sends only the new model parameters, and not the data itself, to the central server. The server performs an aggregation step, where it aggregates all the updates from the clients and produces a better global model. It then sends the model back to the clients, and the cycle repeats. Training continues incrementally until the global model converges to a target performance level or reaches a predetermined number of iterations. This iterative learning paradigm allows FL systems to recursively improve model accuracy while affording strong data privacy guarantees. (Singh et al., 2023).

4.3 Federated Averaging (FedAvg) Algorithm: Mathematical Foundation

Behind Federated Learning lies the FedAvg algorithm, which dictates the aggregation of the local updates from various clients into a new global model. While experimental verification or simulation outcomes are not presented in this chapter, it is beneficial to present the mathematical basis of FedAvg so that the readers can see the underlying logic behind FL coordination theoretically. It also validates the scholarly merit of the chapter and provides a point of reference for researchers contemplating future application (M. Gupta et al., 2023).

FedAvg performs a weighted average of model updates submitted by clients during each training round. Its mathematical formulation is as follows:

$$w_{t+1} = \sum_{k=1}^{K} \frac{n_k}{n} w_t^k \tag{1}$$

In eq. (1), w_{t+1} is global model's updated parameters at round t+1, K is the number of participating clients in the current round, n_k is number of local data samples on client k, $n = \sum_{k=1}^{K} n_k$ is total number of training samples across all selected clients w_t^k is locally updated model parameters from client k at round t. The formula ensures that each client's contribution to the global model is proportional to the volume of its training data. For example, a large urban hospital with 10,000 radiology scans will have more influence than a rural clinic with 1,000 scans, while still protecting both institutions' data privacy.

By formalizing the aggregation mechanism, FedAvg enables distributed learning to approximate the performance of centralized training, without the associated risks of data centralization. Its simplicity and effectiveness have made it the default choice in many real-world FL systems.

4.4 Comparison with Centralized and Decentralized Architectures

To understand the benefits of Federated Learning in healthcare, it is enlightening to compare it with centralized and decentralized machine learning systems:

In centralized learning, all the data is transmitted to a central point where the model is trained. The model here has complete access to data, which would accelerate training and enhance performance. Such systems, however, cause very real problems of data breaches, privacy violation, and non-compliance with regulations, especially when the data concerns patients or images. Decentralized learning, on the other hand, eliminates the central server altogether. Patients are part of a peer-to-peer network, exchanging updates directly with each other. While this architecture maximizes fault tolerance and robustness, it is noted for excessive communication overhead and high coordination complexity. These features limit its realistic use in large-scale, heterogeneous health networks.

Federated Learning provides a reconciliatory solution. It maintains decentralized systems' privacy with data remaining on-device while easing model coordination using a central server. FL also minimizes bandwidth consumption by sending model updates only instead of full datasets. Last but not least, FL is fault-tolerant in nature; missing a few clients in any round does not interfere with global learning (Jain et al., 2024). This decentralized architecture makes FL especially well-suited for medical applications requiring stringent privacy, integration across institutions, and the frequent contexts of infrequent connectivity or fluctuating computational power. By integrating decentralization with centralized coordination, FL mitigates the fundamental challenges that have long plagued efforts to deploy AI in sensitive medical settings.

5. SECURITY AND PRIVACY IN FEDERATED LEARNING

Though Federated Learning (FL) serves the intrinsic concern of centralization of data by ensuring that sensitive records are not let outside the organizational framework, decentralized data per se may not provide robust security or privacy. As discussed earlier, FL provides collective learning between dispersed clients like hospitals or wearables. Still, even with raw data locally preserved, updates of a model, e.g., gradients or parameters, may unwittingly release sensitive data. Thus, an actual privacy-protecting FL system needs to incorporate sophisticated cryptographic and statistical methods to protect both model and data integrity throughout learning (Singh et al., 2021).

This section discusses some of the major techniques that boost the privacy and security of FL in healthcare: the mathematical foundations of differential privacy, secure aggregation protocols, homomorphic encryption, and trusted execution environments. All these elements together constitute the privacy-preserving foundation required for deploying FL in high-risk clinical settings.

5.1 Differential Privacy: Mathematical Modeling

Differential Privacy (DP) offers a mathematical framework for avoiding the inference of a single data point from the model outputs after a model has been trained. In FL, DP is typically achieved through injecting noise into the shared model updates from clients, thus making it statistically challenging for an attacker to infer whether a particular patient's data was used for training. A randomized mechanism M is said to be ϵ\epsilonϵ-differentially private if, for any two neighboring datasets D and D′ (which differ by only one record), and for all possible outputs S, the following condition holds:

$$\Pr[M(D) \in S] \leq e^{\epsilon} \cdot \Pr[M(D') \in S] \tag{2}$$

In Eq. (2), ϵ denotes the privacy budget, which governs the strength of privacy guarantees: lower ϵ values indicate stronger privacy. In healthcare FL applications, such guarantees are critical when training across clinical records, genomic data, or diagnostic imaging, where patient identifiability must be minimized. However, the intentional injection of noise into model updates introduces a tension between privacy and model performance, one that must be carefully managed to preserve diagnostic accuracy.

5.2 Secure Aggregation Protocols

To further ensure client-level privacy, secure aggregation guarantees that the central server merely observes the aggregated result of client updates and never any individual update. Even when raw data is not revealed, exposing per-client model parameters remains privacy threatening, especially in cases with few clients or highly sensitive data. Fig. 2 represent the Multi-Layer Privacy Stack in Federated Learning

Secure aggregation achieves confidentiality by cryptographic masking schemes. Every client masks or encrypts its model update, and only the aggregated result is shared with the server after a synchronized unmasking process. Additive secret sharing and pairwise masking are widely utilized methods. Such protocols are lightweight enough to deploy in healthcare applications, like edge devices or bandwidth-constrained environments.

Figure 2. Multi-Layer Privacy Stack in Federated Learning

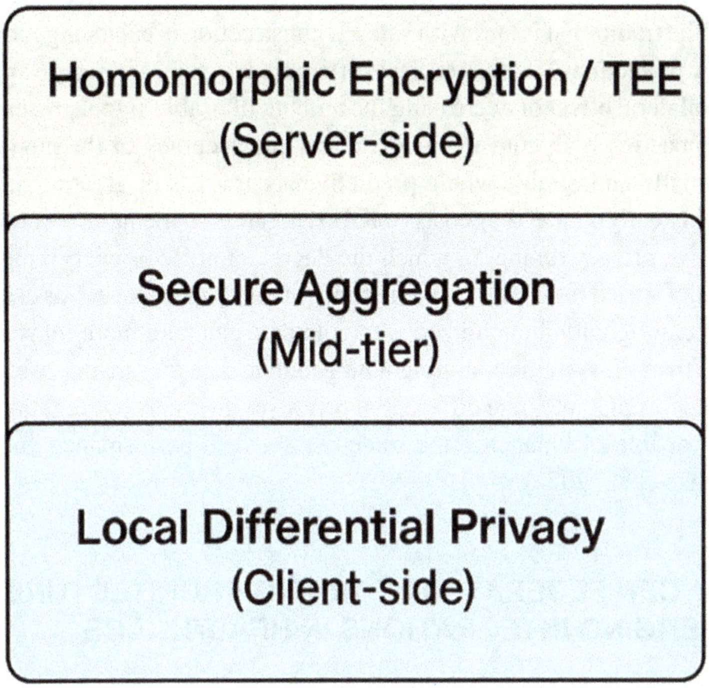

5.3 Homomorphic Encryption and Trusted Execution Environments (TEEs)

In addition to masking, more rigorous cryptographic assurances can be enabled with Homomorphic Encryption (HE). HE allows computations to be executed over encrypted data, so that the central server can compute model updates without ever decrypting them. This provides end-to-end confidentiality even in case of a server compromise. Although fully homomorphic encryption is still computationally costly, partially homomorphic encryption schemes (addition or multiplication) provide a usable compromise in real-world healthcare FL implementations (Almalki et al., 2024).

Alternatively, Trusted Execution Environments (TEEs) offer hardware-level isolation to run sensitive computation securely. In TEEs, e.g., Intel SGX enclaves, model aggregation can be conducted with strong confidentiality assurances, isolated from other system processes and outside attacks. TEEs are being explored more and more in federated medical imaging or cross-institutional EHR learning, though they need prudent provisioning and reliance on hardware integrity.

5.4 The Privacy–Utility Trade-off

One of the traditional issues with safe FL construction is balancing model utility and privacy protection. Methods such as differential privacy and secure aggregation have the collateral effect of decreasing the amount of usable signal present in client updates, impacting both convergence rate and end accuracy of the model. This is often especially undesirable where predictive accuracy is of greatest importance, e.g., in highly early cancer diagnosis or ICU risk score, in medicine. Another method is adaptive privacy tuning, in which the degree of noise or encrypting power is automatically varied based on data sensitivity or task importance. For example, FL systems operating with anonymized wearable data can take more relaxed privacy parameters than FL systems operating with genomic data for rare diseases. Besides, hybrid protocols that integrate differential privacy with secure aggregation or TEEs are better capable of balancing the trade-off between performance and security (Klein Brinke et al., 2024).

6. ADVANCED FEDERATED LEARNING ARCHITECTURES AND EMERGING INTEGRATIONS IN HEALTHCARE

As Federated Learning (FL) grows, its application in healthcare requires innovations to address the sector's complexities, such as data heterogeneity, infrastructure shortages, and stringent privacy requirements. Advanced FL architectures and how they blend with edge technologies are investigated in this section to enhance FL performance in practical applications of healthcare.

6.1 Federated Transfer Learning (FTL) for Heterogeneous Healthcare Data

Data heterogeneity between institutions is likely the most significant impediment to collaborative machine learning in the context of medicine. Hospitals and clinics will likely have different patient populations, modalities provided, and data handling infrastructure. A high-resolution MRI dataset with label structure may be available in a tertiary care hospital, while text-based clinical notes or low-level wearable device biometric readings may be available in a community clinic. This variation of feature space and data distribution is a drawback to the efficacy of standard Federated Learning models, which often presume cooperating clients possess data with similar structures (Ghosh & Ghosh, 2023). Federated Transfer Learning (FTL) leaves this limitation behind by integrating the features of FL and transfer learning. Rather than requiring homogeneity of data within every client, FTL allows institutions to take advantage of ability drawn from a shared world model and adapt it for use within their own data realms by localizing fine-tuning. This is particularly beneficial in rare disease diagnosis environments, in low-resource rural hospitals, or in public health operations between institutions, where data homogeneity could be infinitesimal or zero.

Chen et al., (2020) also introduced FedHealth, an FTL method tailored specifically for personal health monitoring using wearable sensors. They trained their method on the data of a number of diverse clients with unique activity patterns and demonstrated greater flexibility through cross-domain knowledge transfer. Through personalization support with privacy, FTL significantly expands the scope of deployment of FL in practical healthcare applications. It promotes balanced learning, such that even institutions lacking data can tap into global intelligence without losing local relevant information. FTL also presents novel challenges, primarily model alignment, domain adaptation, and debiasing. Robust future research must explore how to align feature representations across institutions and prevent transferred knowledge from exacerbating demographic or institutional bias.

6.2 Adaptive Clinical Decision-Making using FL-RL

Clinical decision-making is typically done in dynamic environments, whose results are achieved through succession of decisions and reactions of patients over time. Conventional supervised learning methods, although highly effective for static classification tasks, fail to adequately model sequential dependencies. Reinforcement Learning (RL), by virtue of its feedback framework, naturally can be applied to such situations. Learning RL agents from sensitive patient interaction data, however, is fraught with serious privacy threats. For this, Federated Reinforcement Learning (FL-RL) uses the power of FL and RL to enable decentralized, privacy-preserving learning among multiple agents or institutions. Agents in a Federated RL system, smart infusion pumps, ICU monitors, or autonomous triage systems, for instance, act locally in their own environments to learn the best policies. These agents sometimes synchronize the learned policies or value functions with a global aggregator, who accumulates the updates and provides a better global policy. This allows learning over multiple clinical workflows while maintaining locality of data.

Qi et al., (2021) presented a detailed explanation of FL-RL, citing its possibility for personalized treatment planning, adaptive therapy recommendation, and predictive hospital resource allocation. They emphasized that FL-RL allows context-aware decision-making in decentralized environments, especially where patient journeys change over time, e.g., managing chronic illness, rehabilitation, or emergency treatment. FL-RL is one of the strengths of an automatic tuning system that is capable of real-time adjustment of strategies as per dynamic patient conditions. Additionally, since the training is on-device or on-premises, it is privacy-friendly without comprising on responsiveness, which is critical for timely healthcare treatment. While FL-RL is an innovative approach, however, it remains computationally expensive and is challenged by stability, convergence, and policy coordination among the agents. Research continues to develop federated policy gradient methods, asynchronous updates, and reward normalization methods suitable for healthcare restrictions.

6.3 Hierarchical and Asynchronous FL for Scalable Collaboration

Healthcare infrastructure is often hierarchical in nature, often spanning from primary care clinics to tertiary hospitals and national research institutions. Hierarchical Federated Learning (HFL) takes advantage of this by offering multi-level model aggregation. Rather than relying on a global server performing coordination of training, HFL assigns intermediate aggregators such as regional data centers that aggregate local client updates first before sending them to a central coordinator. This architecture reduces the bandwidth usage, improves fault tolerance, and allows for region-specific model calibration.

Long et al., (2023) laid out a privacy-conscious HFL framework that has global differential privacy to provide safe aggregation at every level of hierarchy. Their system showed not only communication savings but also robustness against inference attacks that could make use of patterns of updates across layers. Healthcare is one scenario where hierarchical forms are especially applicable in disease surveillance systems, whereby local health facilities provide information regarding endemic diseases and national agencies put together wider patterns. Conversely, Asynchronous Federated Learning tackles the practical limitations of synchronous training since all clients need to do a lock-step in every training round. This assumption is hardly true in actual clinical networks because of heterogeneity in device performance, network access, or local workload. An asynchronous FL setup allows each client to update the global model independently as a function of availability and computational preparedness. This adaptability strongly enhances training efficiency and accommodates resource-limited settings such as rural health posts or mobile diagnostic units.

6.4 Integrating Blockchain for Verifiable Collaboration

Since FL is expanding to cross-institutional collaborations between hospitals, pharmaceutical companies, and research institutions, there is a need for trust and traceability of data. Blockchain technology provides an immutable distributed ledger system in which all transactions or model updates are recorded, thus ensuring verifiability, reproducibility, and non-repudiation in federated processes.

Shahsavari et al. (2024) discussed the incorporation of FL with blockchain frameworks in the healthcare domain and stressed its capability to impose update provenance, defend against tampering, and settle disagreements among actors. Under their suggested architecture, smart contracts regulate model contributions, allowing automatic verification of participation and performance measures. It is especially beneficial in clinical research consortia, wherein institutions have to join hands openly while being in control. In addition, the integration of blockchain with secure multiparty computation or differential privacy mechanisms has the ability to enhance security guarantees, particularly when involving multiple jurisdictions with competing privacy laws. This way, blockchain not only provides a technical enabler but also acts as a governance layer for federated AI ecosystems.

6.5 Explainable Federated Learning for Clinical Transparency

Even with improved model accuracy, the black-box nature of most AI systems holds back adoption in clinical settings. In high-stakes fields such as oncology or neurology, physicians need to understand why a model suggested a given diagnosis or treatment. Explainable AI (XAI) methods, like SHAP (SHapley Additive exPlanations) and LIME (Local Interpretable Model-agnostic Explanations), can provide post-hoc interpretation of model output by pointing out impactful features or decision paths.

Embedding XAI in FL systems, however, is particularly challenging. Local generation of explanations is required, as raw data and model reasoning cannot be transmitted between nodes. A recent work by Shahsavari et al. (2024) introduced a federated XAI framework where explanation modules are trained in parallel with the primary model but isolated to prevent compromising predictive accuracy. This two-path architecture enabled clinicians to see region-based influences on model predictions, like patient age or imaging signs, without revealing patient-level data. Explainable Federated Learning not only increases clinician confidence but also enables regulatory compliance under such requirements as the EU's "right to explanation" provision in automated decision-making. It promotes a culture of responsible AI adoption where transparency, fairness, and accountability are central design considerations.

6.6 FL at the Edge: Real-Time Intelligence from IoT Devices

With the advent of Edge AI—intelligence computed on locally situated devices at the edge of the network, the provision of healthcare services is being revolutionized, especially in settings where latency needs to be avoided or connections are unreliable. Coupled with Federated Learning (FL), Edge AI enables smartwatches, ECG monitors, and handheld ultrasound scanners to learn models on-device from locally collected data. They send encrypted model updates occasionally, as opposed to raw data, to an aggregation server.

In deployment environments, this arrangement allows for real-time risk forecasting, e.g., forecasting cardiac arrhythmias in advance using wearable ECG sensors, without constant interaction with cloud servers. Gupta et al. (2021) showed the feasibility of doing so in remote patient monitoring, where FL-based models learn incrementally from interactions with patients and improve their predictions over time.

Furthermore, edge-based FL designs minimize bandwidth usage and latency, as well as enhance data privacy by limiting sensitive data to the local device. These features are particularly beneficial for remote health centers, mobile diagnostic trailers, or where connectivity is low. At scale, this architecture can enable population-level analysis of health without overloading centralized infrastructure, providing an operational and privacy-preserving solution for public health surveillance, telemedicine, and preventive individualized care.

7. REAL-WORLD CASE STUDIES IN FEDERATED LEARNING FOR HEALTHCARE

While Federated Learning has been widely discussed in theory, its value is best understood through real-world deployments. These case studies demonstrate how FL can be applied in diverse healthcare contexts, balancing privacy with performance.

7.1 EXAM Model for COVID-19 Oxygen Requirement Prediction

During the COVID-19 pandemic, 20 healthcare institutions across North America, Europe, and Asia collaborated to create the EXAM (EMR + Chest X-Ray AI Model). Each site trained the model locally on its own electronic medical records and chest X-ray data, sharing only encrypted weight updates with a central aggregator. The federated model achieved an average area under the curve (AUC) greater than 0.92, outperforming individual site models by 16% and improving generalizability by 38% across different populations. This project showed how FL can accelerate the development of clinically relevant AI tools in crisis situations while complying with strict data protection laws (Dayan et al., 2021; NVIDIA, 2021).

7.2 Federated Detection of COVID-19 on Chest CT Imaging

A multinational consortium of seven hospitals trained an FL model to detect COVID-19-related lung abnormalities from chest computed tomography (CT) scans. By keeping all patient data on-premises and sharing only secure model updates, the team preserved patient privacy while achieving high diagnostic accuracy (AUC > 0.90) across institutions with different scanner types and imaging protocols. The study proved that FL can deliver robust and scalable diagnostic solutions, even in highly heterogeneous radiology environments (Xu et al., 2021).

7.3 NVIDIA Clara for Multi-Institutional Medical Image Segmentation

The NVIDIA Clara Train SDK has been deployed in collaborative brain tumor segmentation projects involving MRI data from multiple hospitals. Each site trained its local model independently, with secure socket layer (SSL) encryption ensuring safe transmission of model parameters to the central server. Compared to single-site models, the federated approach achieved significantly higher Dice similarity scores, benefiting from the diversity of datasets across institutions without compromising data privacy. This case demonstrates the operational readiness of FL frameworks for real-world medical imaging applications (Sheller et al., 2020).

8. CHALLENGES AND FUTURE DIRECTIONS

Despite the growing popularity and applicability of Federated Learning (FL) in medicine, various open issues still prevent it from being universally adopted in real-world clinical systems. As FL transitions from prototype research to real medical implementations, it must not only overcome technical limitations but also meet the demands of personalization, legal limitations, and infrastructural inconsistencies. This section outlines two of the most important challenges, model drift and personalization, and regulatory interoperability, and offers future directions that can guide the creation of robust, compliant, and equitable federated healthcare ecosystems.

8.1 Challenges in Regulatory Compliance and Interoperability

As FL is used more and more at scale and across borders within the healthcare context, it must function within a complex landscape of data protection law and institutional regulation. Regulations such as the Health Insurance Portability and Accountability Act (HIPAA) in the United States and General Data Protection

Regulation (GDPR) in the European Union impose stringent rules for dealing with sensitive health information. Although FL minimizes raw data transmission, model gradients or weight updates transfer can still be interpreted as sensitive in certain legal contexts, creating regulatory uncertainty that can hinder deployment.

Furthermore, technical interoperability remains one of the primary barriers to collaborative learning. Variations in data formats, coding practices, and health ontologies across institutions pose impediments to transparent model training deployment. Without secure communication and standard data representation, FL cannot take advantage of its decentralized nature. For FL to be forced into compliant and interoperable practice, multi-stakeholder cooperation is required. There is a requirement for synchronized action from regulators, AI developers, and health providers to create federated learning standards reconciled with privacy regulations, ethical AI standards, and clinical operational needs. Future research priorities should emphasize legal alignment mechanisms, safe model update paradigms, and open technical standards to enable federated AI adoption in global health systems.

8.2 Resource Efficiency and Infrastructure Constraints

Even though FL reduces data transmission, it also brings other computation and communication overhead. Clients will need to support local training loops, regularly synchronize with the server, and possibly employ cryptographic methods such as differential privacy or secure aggregation. Such requirements are unsustainable for clients that have constrained resources such as community clinics or low-end edge devices with scarce memory, computing capabilities, or battery life.

Bandwidth constraints and intermittent connectivity can also further compound these problems, particularly in rural or low-resource environments. Asynchronous training and gradient compression methods are being investigated to help alleviate these costs, but energy-efficient real-time FL is still an open engineering problem, especially for such applications as mobile health monitoring or emergency response systems.

8.3 Federated AI Marketplaces and Collaborative Ecosystems

The future direction that promises to be most compelling is the development of federated AI marketplaces whereby hospitals, clinics, research centers, and even private entities contribute to collaborative models in return for utility or incentives. The ecosystems would potentially democratize access to highly capable healthcare

AI through the provision of global intelligence to institutions with limited data or capabilities, while still enabling value input through special datasets.

Such shared marketplaces would most probably employ blockchain or other decentralized trust schemes to record contributions, ensure data integrity, and manage incentives transparently. However, building such systems raises new issues of governance, consensus frameworks, and equitable participation, particularly where competition or cross-jurisdictional markets exist. However, the possibility of integrating fragmented health systems into a worldwide integrated AI network is exciting and promising.

9. CONCLUSION

This chapter has provided an extensive overview of FL and its increasing importance in the advancement of healthcare by means of privacy-preserving, collective intelligence. Starting with the building blocks i.e., FL's framework, communication process, and fundamental algorithms such as Federated Averaging, we discussed how FL facilitates collaborative training of a model over distributed healthcare organizations without jeopardizing patient confidentiality and transgressing data protection laws.

Expanding on this, the chapter examined how FL is further developing with new architectures, such as Federated Transfer Learning, Federated Reinforcement Learning, Hierarchical FL, and Asynchronous frameworks. These were placed in the context of contemporary healthcare realities, where data are heterogeneous, infrastructures differ, and connectivity is sometimes inconsistent or intermittent. Concurrently, we explained how incorporating new-age technologies like blockchain, XAI, and Edge AI still enhances FL's ability further with safe, open, and real-time deployment in even resource-deprived or decentralized settings. Fundamentally, FL's strength is in its multi-layered privacy protections of differential privacy, secure aggregation, and homomorphic encryption, which collectively protect against data leakage and inference attacks. Additionally, the chapter faced key design trade-offs, specifically, the need to balance privacy and utility, model drift management, and enabling personalized model adaptation across varied clinical settings.

Looking to the future, Federated Learning has the potential to significantly enhance digital healthcare systems. It provides a vision of decentralized intelligence honoring patient autonomy, facilitating institutional independence, and allowing for collaboration at scale, all while meeting ethical and legal requirements. But this promise can only be fulfilled by overcoming long-standing barriers: regulatory fragmentation, unequal technical capacity, and the necessity of scalable, interoperable infrastructure. Unlocking the complete potential of FL requires a joint effort across fields. Researchers, engineers, and policymakers need to collaborate to develop flexible frameworks, optimize algorithms for practical limitations, and create incentives that facilitate cross-institutional collaboration. With intentional application, Federated Learning has the potential to enable in a new age of intelligent, fair, and secure healthcare, supported by collaborative medical knowledge frameworks rather than centralized authority.

REFERENCES

Adnan, M., Syed, M. H., Anjum, A., & Rehman, S. (2025). *A Framework for privacy-preserving in IoV using Federated Learning with Differential Privacy*. IEEE., DOI: 10.1109/ACCESS.2025.3526934

Almalki, J., Alshahrani, S. M., & Khan, N. A. (2024). A comprehensive secure system enabling healthcare 5.0 using federated learning, intrusion detection and blockchain. *PeerJ. Computer Science*, *10*, e1778. Advance online publication. DOI: 10.7717/peerj-cs.1778 PMID: 38259900

Chen, Y., Qin, X., Wang, J., Yu, C., & Gao, W. (2020). FedHealth: A Federated Transfer Learning Framework for Wearable Healthcare. *IEEE Intelligent Systems*, *35*(4), 83–93. DOI: 10.1109/MIS.2020.2988604

Dayan, I., Roth, H. R., Zhong, A., Harouni, A., Gentili, A., Abidin, A. Z., Lui, Y. W., Costa, A. B., Wood, B. J., Tsai, C. S., Li, K., Cheng, Y., McKenzie, S., Liu, A., Costa, A. F., Gidwani, M., Patel, V., Balachandar, N., Zhao, C., & Xu, D. (2021). Federated learning for predicting clinical outcomes in patients with COVID-19. *Nature Medicine*, *27*(10), 1735–1743. DOI: 10.1038/s41591-021-01506-3 PMID: 34526699

Elayan, H., Aloqaily, M., & Guizani, M. (2022). Sustainability of Healthcare Data Analysis IoT-Based Systems Using Deep Federated Learning. *IEEE Internet of Things Journal*, *9*(10), 7338–7346. DOI: 10.1109/JIOT.2021.3103635

Ghosh, S., & Ghosh, S. K. (2023). FEEL: FEderated LEarning Framework for ELderly Healthcare Using Edge-IoMT. *IEEE Transactions on Computational Social Systems*, *10*(4), 1800–1809. DOI: 10.1109/TCSS.2022.3233300

Gupta, D., Kayode, O., Bhatt, S., Gupta, M., & Tosun, A. S. (2021). Hierarchical Federated Learning based Anomaly Detection using Digital Twins for Smart Healthcare. *Proceedings - 2021 IEEE 7th International Conference on Collaboration and Internet Computing, CIC 2021*, 16–25. DOI: 10.1109/CIC52973.2021.00013

Gupta, M., Singh, M., Sharma, A., Sukhija, N., Aggarwal, P. K., & Jain, P. (2023). Unification of machine learning and blockchain technology in healthcare industry. In *Innovations in Healthcare Informatics: From interoperability to data analysis* (pp. 185–206). Institution of Engineering and Technology. DOI: 10.1049/PBHE041E_ch6

Hakak, S., Ray, S., Khan, W. Z., & Scheme, E. (2020). A Framework for Edge-Assisted Healthcare Data Analytics using Federated Learning. *Proceedings - 2020 IEEE International Conference on Big Data, Big Data 2020*, 3423–3427. DOI: 10.1109/BigData50022.2020.9377873

Jain, P., Sharma, S., Arora, S., Shokeen, V., Aggarwal, P. K., & Singh, M. (2024). Edge computing-based design for IoT security. In *Network Optimization in Intelligent Internet of Things Applications: Principles and Challenges* (pp. 298–309). CRC Press. DOI: 10.1201/9781003405535-22

Klein Brinke, J., Van Der Linden, M., & Havinga, P. (2024). Using Federated Learning and Channel State Information-Based Sensing for Scalable and Realistic At-Home Healthcare. *ACM International Conference Proceeding Series*, 186–193. DOI: 10.1145/3655693.3660254

Kumar, S., Lakshminarayanan, A., Chang, K., Guretno, F., Mien, I. H., Kalpathy-Cramer, J., Krishnaswamy, P., & Singh, P. (2022). Towards More Efficient Data Valuation in Healthcare Federated Learning Using Ensembling. *Lecture Notes in Computer Science (Including Subseries Lecture Notes in Artificial Intelligence and Lecture Notes in Bioinformatics), 13573 LNCS*, 119–129. DOI: 10.1007/978-3-031-18523-6_12

Li, K. (2025). A Blockchain-Integrated Federated Learning Approach for Secure Data Sharing and Privacy Protection in Multi-Device Communication. *Applied Artificial Intelligence*, *39*(1), 2442770. Advance online publication. DOI: 10.1080/08839514.2024.2442770

Long, Y., Zhang, J., Wang, G., & Fu, J. (2023). Hierarchical federated learning with global differential privacy. *Electronic Research Archive*, *31*(7), 3741–3758. DOI: 10.3934/era.2023190

Mathew, U. O., Rodriguez, D. Z., Rosa, R. L., Ayub, M. S., & Adasme, P. (2024). Advancing Healthcare 5.0 through Federated Learning: Opportunity for Security Enforcement using Blockchain. *2024 32nd International Conference on Software, Telecommunications and Computer Networks, SoftCOM 2024*. DOI: 10.23919/SoftCOM62040.2024.10722012

Muazu, T., Mao, Y., Muhammad, A. U., Ibrahim, M., Kumshe, U. M. M., & Samuel, O. (2024). A federated learning system with data fusion for healthcare using multi-party computation and additive secret sharing. *Computer Communications*, *216*, 168–182. DOI: 10.1016/j.comcom.2024.01.006

Narwaria, M., & Jaiswal, S. (2024). Multicriteria client selection model using class topper optimization based optimal federated learning for healthcare informatics. *Cluster Computing*, *27*(8), 10325–10342. DOI: 10.1007/s10586-024-04466-8

Natarajan, R., Krishna, S., & Ranjith, C. P. (2025). A Novel Federated Learning Framework for Healthcare Applications Using Wearable Devices. *2025 IEEE 4th International Conference on AI in Cybersecurity, ICAIC 2025*. https://doi.org/DOI: 10.1109/ICAIC63015.2025.10848974

NVIDIA. (2021, October 20). *Federated learning helps hospitals predict COVID patients' oxygen needs*. NVIDIA Blog. https://blogs.nvidia.com/blog/federated-learning-covid-oxygen-needs/

Purohit, R. M., Verma, J. P., Jain, R., & Kumar, A. (2025). FedBlocks: Federated learning and blockchainbased privacy-preserved pioneering framework for IoT healthcare using IPFS in web 3.0 era. *Cluster Computing*, *28*(2), 139. DOI: 10.1007/s10586-024-04738-3

Qi, J., Zhou, Q., Lei, L., & Zheng, K. (2021). Federated reinforcement learning: techniques, applications, and open challenges. In *Intelligence and Robotics* (Vol. 1, pp. 18–57). OAE Publishing Inc., DOI: 10.20517/ir.2021.02

Shahsavari, Y., Dambri, O. A., Baseri, Y., Hafid, A. S., & Makrakis, D. (2024). *Integration of Federated Learning and Blockchain in Healthcare: A Tutorial.*

Sheller, M. J., Edwards, B., Reina, G. A., Martin, J., Pati, S., Kotrotsou, A., Milchenko, M., Xu, W., Marcus, D., Colen, R. R., Bakas, S., & Davatzikos, C. (2020). Federated learning in medicine: Facilitating multi-institutional collaborations without sharing patient data. *Scientific Reports*, *10*(1), 12598. DOI: 10.1038/s41598-020-69250-1 PMID: 32724046

Singh, M., Gupta, M., Sharma, A., Jain. Parita, & Aggarwal, P. (2023). *Role of Deep Learning in Healthcare Industry: Limitations, Challenges and Future Scope* (Vol. 11). BENTHAM SCIENCE PUBLISHERS. DOI: 10.2174/97898150802301230201

Singh, M., Sukhija, N., Sharma, A., Gupta, M., & Aggarwal, P. K. (2021). Security and Privacy Requirements for IoMT-Based Smart Healthcare System: Challenges, Solutions, and Future Scope. In *Big Data Analysis for Green Computing*. Concepts and Applications., DOI: 10.1201/9781003032328-2

Ullah, F., Srivastava, G., Xiao, H., Ullah, S., Lin, J. C. W., & Zhao, Y. (2024). A Scalable Federated Learning Approach for Collaborative Smart Healthcare Systems with Intermittent Clients Using Medical Imaging. *IEEE Journal of Biomedical and Health Informatics*, *28*(6), 3293–3304. DOI: 10.1109/JBHI.2023.3282955 PMID: 37279135

Xu, J., Glicksberg, B. S., Su, C., Walker, P., Bian, J., & Wang, F. (2021). Federated learning for healthcare informatics. *Journal of Healthcare Informatics Research, 5*(1), 1–19. DOI: 10.1007/s41666-020-00082-4 PMID: 33204939

Yaqoob, M. M., Alsulami, M., Khan, M. A., Alsadie, D., Saudagar, A. K. J., AlKhathami, M., & Khattak, U. F. (2023). Symmetry in Privacy-Based Healthcare: A Review of Skin Cancer Detection and Classification Using Federated Learning. *Symmetry, 15*(7), 1369. DOI: 10.3390/sym15071369

Chapter 3
AI-Based Low-Cost Insulin Pump for Diabetes Management

Sanskruti Chhagan Chandankar
https://orcid.org/0009-0002-2813-752X
G H Raisoni College of Engineering, Nagpur, India

Vibha Rajesh Bora
https://orcid.org/0000-0002-7550-3409
G H Raisoni College of Engineering, Nagpur, India

Sanket Suresh Somkuwar
https://orcid.org/0009-0003-1308-2471
G H Raisoni College of Engineering, Nagpur, India

Manthan Ghosh
https://orcid.org/0000-0002-2020-0670
G H Raisoni College of Engineering, Nagpur, India

ABSTRACT

Diabetes is a chronic condition that demands continuous monitoring and precise control of blood glucose levels. This study introduces a low-cost, AI-driven insulin pump system that employs an electrochemical cell combined with a peristaltic pump for automated insulin delivery. Central to the system is a custom-designed potentiostat that measures glucose levels in simulated sugar solutions using electrochemical sensing techniques. The resulting voltage signals are analyzed to estimate glucose concentration, which then informs insulin dosing recommendations through a regression-based AI model. These recommendations are transmitted to a mobile application, which displays the suggested insulin dose and offers a manual override

DOI: 10.4018/979-8-3373-3306-9.ch003

option if needed. An ESP32 microcontroller manages both data acquisition and insulin administration, delivering an affordable and accessible solution for diabetes care. This system aims to provide a cost-effective alternative to commercial insulin pumps, making advanced diabetes management more accessible to underserved populations.

INTRODUCTION

Diabetes mellitus is a long-term metabolic disorder marked by elevated blood glucose levels, typically due to inadequate insulin production or the body's inability to effectively use insulin. This chronic condition affects millions globally and, if not managed properly, can lead to severe complications like cardiovascular disease, nerve damage, vision impairment, and kidney failure. According to the International Diabetes Federation (IDF), over 537 million adults are currently living with diabetes, and this number is expected to rise sharply in the coming years. Effective management requires regular monitoring and timely insulin administration, which is not always feasible for every patient due to financial or technological constraints.

Continuous Glucose Monitoring (CGM) systems (Ribet, Stemme, & Roxhed, 2018; Joshi, Jain, & Mohanty, 2020; Chien, Chen, Bai, & Huang, 2022; Liu, Yu, Luo, Yang, & Cui, 2021) have become a breakthrough in diabetes care by providing real-time tracking of blood glucose levels, significantly improving response and control. Similarly, insulin pumps automate insulin delivery and reduce the need for frequent injections. However, both technologies remain prohibitively expensive for many, particularly in developing or low-resource settings. As a result, there is a pressing need for an affordable solution that can offer both glucose monitoring and automated insulin delivery without compromising functionality.

In this chapter, we have developed a low-cost integrated insulin pump system that combines electrochemical glucose sensing with automated insulin delivery. The system employs a potentiostat-based setup to detect glucose levels by measuring voltage changes, which are translated into glucose concentrations using a linear regression model. These values are processed using an ESP32 microcontroller and displayed via a web server, enabling real-time monitoring. A peristaltic pump handles insulin delivery based on either manually entered doses or AI-generated predictions, ensuring timely and precise insulin administration.

This solution uses fundamental electrochemical principles to eliminate the need for expensive CGM sensors. The integration of AI helps personalize treatment by estimating required insulin doses, and the system distinguishes between basal and bolus insulin needs.

LITERATURE REVIEW

The author offers a comprehensive examination of the historical evolution, current utilization, and future trajectory of insulin pump therapy. The paper emphasizes the critical impact of the Diabetes Control and Complications Trial (DCCT) in establishing the clinical significance of intensive insulin therapy. It also highlights the shift from rudimentary pumps to advanced systems that provide more physiologic insulin delivery, enhanced flexibility, and improved glycemic control—especially for individuals with type 1 diabetes (T1D) (Berget, Messer, & Forlenza, 2019). The increasing application of CSII in type 2 diabetes (T2D) is noted, with supporting evidence demonstrating improved glycemic outcomes and reduced insulin needs. Furthermore, the review effectively differentiates among various pump technologies—including conventional, patch, and sensor-augmented pumps—and addresses innovations like hypoglycemia suspension features, offering practical insights for clinicians and patients alike.

Building on the progression of pump technology, the study by Keith-Hynes et al. (Berget, Lange, Messer, & Forlenza, 2020) focuses on a specific commercial device that exemplifies modern advancements in automated insulin delivery. The t:slim X2, a hybrid closed-loop system integrated with the Dexcom G6 continuous glucose monitor (CGM), offers predictive low glucose suspend (Basal-IQ) and automated insulin adjustment with correction boluses (Control-IQ). These features have demonstrated significant improvements in time-in-range and reduced incidence of hypoglycemia, with clinical trials supporting their efficacy over traditional sensor-augmented pump therapy. The t:slim X2's ability to receive remote software updates also positions it as a dynamic, future-ready device within the evolving insulin pump landscape.

Parallel to these developments in insulin delivery are substantial advances in glucose sensing technologies. Paper (Hassan, Vyas, Grieve, & Bartolo, 2021) reviews the mechanisms, materials, and innovations in glucose sensors, focusing on both enzymatic systems—particularly those utilizing glucose oxidase (GOx)—and emerging non-enzymatic approaches. While enzymatic sensors offer high selectivity and bioactivity, they suffer from enzyme instability. Non-enzymatic sensors, which rely on noble metal catalysts, provide enhanced durability but face challenges with selectivity and electrode fouling. The paper emphasizes how recent material innovations, such as carbon nanotubes and molecularly imprinted polymers, have improved sensor performance, though the need for greater stability and accuracy remains critical.

Complementing this perspective, it provides an in-depth analysis of the application and evolution of electrochemical glucose sensing technologies. The review traces developments from laboratory analyzers to portable blood glucose meters and continuous glucose monitors (CGMs) (Heller & Feldman, 2008). It explores enzyme-based detection methods and highlights issues such as hematocrit interference and calibration challenges in home test strips. The authors underline the transformative impact of continuous monitoring on diabetes management and anticipate future directions focused on sensor miniaturization, biocompatibility, and implantable systems with integrated power sources.

Expanding the scope of glucose monitoring, the study introduces an innovative application of biosensor technology in aqua culture (Yonemori, Takahashi, Ren, Hayashi, & Endo, 2009). The authors propose using the eyeball scleral interstitial fluid (EISF) in fish as an alternative medium for glucose sensing, demonstrating high correlation with blood glucose levels. A flexible, needle-type enzyme sensor with glucose oxidase is implanted in the EISF and validated through continuous monitoring experiments. This research illustrates the broader utility of electrochemical biosensing beyond human medicine, with implications for sustainable aquaculture practices.

From a hardware development standpoint, it presents a low-cost, Arduino-based potentiostat for electrochemical experiments (Meloni, 2016). Designed for educational settings, the device supports techniques like cyclic voltammetry and chronoamperometry, enabling students to understand electrochemistry and instrumentation hands-on. Despite its simplicity, the device demonstrates accurate performance and provides a customizable, accessible tool for teaching and innovation in low-resource environments.

While technological advancements offer promising pathways for diabetes management, psychological and systemic barriers continue to hinder timely initiation of insulin therapy, particularly in type 2 diabetes. The paper addresses patient-level fears (hypoglycemia, injections, stigma), provider hesitance (therapeutic inertia), and structural obstacles (Galdón Sanz-Pastor, Justel Enríquez, Sánchez Bao, & Ampudia-Blasco, 2024). The authors advocate for patient education, provider training, and adoption of newer, user-friendly insulin formulations—such as once-weekly basal insulins (e.g., insulin icodec)—to mitigate these barriers and improve patient adherence and outcomes.

A foundational understanding of diabetes mellitus and the pivotal role of insulin is critical for evaluating the current innovations in insulin delivery systems. It presents a thorough examination of the pathophysiology, diagnosis, and management of diabetes, starting with a historical perspective—from early descriptions in Egyptian and Indian medical texts to the landmark discovery of insulin in the 20th century (Mohiddin, 2022). The author emphasizes the global burden of diabetes, predicting a rise in cases from over 350 million to 438 million by 2030, with India being one of the most affected countries. The paper provides detailed insights into the physiological role of insulin in glucose metabolism, explaining how it facilitates glucose uptake through GLUT4 transporters and regulates hepatic glucose production.

Building upon this foundation the author explores recent advances aimed at improving insulin delivery and patient adherence. The authors underscore that despite its therapeutic importance, insulin therapy—particularly in Type 2 diabetes—is often delayed due to psychological resistance, injection burden, and complexity of regimens. The paper reviews the evolution from traditional human insulin to advanced analogs, including ultra-long-acting, ultra-rapid-acting, hepato-preferential insulins, biosimilars, and fixed-ratio combinations (Nkonge, Nkonge, & Nkonge, 2023). A major focus is placed on novel delivery modalities such as once-weekly basal insulin and non-injectable routes, especially inhaled and oral insulins, which show potential to enhance convenience and treatment compliance. Clinical trials cited in the review suggest that these formulations not only simplify therapy but also improve glycemic outcomes and patient satisfaction. By reducing injection frequency and providing more physiologic insulin profiles, these innovations address critical barriers to effective diabetes management.

With rapid advancements in diabetes technology, understanding the progress and diversity of insulin delivery methods has become increasingly important. This provides an in-depth review of the development, classification, and comparative performance of insulin pump technologies. The authors trace the journey from early animal-derived insulins and multiple daily injections to the introduction of continuous subcutaneous insulin infusion (CSII) and the modern pursuit of artificial pancreas systems (Rimon, Hasan, Hassan, & Cesmeci, 2024). The review categorizes insulin pumps into conventional, patch, and implantable types, detailing their unique features, delivery mechanisms, and integration with continuous glucose monitoring (CGM). It presents a comprehensive comparison of commercially available pumps, analyzing specifications such as basal and bolus dosing capabilities, reservoir size, user interface, portability, and compatibility with other diabetes care tools. The paper highlights the significant progress in pump design, automation, and user-friendliness, emphasizing how advanced hybrid closed-loop systems and do-it-yourself (DIY) artificial pancreas solutions are transforming glycemic control and patient quality of life.

The authors explain the significance of tight glycemic control in diabetes management through their landmark study which presents findings from the Diabetes Control and Complications Trial (DCCT). This pivotal clinical trial assessed whether intensive diabetes management reduces the risk of long-term complications in individuals with type 1 diabetes. The DCCT enrolled 1,441 participants aged 13–39 with insulin-dependent diabetes mellitus (IDDM) and followed them for an average of 6.5 years (Manov et al., 2023). Participants were randomized to receive either intensive therapy—aimed at maintaining blood glucose levels as close to normal as possible—or conventional therapy, which focused on preventing symptomatic hyperglycemia and hypoglycemia without specific glucose targets. The findings demonstrated that intensive therapy dramatically reduced the risk of diabetes-related complications. Specifically, intensive treatment reduced the onset of retinopathy by 76%, and slowed its progression by 54% compared to conventional treatment. Similarly, the risk of microalbuminuria and clinical nephropathy was reduced by 39% and 54%, respectively. Additionally, intensive therapy reduced the incidence of neuropathy by 60%.These benefits were closely linked to improved glycemic control, as participants in the intensive group maintained a significantly lower mean hemoglobin A1c (HbA1c) level (7.2%) compared to those in the conventional group (9.1%). However, intensive treatment also led to a threefold increase in the risk of severe hypoglycemia.

Extending the conversation around barriers to successful adoption of advanced diabetes technologies, Tanenbaum et al. explore the psychological and demographic factors influencing the uptake of insulin pumps and continuous glucose monitors (CGMs) in their 2017 study (Tanenbaum et al., 2017). Drawing data from 1,503 adult participants in the T1D Exchange registry, the study aims to identify modifiable barriers that could be addressed through clinical or behavioral interventions. While the clinical benefits of devices like insulin pumps and CGMs are well-documented, the study found device usage remains suboptimal, particularly among younger adults. The most commonly reported modifiable barriers included the hassle of wearing devices (47%) and discomfort or dislike of having devices on the body (35%). Cost-related factors, although non-modifiable, were also widely cited. Notably, the 18–25 age group had the lowest device uptake, the highest HbA1c levels (average 8.3%), and the highest levels of diabetes distress. These younger participants were also more likely to cite social concerns such as appearance and fear of judgment. Women were more likely than men to use insulin pumps, but also reported higher distress and more body image-related concerns.

Complementing previous findings on glycemic control and long-term risks in diabetes management, Fatourechi et al. (2009) present a systematic review and meta-analysis.This review evaluates the effectiveness of continuous subcutaneous insulin infusion (CSII) compared to multiple daily injections (MDI) in reducing hypoglycemia and improving glycemic outcomes (Fatourechi et al., 2009). The analysis included 15 randomized controlled trials published after 2002, comprising both type 1 and type 2 diabetes populations. In patients with type 1 diabetes, CSII modestly lowered HbA1c by an average of 0.2% compared to MDI. However, the impact on hypoglycemia was less clear. There was no statistically significant reduction in severe or nocturnal hypoglycemia overall, although a slight trend favored CSII. Interestingly, trial results varied by age group and design. While adolescents and adults in crossover trials saw a slight, non-significant reduction in minor hypoglycemia episodes with CSII, children in parallel trials experienced more such episodes with CSII than MDI. For type 2 diabetes, no significant differences in either HbA1c or hypoglycemia rates were observed between the two insulin delivery methods (Wilson & Castle, 2020). The authors noted that most trials excluded patients at high risk of hypoglycemia, limiting conclusions for those with hypoglycemia unawareness or frequent severe episodes.

MATERIALS AND METHODS

Materials

1.ESP32 Microcontroller

The ESP32 is a powerful, low-cost system-on-chip microcontroller featuring integrated Wi-Fi and Bluetooth, making it the core processing unit of the entire insulin delivery system. It reads voltage signals from the potentiostat circuit, performs real-time calculations to estimate glucose concentration, and wirelessly transmits this data to the control interface. It also executes the logic for insulin dose delivery by activating the appropriate components. Due to its strong computational capabilities and versatile wireless communication, the ESP32 is well-suited for biomedical and IoT-based applications like continuous glucose monitoring and smart insulin administration.

2.Electrochemical Cell (Glucose Sensor)

The electrochemical glucose sensor functions using a three-electrode configuration—working electrode (WE), reference electrode (RE), and counter electrode (CE). The WE is coated with glucose oxidase (GOx), which catalyzes the oxidation of glucose to produce gluconolactone and hydrogen peroxide. The hydrogen peroxide is then electrochemically oxidized at the WE, releasing electrons and generating a current that is directly proportional to the glucose concentration. The RE maintains a stable reference potential, while the CE completes the circuit and ensures current flow. These sensors are categorized into enzymatic and non-enzymatic types; enzymatic sensors, such as the one used in this setup, offer high specificity due to the enzyme's selectivity toward glucose, making them suitable for real-time glucose monitoring applications.

Three-Electrode System:

The three-electrode system is a fundamental configuration used in electrochemical measurements, especially for biosensing applications like glucose detection. This system consists of three distinct electrodes: the **Working Electrode (WE)**, the **Reference Electrode (RE)**, and the **Counter Electrode (CE)**. Each electrode serves a specific role in maintaining controlled electrochemical reactions and accurately measuring the resulting signals.

Working Electrode (WE)

The working electrode is the primary site where the electrochemical reaction of interest takes place. In the context of glucose sensing, for example, the working electrode is coated with an enzyme such as glucose oxidase. When glucose molecules come in contact with this electrode, they undergo oxidation, producing by-products such as hydrogen peroxide (H_2O_2). The oxidation of H_2O_2 at the electrode surface releases electrons, which generates a current. This current is proportional to the concentration of glucose in the solution. The material used for the working electrode is typically carbon, platinum, or gold due to their conductive and electrochemically stable properties.

Reference Electrode (RE)

The reference electrode provides a stable and known voltage against which the potential of the working electrode is controlled. It does not pass any current during the measurement process, which helps it maintain a constant potential. The accuracy and stability of the reference electrode are crucial because it ensures that the voltage applied to the working electrode remains precise throughout the experiment. Common reference electrodes include the silver/silver chloride (Ag/AgCl) electrode and the saturated calomel electrode (SCE). In miniaturized systems, pseudo-reference electrodes are also used, although they are less stable over time.

Counter Electrode (CE)

The counter electrode, also known as the auxiliary electrode, serves to complete the electrical circuit by allowing current to flow from the working electrode through the electrolyte. It is connected to the output of the potentiostat's control amplifier and is responsible for supplying or accepting electrons to balance the current generated at the working electrode. The counter electrode is typically made of an inert, conductive material such as platinum or carbon. Its size is generally larger than the working electrode to ensure that it can handle all the current without affecting the electrochemical process at the working electrode.

3.Potentiostat Circuit / Galvanostat

A potentiostat/galvanostat (Dobbelaere, Vereecken, & Detavernier, 2017) is an essential electronic instrument used in electrochemical experiments, especially for biosensing applications like glucose monitoring. It controls the voltage between the working and reference electrodes while measuring the resulting current between the working and counter electrodes. This current is directly proportional to the concentration of the target analyte such as glucose in a given solution.

4.Peristaltic Pump

The peristaltic pump plays a vital role in the sterile and accurate delivery of insulin. It operates by compressing and releasing a flexible tube using rotating rollers, ensuring that the insulin flows through without coming into contact with the internal mechanical parts of the pump. The Kamoer NKP-S06 is a compact, medical-grade peristaltic pump used for precise insulin delivery in this project. It operates using a roller-based compression mechanism and supports medical-grade silicone or Teflon tubing to ensure sterile, non-reactive fluid handling. The flow rate is programmable based on control duration, allowing accurate microdosing. In this setup, the pump is controlled by an ESP32 through a 5V relay module and is calibrated to deliver exact insulin units based on AI-driven dose recommendations, making it highly suitable for reliable and contactless insulin therapy.

Figure 1. Figure 1. (a) Electrochemical Cell (b) Galvanoplot GX102 (c) Peristaltic Pump

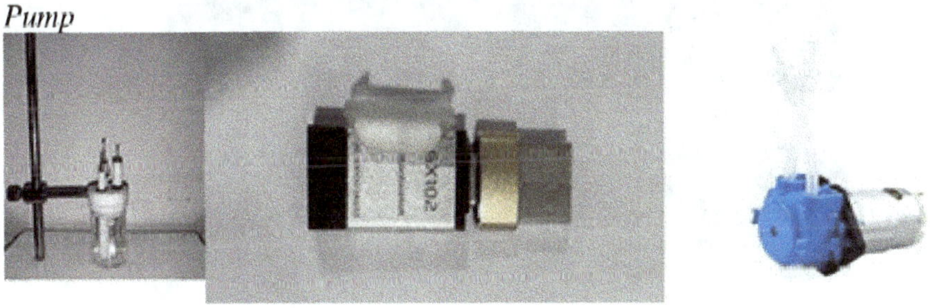

5.Galvanoplot Suite

The Galvanostat Suite software is a sophisticated tool used for controlling and analyzing electrochemical experiments conducted with a galvanostat. In the context of this continuous glucose monitoring (CGM) project, the software provides a user-friendly interface for setting up and managing electrochemical tests. It allows users to configure various parameters such as current, voltage, and timing to precisely control the experiments. The software collects data from the galvanostat and provides real-time monitoring and visualization of electrochemical processes, enabling detailed analysis and interpretation of results. Advanced features may include automated data logging, graphical plotting of results, and statistical analysis, which are crucial for optimizing sensor performance and ensuring accurate glucose measurements. By using Galvanostat Suite, researchers can streamline their workflow, enhance data accuracy, and gain deeper insights into the electrochemical behavior of the glucose sensors used in the CGM device. The Galvanostat Suite software is designed to be compatible with various types of galvanostats and potentiostats, offering extensive flexibility and customization for different experimental needs. It supports a range of electrochemical techniques such as cyclic voltammetry, chronoamperometry, and impedance spectroscopy, making it a versatile tool for comprehensive sensor evaluation. Users can program complex experimental sequences and automate repetitive tasks, significantly enhancing efficiency

and reproducibility. The software also features robust data management capabilities, including data export options in multiple formats for further analysis and reporting.

Figure 2. Galvanoplot Suite

How To Take Insulin Doses?

Managing diabetes effectively requires accurate insulin dosing. Whether you're on multiple daily injections (MDI) or using an insulin pump, understanding how to calculate and adjust insulin doses is essential for maintaining optimal blood glucose levels. Following is the Standard sliding scale Insulin dosage chart:-

Table 1. Relationship between Blood Glucose Concentration and Insulin Dose

Blood Glucose (mg/dl)	Insulin (units)
61 – 150	0
151 – 200	3
201 – 250	5
251 – 300	8
301 – 350	10
351 – 400	12
> 400	15 a

The following will explain the three primary types of insulin doses—**basal**, **bolus**, and **correction**—along with the formulas, dosage charts, and common questions people ask.

Basal Insulin: Long-Acting Background Dose

Basal insulin is the long-acting insulin that keeps your blood sugar stable between meals and overnight. It mimics the background insulin secretion of a healthy pancreas. People typically take basal insulin once or twice a day, depending on the type prescribed (e.g., Lantus, Levemir, Tresiba).

How to Calculate Basal Dose

The basal dose typically accounts for **40% to 50%** of your Total Daily Insulin Dose (TDID).

Formula:

Basal Dose = TDID × 50%

Example:

If your total insulin requirement per day is 40 units:

40 × 0.5 = 20 units of basal insulin

This dose is often taken once daily (morning or bedtime) or split into two equal doses depending on your endocrinologist's guidance.

Bolus Insulin: Mealtime Coverage

Bolus insulin is short- or rapid-acting insulin (like Novolog, Humalog) that is taken before meals to cover the rise in blood glucose caused by carbohydrates. The amount needed depends on the number of carbohydrates you plan to eat and your Insulin-to-Carbohydrate Ratio (ICR).

Bolus Dose Formula

Formula:

Bolus Dose = Total Carbohydrates in Meal (grams) ÷ ICR

Example:

If you're eating 60 grams of carbs and your ICR is 1:10, then:

60 ÷ 10 = 6 units of bolus insulin

Your ICR is determined through personal observation or testing, usually under the supervision of a doctor or diabetes educator.

Table 2. Recommended Insulin Doses for Varying Levels of Carbohydrate Intake

Carbohydrates in Meal (g)	Rapid-Acting Insulin Units
0-15	1 unit
16-30	2 units
31-45	3 units
46-60	4 units

Correction Dose: High Blood Sugar Adjustment

Sometimes, your blood glucose may spike above the target range. In such cases, a **correction dose** of insulin is needed to bring it back to normal. This is also known as the "insulin sensitivity correction."

Correction Dose Formula

Formula:

Correction Dose = (Current BG – Target BG) ÷ Correction Factor (CF)

The Correction Factor (also called Insulin Sensitivity Factor or ISF) tells you how much 1 unit of insulin will lower your blood sugar. A common starting point for adults is a CF of 50 (i.e., 1 unit of insulin lowers glucose by 50 mg/dL).

Example:

- Current Blood Sugar: 220 mg/dL
- Target Blood Sugar: 120 mg/dL
- Correction Factor: 50
- Calculation: (220 – 120) ÷ 50 = 2 units of insulin

Methods

Figure 3. Block Diagram of Insulin Pump

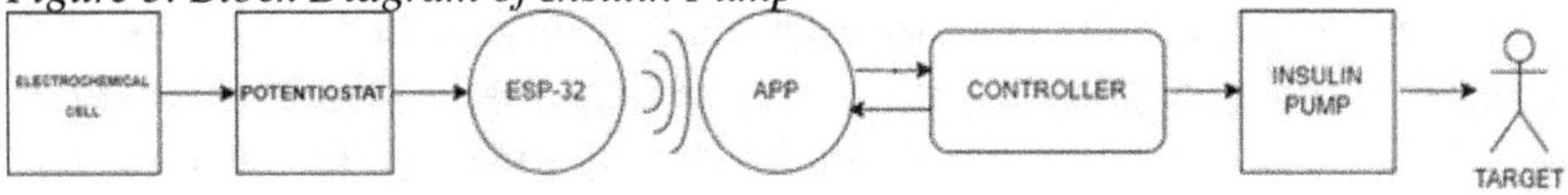

Fig.5 represents a low-cost, AI-driven solution for real-time diabetes management by integrating an electrochemical cell/continuous glucose monitoring (CGM) sensor with an insulin pump (Madsen et al., 2023; Naranjo, Tanenbaum, Iturralde, & Hood, 2016; Benkhadra et al., 2017; Thomas et al., 2021; Andersen, Hangaard, Hommel, & Ridderstråle, 2018; Clements et al., 2015) controlled via a custom local website. The architecture involves seamless data acquisition, transmission, analysis, and actuation components that collectively form a closed-loop insulin delivery system.

An electrochemical glucose sensor in an insulin pump is a device that detects and quantifies glucose levels using electrochemical reactions, specifically the oxidation or reduction of glucose at electrodes, to generate a measurable electrical signal. This signal is then converted into a glucose reading. The sensor typically consists of a working electrode (where the reaction occurs), a reference electrode (which provides a stable potential), and a counter electrode (to complete the circuit). Many of these sensors are based on glucose oxidase (GOx), an enzyme that catalyzes the oxidation of glucose, enabling real-time and continuous glucose monitoring for precise insulin management.

The potentiostat functions as the analog front-end, maintaining the desired potential between electrodes and amplifying the signal. It converts the electrochemical response into a stable analog output. This output is passed on to the ESP32 module, which acts as the data transmission unit.

The ESP32 is a low-cost microcontroller with integrated Wi-Fi and Bluetooth, responsible for sending glucose level data from the potentiostat to the user's mobile application. Communication occurs wirelessly via Bluetooth (preferred for stability and IP independence). The mobile app serves as the brain of the system, integrating a trained AI model (e.g., regression, neural network) that analyzes trends in glucose levels and predicts future readings.

Based on real-time glucose data and optionally user-input information (like meals, activity), the AI engine calculates personalized insulin dosage recommendations—including basal (continuous) and bolus (meal-based) doses. These recommendations are transmitted to a controller module.

The controller, typically an embedded system or microcontroller, receives instructions from the mobile app and triggers the insulin pump accordingly. The insulin pump is a small body-mounted device (e.g., peristaltic or piston-based), capable of delivering precise quantities of insulin subcutaneously to the target, i.e., the diabetic patient.

This entire architecture forms a feedback-controlled, AI-guided, wearable system that enables continuous, intelligent, and automated glucose management (Ghosh & Bora, 2025). The integration of real-time biosensing, wireless IoT communication, AI-based prediction, and insulin actuation offers a promising, scalable, and affordable solution for diabetic patients.

This approach leverages the fundamentals of electrochemistry to eliminate the need for expensive sensors. Additionally, the integration of AI for glucose prediction and dose recommendation enhances the accuracy and effectiveness of the insulin administration process. The system also differentiates between basal and bolus doses to support personalized and timely treatment. This chapter delves into the detailed hardware setup, software implementation, method of execution, results obtained from experimental trials, safety considerations, comparison with commercial systems, calibration and validation protocols, and the broader implications of this innovation.

The experimental setup began with meticulous preparation of glucose solutions to simulate a wide range of sugar levels for both sensor calibration and validation testing. A total of seven individual solutions were prepared by dissolving varying amounts of dextrose (a form of glucose) in 20 ml of distilled water per container. The exact amounts of dextrose added were 0.1 g, 0.2 g, 0.3 g, 0.4 g, 0.5 g, 0.6 g, and 0.7 g, representing glucose concentrations ranging from very low to significantly high levels. Each quantity of dextrose was carefully measured using a precision electronic balance to ensure accuracy. The dextrose was then added to the distilled water in individual containers. To ensure complete dissolution and achieve a homogeneous solution, each container was stirred thoroughly using a magnetic stirrer. This equipment uses a rotating magnetic field to spin a stir bar immersed in the liquid, allowing for consistent and uniform mixing without manual intervention. Once the dextrose was fully dissolved, the solutions were clearly labeled according to their respective concentrations for easy identification in subsequent phases.

Out of these seven prepared solutions, four solutions containing 0.1 g, 0.2 g, 0.3 g, and 0.4 g of dextrose were designated for the calibration phase of the electrochemical sensor. These known concentrations were used to establish a reliable correlation between the sensor's electrical response and actual glucose levels. The remaining three solutions containing 0.5 g, 0.6 g, and 0.7 g of dextrose were reserved for the testing phase, where the sensor's accuracy and predictive ability were validated against unseen concentrations.

Figure 4. Dextrose Preparation using Magnetic Stirrer

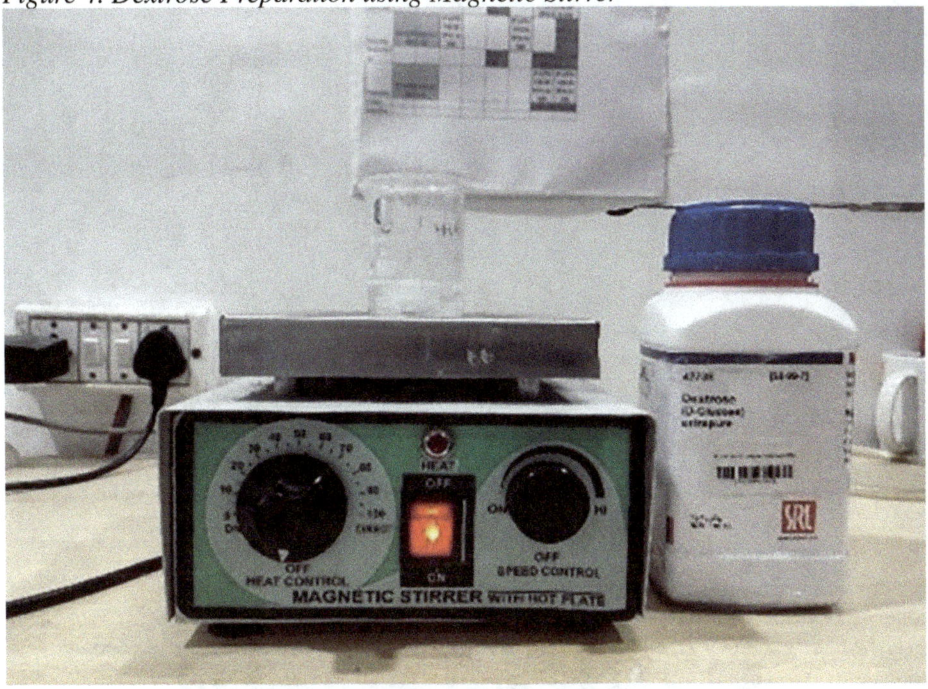

Next, the glucose sensor strips were coated with glucose oxidase and allowed to dry completely. After drying, the sensor was dipped into each prepared glucose solution. The glucose sensor was connected to the galvanoplot suite via a galvanostat for electrochemical measurements. In the galvanoplot suite, chronoamperometry was selected as the testing technique with a voltage range set from -400 mV to +400 mV, a scan rate of 100 mV/s, and a measurement time of 5 seconds. After pressing the start button, a current versus time graph was generated. The peak current value observed on this graph was noted as the maximum current, which is directly related to the glucose concentration.

Table 3. Values of Current corresponding to Sugar Concentration

Dextrose in 40ml distilled water	Current (in micro-ampere)
0.1 g	4.63
0.2 g	5.86
0.3 g	7.23
0.4 g	9.21

Figure 5. Figure 5. (a) Dense Solution of Glucose Oxidase (GOx) (b)Electrochemical Cell connected with Galvanostat

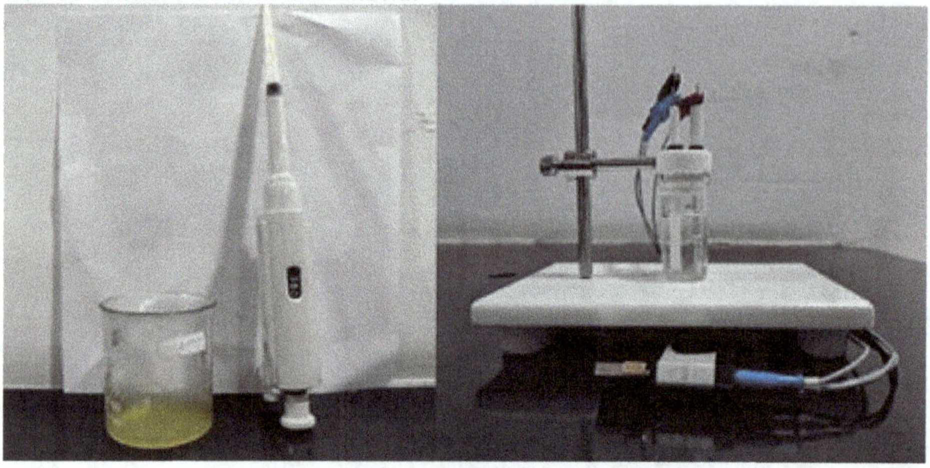

Figure 6. Figure 6. Peak Current for 0.4 grams of Glucose Solution

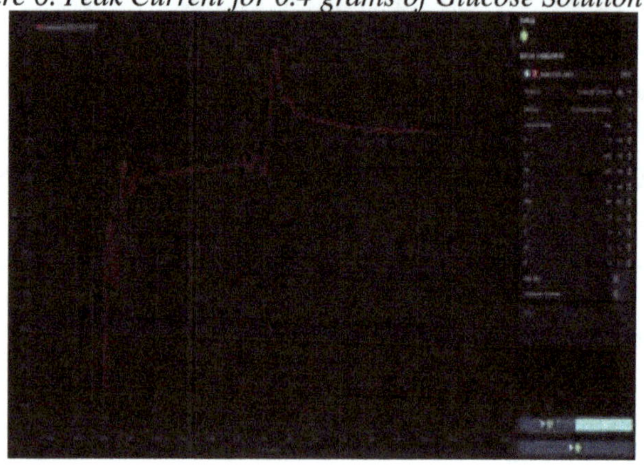

Figure 7. Excel Sheet with the Peak Current generated with help of Galvanoplot Suite

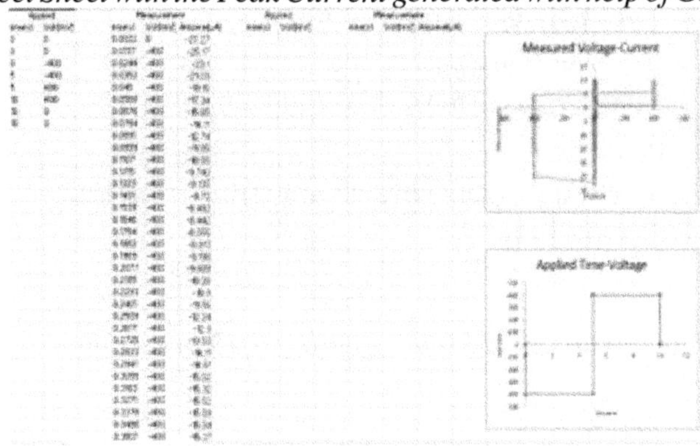

Calculations:

Step 1: Linear Regression Model

Current = m × Dextrose + c

where m = slope and c = intercept

Step 2: Formulae

$m = (N \sum(xy) - \sum x \sum y) / (N \sum x2 - (\sum x)2$

$c = (\sum y - m \sum x) / x$

Step 3: Data Table & Sums

Table 4. Calculations

Dextrose (x)	Current (y)	x * y	x^2
0.1	4.63	0.463	0.01
0.2	5.86	1.172	0.04
0.3	7.23	2.169	0.09
0.4	9.20	3.680	0.16
Sum	26.92	7.484	0.30

Following data collection, a regression model was developed to correlate the peak current to glucose concentration. This model allows the prediction of glucose levels for unknown samples by dipping the sensor into an unknown solution, measuring the peak current, and applying the regression equation to estimate the glucose concentration.

Step 4: Calculate Slope (m)

$m = (4 \times 7.484 - 1.0 \times 26.92) / (4 \times 0.3 - (1.0)\ 2)$

$m = 15.08$

Step 5: Calculate Intercept (c)

C = 26.92 – (15.08×1.0) / 4 = 11.844 = 2.96

Step 6: Final Regression Equation

Current = 15.08 × Dextrose + 2.96

Step 7: Use for Prediction

To find Dextrose from unknown current value III:

Dextrose = (I – 2.96) / 15.08

Figure 8. Linear Regression of Current vs Dextrose Concentration

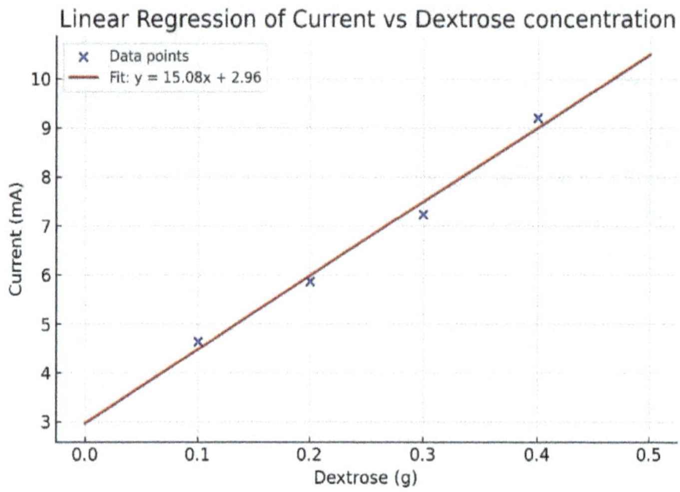

To align the lab-based electrochemical sensor data with clinically relevant glucose levels, a linear transformation was applied to the input dextrose concentrations. The original data, expressed in grams (g) of dextrose per 100 mL solution, represents high concentrations not directly comparable to glucose levels, which are typically measured in mg/dL. For instance, 0.1 g in 100 mL equates to 1000 mg/dL, far exceeding the human physiological range. Therefore, to simulate realistic glucose conditions, the concentration values ranging from 0.0 to 0.4 g were linearly scaled to the range of 151–350 mg/dL. This transformed scale reflects common blood glucose levels observed in diabetic individuals, allowing the regression model to meaningfully correlate sensor current (in mA) with realistic glucose readings. This step is crucial to ensure that the developed system remains clinically relevant and suitable for integration with AI-based prediction models or decision-making algorithms for diabetes management.

To convert the scale from 0.0g - 0.5g to 151mg/dl – 400mg/dl

Step 1: Transform X-axis from [0.0–0.5] to [151–350]

We use linear scaling formula:

Xnew = a – { (x – x min) / (xmax – x min) } * (b * a)

where x = (0.0 to 0.5), a = 151, b = 350, xmin = 0.0, xmax=0.5

xnew = 151+ (x / 0.5) * 199

Step 2: New Dataset (After Transformation)

Table 5. Relationship between Scaled Dextrose Concentration and Measured Current

Dextrose (scaled)	Current (mA)
151.0	3.0
190.8	4.6
230.6	5.9
270.4	7.4
310.2	9.2

Step 3: Linear Regression

We use scikit-learn to fit the linear regression, we got **Slope (m)** ≈ 0.0382 , **Intercept (c)** ≈ -2.79

So the final regression equation is:

Y = 0.0382 x – 2.79

Figure 9. Linear Regression of Current vs Transformed Dextrose Concentration

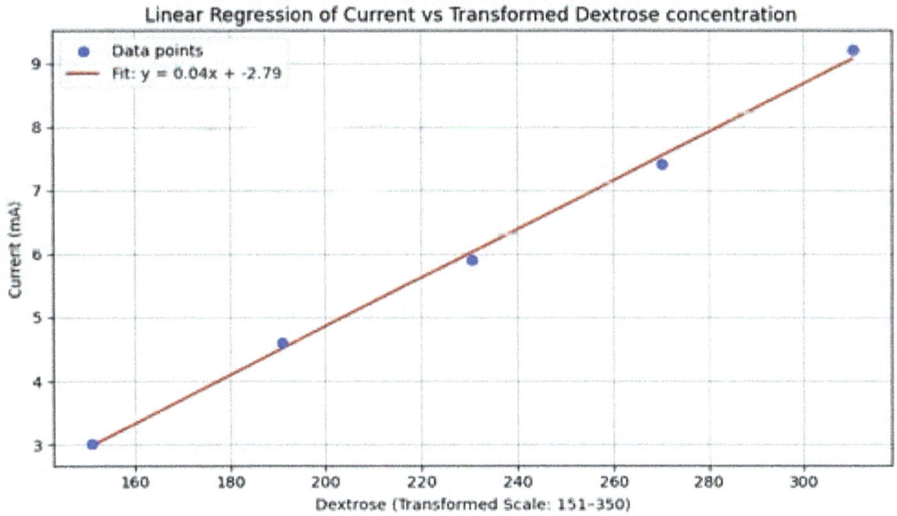

Finally, this glucose concentration value is sent to an ESP32 microcontroller via a web server. The ESP32 Arduino code already contains a predefined mapping of glucose concentration ranges to the required insulin dose. Based on the received glucose value, the ESP32 sends commands via a relay to control a motor that dispenses the corresponding amount of insulin units. This automated process ensures that the precise insulin dose is delivered according to the measured glucose concentration, completing the closed-loop system for diabetes management.

Web-Based Interface

As part of the IoT-enabled insulin delivery system, a custom browser-based interface was developed using Flask (Python), HTML, and CSS. Instead of relying on a native mobile application, this solution offers a lightweight, accessible alternative that can run locally in any web browser. The interface is designed to be intuitive and user-friendly, allowing patients or caregivers to monitor real-time glucose levels and wirelessly control insulin dosage using a laptop or mobile browser. This approach improves accessibility and eliminates dependency on platform-specific mobile environments.

Figure 10. Web Based Interface

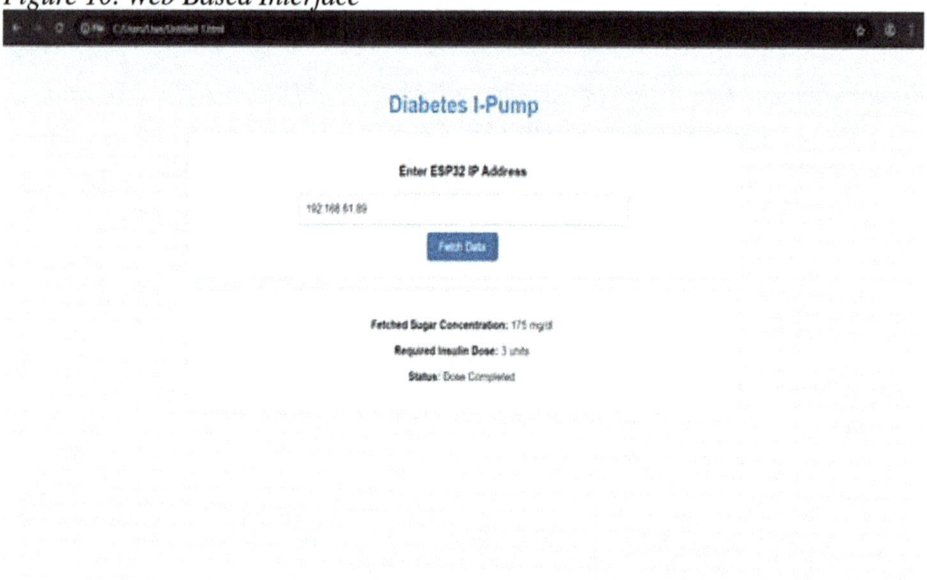

The web interface communicates with the ESP32 microcontroller over a local Wi-Fi network using HTTP protocol. The ESP32 hosts a server that exposes endpoints for glucose data retrieval and insulin delivery commands. On the client side, the Flask server manages user interactions and handles request routing. When a user enters the ESP32's IP address and clicks the "" button, a GET request is sent to the ESP32 to retrieve the latest glucose value. The response is displayed on the screen dynamically. Similarly, users can select a predefined insulin dose or manually input a custom value, which is then sent as a POST request to the ESP32 via the Flask backend for delivery via a peristaltic pump.

The user interface is constructed with standard HTML elements, styled using CSS to ensure readability and responsiveness. Key features include input fields for IP configuration, buttons to retrieve sensor data, fields to input insulin dosage, and a live feedback area to confirm data transmission or dosage status. The overall system follows a client-server architecture, where the browser acts as the client and the ESP32 microcontroller functions as the server, offering a closed-loop control mechanism for insulin delivery.

By using a web-based platform rather than a mobile application, the solution achieves flexibility, cross-platform compatibility, and reduced deployment complexity. This is especially beneficial in resource-constrained environments where smartphone availability or app installation may pose challenges. The local website-based approach maintains functionality while remaining cost-effective and technically efficient.

System Architecture

The local web interface developed using Flask (Python), HTML, and CSS acts as the client, whereas the ESP32 functions as a server. The system follows a Client-Server architecture over a shared Wi-Fi network. The website allows users to monitor real-time glucose readings and send insulin dosage commands to the ESP32-controlled peristaltic pump using HTTP GET and POST methods. This lightweight approach eliminates the need for a dedicated mobile app while ensuring real-time interaction through any web browser.

Security Considerations

Although the current prototype operates over plain HTTP on a local network, the following security enhancements are suggested for future deployments:

- *HTTPS Integration*: To enable secure medical data transmission.
- *User Authentication*: To ensure only verified individuals can access and control the insulin delivery system.
- *Dose Validation Algorithms*: To block unsafe insulin dosages based on patient history and physiological constraints.

Pump Calibration & Control Logic

The peristaltic pump was calibrated by mapping activation duration to insulin volume dispensed. For calibration:

- The pump was operated for various time intervals.
- Output volume was measured using a precision syringe.
- A lookup table was created linking duration (ms) with insulin units (IU).
- This table was integrated into the ESP32 firmware.

When the Flask website sends a dose command (entered manually or computed by the AI), the ESP32 retrieves the appropriate pump duration from the table and activates the pump via a relay module. This ensures accurate and consistent insulin delivery.

Safety Mechanisms

To prevent failure or over-delivery, the following safety layers were added:

- Timeout Function: Terminates pump activity if the run-time exceeds expected thresholds.
- Voltage and Sensor Monitoring: Continuously monitors sensor voltages and glucose readings. If abnormal values are detected, alerts are triggered on the local web interface.
- Future Feedback Loop (Optional): A flow sensor or secondary glucose probe can be added for real-time delivery verification and failure detection.

Validation & Performance Testing

1.*Calibration Verification*

Five glucose solutions with known concentrations were tested with the potentiostat and ESP32 setup. The system's predicted glucose values were compared with actual concentrations to assess:

- Precision: Reproducibility across multiple trials.
- Accuracy: Alignment with the true concentration.

Most readings were within an acceptable error margin, showing high reliability.

2. *Dynamic Testing*

Simulated glucose variations were introduced over time to test the system's responsiveness. Observations:

- The system responded in real-time to glucose changes.
- Correct dose recommendations were generated.
- Pump was triggered appropriately via website control.

These tests confirmed the robustness of the AI model and the mechanical control system, validating end-to-end performance.

RESULTS

The electrochemical sensor gave consistent voltage readings for each known dextrose concentration. A clear linear relationship was observed between the voltage output and the glucose concentration. The linear regression model generated from this data accurately mapped voltage to glucose levels within the experimental range.

The ESP32 microcontroller successfully processed the analog voltage signals in real-time and converted them into glucose concentration values using the regression equation. There was minimal delay in response, and the system maintained stability throughout testing.

Figure 11. Experimental Setup of Potentiostat

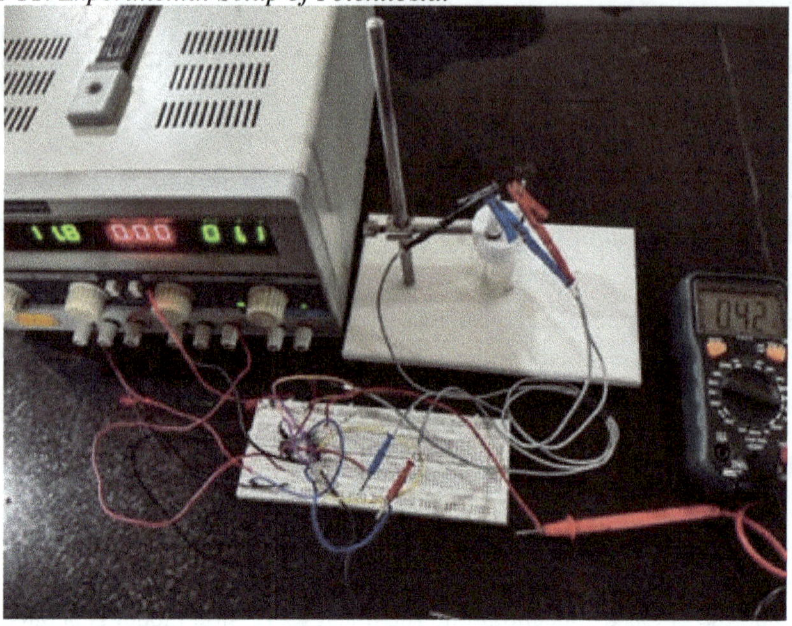

Figure 14 represents a circuit of potentiostat and electrochemical cell. A multimeter is used here to get the readings of the voltage derived through the circuit.

In this experiment, we worked with three unknown liquid samples to estimate their sugar concentration using an electrochemical sensing method. Each sample was carefully **placed into an electrochemical cell**, where a chemical reaction occurred, resulting in the generation of an electric current. The current produced during this process was accurately measured using the *Galvanoplot Suite* software.

Figure 12. Experimental Setup of Electrochemical Cell

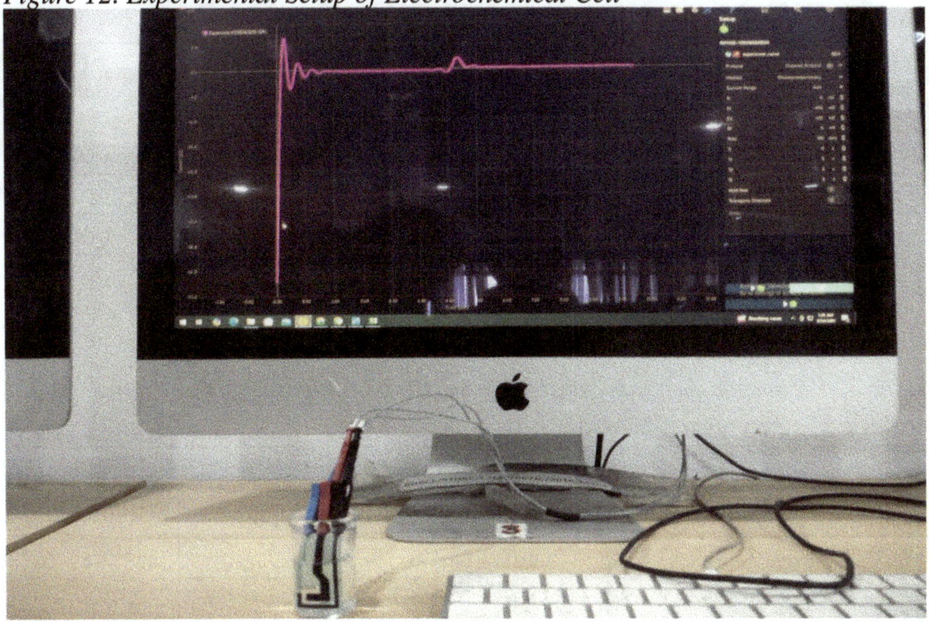

The recorded current values served as the basis for calculating the sugar concentration present in each sample. Using a predefined calibration curve or mathematical model, we computed the predicted sugar concentration in two commonly used units: milligrams per deciliter (mg/dl) and grams (g).

Once the predicted values were obtained, we compared them with the actual sugar concentrations of the samples, which were determined through a standard reference method. This comparison was essential to assess how accurately the electrochemical technique could predict sugar levels.

To quantify the prediction accuracy, we calculated the Mean Squared Error (MSE) between the predicted and actual values. The MSE is a widely used statistical measure that indicates how close the predicted values are to the true values. It is calculated by taking the average of the squared differences between each predicted and actual value.

For this set of three samples, the Mean Squared Error (MSE) was found to be approximately 0.00163. This relatively low MSE value suggests that the prediction model performed well, and the estimated sugar concentrations were closely aligned with the actual values.

Table 6. Prediction Accuracy of Unknown Glucose Samples Using Galvanostatic Measurements

Unknown Samples	Value of current through galvanoplot	Predicted value (mg/dl)	Predicted value (g)	Actual value (g)	Mean Square Error
Sample 1	5.22	210.7	0.15	0.13	0.00163
Sample 2	8.53	298.26	0.37	0.34	0.00163
Sample 3	12.30	397.76	0.62	0.68	0.00163

Table 7. Prediction Accuracy of Real-Time Blood Glucose Sample Using Galvanostatic Measurements

Patient ID	Galvanoplot current value (nA)	Predicted value (mg/dl)	Actual Glucose Concentration (Accu-Check) (mg/dl)	Percentage Error (%)
001	7.42	180	176	6.5
002	6.23	166	147	8.6

Correction Dose = (180 – 90) ÷ 50
= 1.8
Where,
Current BG=180 mg/dL, Target BG= 90 mg/dL, Correction Factor (CF)= 50

After calculating the glucose concentration (Table 7) from the current value, this information was sent to the ESP32 microcontroller over a web server. The ESP32 processed this data using a predefined sliding scale to determine the necessary insulin dosage. Based on this dosage, the ESP32 activated a relay that controlled a motor responsible for dispensing insulin. For example, a glucose concentration corresponding to 280 mg/dl would trigger an insulin dose of 8 units. This closed-loop automation, from detection to delivery, ensures prompt and precise insulin administration, offering a potential breakthrough in affordable diabetes care.

Table 8. Post Insulin delivery chart

Patient ID	Predicted value (mg/dl)	Pre- Insulin Actual Glucose Concentration (Accu-Check) (mg/dl)	Dosage	Post-Insulin Actual Glucose Concentration (Accu-Check) (mg/dl)
001	180	176	1.8	101
002	166	147	1.5	91

Figure 13. Experimental Setup of Low-Cost Insulin Pump

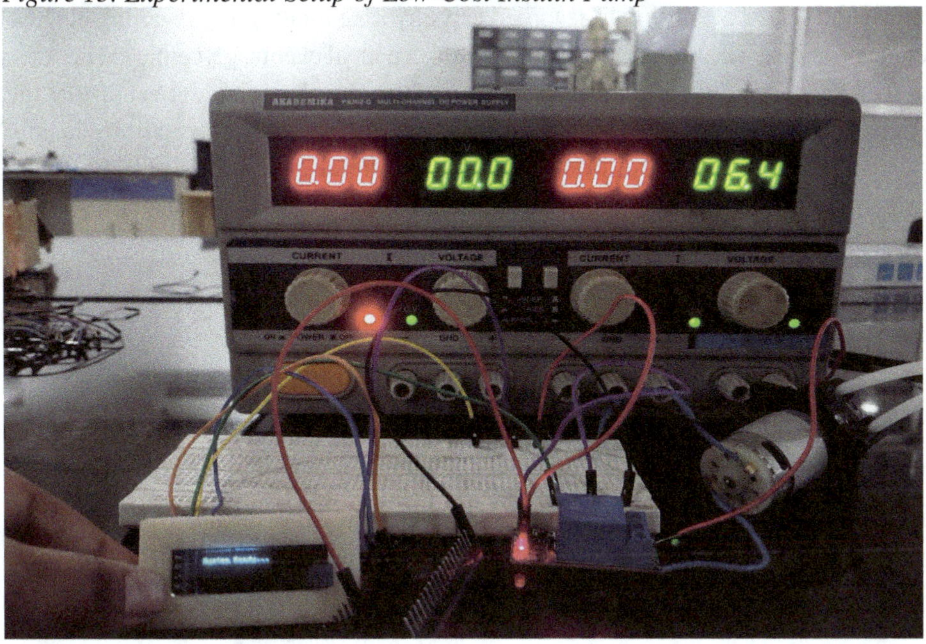

The website interface displayed real-time glucose readings and suggested appropriate insulin doses based on the mapped values. The user interface was simple and responsive. The peristaltic pump delivered insulin accurately based on calculated doses. The error margin in delivery was within ±5%, and both basal and bolus dose types were tested and worked properly. Table 8 shows the pre and post blood glucose concentration of insulin delivery.

Key Observations:

- Voltage output was stable across all tested concentrations.
- Regression mapping was consistent and accurate.
- ESP32 handled real-time data processing without lag.
- Website showed correct values and responded well.
- Insulin pump delivered near-exact amounts with minimal deviation.

This dataset provides real-time evidence of the dynamic interplay between glucose variability, insulin dosing, and meal intake in an individual with diabetes managed by an AI-assisted insulin delivery system over a 48-hour monitoring period (Figure.14). The continuous glucose data capture expected postprandial excursions and subsequent normalization within the recommended target range, demonstrating the effectiveness of the system in maintaining glycemic stability. Basal insulin delivery ensured background metabolic control, while bolus doses were precisely timed and scaled according to recorded carbohydrate intake and prevailing glucose concentrations. The temporal alignment between meal events, glycemic excursions, and corrective insulin administration underscores the physiological validity of the dataset and highlights the capacity of real-time data integration to optimize insulin therapy. Collectively, these findings exemplify the clinical utility of closed-loop systems in achieving individualized and adaptive diabetes management.

Figure 14. Glucose concentration and insulin administration over a 48-hour period with annotated meal and bolus events

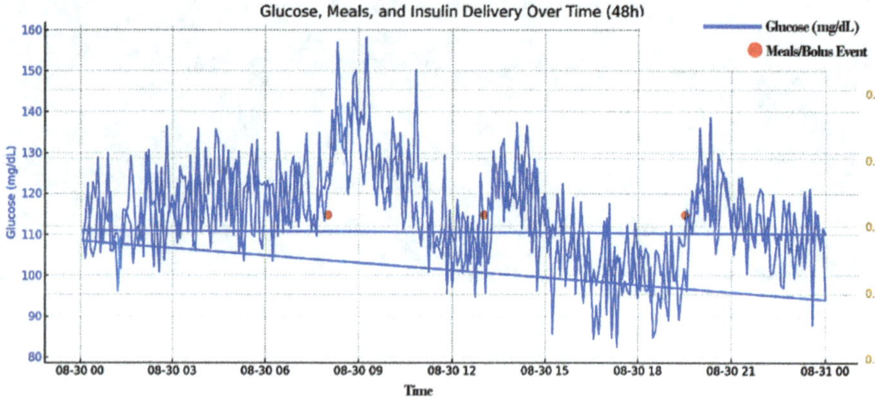

Comparison with Commercial Systems

Commercial systems like Dexcom, Freestyle Libre, and Medtronic offer sophisticated CGM and insulin delivery mechanisms. However, these systems are cost-intensive and require regular consumables. Our system:

- Operates on a fraction of the cost.
- Uses easily available components.
- Supports AI-based dose prediction.
- Allows integration with Android-based applications.

While commercial systems offer higher integration and professional calibration, the proposed model provides a highly accessible alternative suitable for education, research, and eventual clinical adaptation.

CONCLUSION

The proposed insulin pump system represents a significant step toward democratizing diabetes care. By leveraging low-cost hardware, electrochemical sensing, and AI-based analysis, this system makes real-time glucose monitoring and insulin delivery accessible to a broader population. The use of a potentiostat for glucose measurement enables a simplified and economical CGM alternative, while the integration of an ESP32 microcontroller and mobile application ensures a user-friendly experience.

The dual-mode insulin delivery (basal and bolus), real-time monitoring, and personalized dose recommendation collectively improve patient outcomes and compliance. Moreover, the ability for users to manually control dosage enhances adaptability for varying lifestyle needs. Future improvements could include miniaturization, integration of wearable sensors, closed-loop control with feedback, and real blood testing validation.

Ultimately, this project highlights the power of interdisciplinary innovation — combining biomedical engineering, embedded systems, AI, and user-centric design to create impactful healthcare solutions.

REFERENCES

Andersen, H. U., Hangaard, S., Hommel, E., & Ridderstråle, M. (2018). Six-year follow-up after insulin pump initiation: HbA1c is significantly reduced without weight gain. *Journal of Diabetes Science and Technology*, *12*(2), 535–536. DOI: 10.1177/1932296817731424 PMID: 28927286

Benkhadra, K., Alahdab, F., Tamhane, S. U., McCoy, R. G., Prokop, L. J., & Murad, M. H. (2017). Continuous subcutaneous insulin infusion versus multiple daily injections in individuals with type 1 diabetes: A systematic review and meta-analysis. *Endocrine*, *55*(1), 77–84. DOI: 10.1007/s12020-016-1039-x PMID: 27477293

Berget, C., Lange, S., Messer, L., & Forlenza, G. P. (2020). A clinical review of the t:slim X2 insulin pump. *Expert Opinion on Drug Delivery*, *17*(12), 1675–1687. DOI: 10.1080/17425247.2020.1814734 PMID: 32842794

Berget, C., Messer, L. H., & Forlenza, G. P. (2019). A clinical overview of insulin pump therapy for the management of diabetes: Past, present, and future of intensive therapy. *Diabetes Spectrum*, *32*(3), 194–204. DOI: 10.2337/ds18-0091 PMID: 31462873

Chien, M. N., Chen, Y. J., Bai, C. H., & Huang, J. T. (2022). Continuous glucose monitoring system based on percutaneous microneedle array. *Micromachines*, *13*(3), 478. DOI: 10.3390/mi13030478 PMID: 35334773

Clements, M., Matuleviciene, V., Attvall, S., Ekelund, M., Pivodic, A., Dahlqvist, S., Fahlén, M., Haraldsson, B., & Lind, M. (2015). Predicting the effectiveness of insulin pump therapy on glycemic control in clinical practice: A retrospective study of patients with type 1 diabetes from 10 outpatient diabetes clinics in Sweden over 5 years. *Diabetes Technology & Therapeutics*, *17*(1), 21–28. DOI: 10.1089/dia.2014.0139 PMID: 25470010

Dobbelaere, T., Vereecken, P., & Detavernier, C. (2017). A USB-controlled potentiostat/galvanostat for thin-film battery characterization. *HardwareX*, *2*, 34–49. DOI: 10.1016/j.ohx.2017.08.001

Fatourechi, M. M., Kudva, Y. C., Murad, M. H., Elamin, M. B., Tabini, C. C., & Montori, V. M. (2009). Clinical review: Hypoglycemia with intensive insulin therapy: A systematic review and meta-analyses of randomized trials of continuous subcutaneous insulin infusion versus multiple daily injections. *The Journal of Clinical Endocrinology and Metabolism*, *94*(3), 729–740. DOI: 10.1210/jc.2008-1415 PMID: 19088167

Galdón Sanz-Pastor, A., Justel Enríquez, A., Sánchez Bao, A., & Ampudia-Blasco, F. J. (2024). Current barriers to initiating insulin therapy in individuals with type 2 diabetes. *Frontiers in Endocrinology, 15*, 1366368. DOI: 10.3389/fendo.2024.1366368 PMID: 38559691

Ghosh, M., & Bora, V. R. (2025). Evolution in blood glucose monitoring: A comprehensive review of invasive to non-invasive devices and sensors. *Discovery Medicine*, *2*(1), 74. DOI: 10.1007/s44337-025-00273-1

Hassan, M. H., Vyas, C., Grieve, B., & Bartolo, P. (2021). Recent advances in enzymatic and non-enzymatic electrochemical glucose sensing. *Sensors (Basel)*, *21*(14), 4672. DOI: 10.3390/s21144672 PMID: 34300412

Heller, A., & Feldman, B. (2008). Electrochemical glucose sensors and their applications in diabetes management. *Chemical Reviews*, *108*(7), 2482–2505. DOI: 10.1021/cr068069y PMID: 18465900

Joshi, A. M., Jain, P., & Mohanty, S. P. (2020, July). Secure-iGLU: A secure device for noninvasive glucose measurement and automatic insulin delivery in IoMT framework. In 2020 IEEE Computer Society annual symposium on VLSI (ISVLSI) (pp. 440-445). IEEE. https://doi.org/DOI: 10.1109/ISVLSI49217.2020.00-17

Liu, Y., Yu, Q., Luo, X., Yang, L., & Cui, Y. (2021). Continuous monitoring of diabetes with an integrated microneedle biosensing device through 3D printing. *Microsystems & Nanoengineering*, *7*(1), 75. DOI: 10.1038/s41378-021-00302-w PMID: 34631143

Madsen, K. P., Olsen, K. R., Rytter, K., Willaing, I., Pedersen-Bjergaard, U., Schmidt, S., Nørgaard, K., & Kjær, T. (2023). Effects of initiating insulin pump therapy in the real world: A nationwide, register-based study of adults with type 1 diabetes. *Diabetes Research and Clinical Practice*, *196*, 110225. DOI: 10.1016/j.diabres.2022.110225 PMID: 36535513

Manov, A. E., Chauhan, S., Dhillon, G., Dhaliwal, A., Antonio, S., Donepudi, A., Jalal, Y. N., Nazha, J., Banal, M., & House, J. (2023). The effectiveness of continuous glucose monitoring devices in managing uncontrolled diabetes mellitus: A retrospective study. *Cureus*, *15*(7), e42545. DOI: 10.7759/cureus.42545 PMID: 37637581

Meloni, G. N. (2016). Building a microcontroller-based potentiostat: An inexpensive and versatile platform for teaching electrochemistry and instrumentation. *Journal of Chemical Education*, *93*(7), 1320–1322. DOI: 10.1021/acs.jchemed.5b00961

Mohiddin, A. (2022). Insulin and diabetes mellitus [Review]. *International Journal of Science and Research (Raipur, India), 11*(12), 1299–1302. DOI: 10.21275/MR22125112434

Naranjo, D., Tanenbaum, M. L., Iturralde, E., & Hood, K. K. (2016). Diabetes technology: Uptake, outcomes, barriers, and the intersection with distress. *Journal of Diabetes Science and Technology, 10*(4), 852–858. DOI: 10.1177/1932296816650900 PMID: 27234809

Nkonge, K. M., Nkonge, D. K., & Nkonge, T. N. (2023). Insulin therapy for the management of diabetes mellitus: A narrative review of innovative treatment strategies. *Diabetes Therapy : Research, Treatment and Education of Diabetes and Related Disorders, 14*(11), 1801–1831. DOI: 10.1007/s13300-023-01468-4 PMID: 37736787

Ribet, F., Stemme, G., & Roxhed, N. (2018). Real-time intradermal continuous glucose monitoring using a minimally invasive microneedle-based system. *Biomedical Microdevices, 20*(4), 101. DOI: 10.1007/s10544-018-0349-6 PMID: 30523421

Rimon, M. T. I., Hasan, M. W., Hassan, M. F., & Cesmeci, S. (2024). Advancements in insulin pumps: A comprehensive exploration of insulin pump systems, technologies, and future directions. *Pharmaceutics, 16*(7), 944. DOI: 10.3390/pharmaceutics16070944 PMID: 39065641

Tanenbaum, M. L., Hanes, S. J., Miller, K. M., Naranjo, D., Bensen, R., & Hood, K. K. (2017). Diabetes device use in adults with type 1 diabetes: Barriers to uptake and potential intervention targets. *Diabetes Care, 40*(2), 181–187. DOI: 10.2337/dc16-1536 PMID: 27899489

Thomas, M. G., Avari, P., Godsland, I. F., Lett, A. M., Reddy, M., & Oliver, N. (2021). Optimizing type 1 diabetes after multiple daily injections and capillary blood monitoring: Pump or sensor first? A meta-analysis using pooled differences in outcome measures. *Diabetes, Obesity & Metabolism, 23*(11), 2521–2528. DOI: 10.1111/dom.14498 PMID: 34286892

Wilson, L. M., & Castle, J. R. (2020). Recent advances in insulin therapy. *Diabetes Technology & Therapeutics, 22*(12), 929–936. DOI: 10.1089/dia.2020.0065 PMID: 32310681

Yonemori, Y., Takahashi, E., Ren, H., Hayashi, T., & Endo, H. (2009). Biosensor system for continuous glucose monitoring in fish. *Analytica Chimica Acta, 633*(1), 90–96. DOI: 10.1016/j.aca.2008.11.023 PMID: 19110121

Chapter 4
Collaborative Health Intelligence:
Federated Learning and the Future of AI-Driven Medical Care

B. Yamini
https://orcid.org/0000-0003-3531-108X
SRM Institute of Science and Technology, India

Siva Subramanian R.
https://orcid.org/0000-0002-7509-9223
SRM Institute of Science and Technology, India

T. Thilagam
https://orcid.org/0000-0002-7657-0726
Vel Tech Rangarajan Dr. Sagunthala R&D Institute of Science and Technology, India

Anish T. P.
https://orcid.org/0000-0002-4308-9645
R.M.K. College of Engineering and Technology, India

ABSTRACT

Federated Learning (FL) is emerging as a transformative approach to AI-driven medical care, allowing for decentralized, privacy-preserving model training across multiple healthcare institutions. This chapter explores the potential of FL in enhancing healthcare systems, from personalized treatment recommendations to improving disease prediction accuracy. By enabling the secure sharing of healthcare data while ensuring patient privacy, FL has the capacity to address critical challenges such as data silos and biased models. However, challenges remain in areas like

DOI: 10.4018/979-8-3373-3306-9.ch004

model convergence, communication efficiency, and data heterogeneity. Further the chapter discuss the ethical, regulatory, and collaborative dimensions necessary for the successful deployment of FL in healthcare. The future of AI-driven medical care hinges on advancements in FL techniques, integration with IoMT, and interdisciplinary collaboration for more efficient, transparent, and personalized healthcare.

1. INTRODUCTION

Healthcare industry is considered as one of the most promising fields for the implementation of AI. AI technologies are gaining their place in medical field as a tool to increase the effectiveness, speed and efficiently of the healthcare services (Mangairkarasi et al., 2025). The new techniques of working together and sharing data are appearing as the AI progresses, which can open up more possibilities for enhancing patients' lives and medical science. FL is a decentralized learning approach that can analyze the data without the need to share the medical data of the patients. This chapter aims at discussing the emerging concept of Collaborative Health Intelligence with the emphasis on the application of FL and its impact on the development of AI in medicine (Saraswat et al 2022).

1.1. Overview of AI in Healthcare

It is the use of AI & ML techniques in the healthcare industry with the aim of enhancing the quality of human health(Gopi et al 2024). AI has a broad application in medical care, for example, in diagnosis, treatment, patient-specific medicine, and healthcare management. AI systems are capable of dealing with large medical data such as patient's records, medical images, genetics data, and even data from wearable devices(Khang 2023). These data sources enable the AI to help the healthcare professionals in the formulation of the right diagnosis, prognosis and the best treatment methodologies to be taken. The historical development of AI in healthcare can be dated back to the 1970s with the development of expert systems that were aimed at emulating the decision-making process of health care professionals. These early systems, such as MYCIN, were designed to offer diagnostic advice in accordance with rules of medicine. But it was only when researchers obtained access to better computational tools and when algorithms of machine learning appeared that AI was able to demonstrate high potential in the sphere of medicine(Indu V et al., 2026). Due to the advancement of deep learning especially CNN, there has been significant improvement of medical image analysis where the AI systems can make diagnosis as accurate as a human expert in fields like radiology and dermatology(Keerthika et al 2023).

1.2. Rise of Collaborative Health Intelligence

The concept of Collaborative Health Intelligence refers to the collective effort of multiple healthcare entities such as hospitals, research institutions, and healthcare providers working together to leverage AI for better patient care. This approach is different from the more conventional systems where all the data is collected to a central system for analysis(Boopathi, S., & Khang, A. 2023). It does not promote the models that require the sharing of the patient data and information but supports the distributed models that allow the learning to be done in parallel. These are some of the factors that are likely to have contributed to the development of the collaborative health intelligence: the need for sharing information across institutions. In the healthcare industry, there is a major issue of data disintegration. These multiple centers including hospitals, clinics and health systems have patient data that are not well integrated hence it is challenging to develop AI models that can utilize the full range of healthcare data. Collaborative health intelligence helps in overcoming these barriers and helps in building better and generalized models of AI. With collaborative intelligence, it is possible to enhance the coverage and effectiveness of AI applications in different areas of healthcare sector through cooperation between providers while keeping the providers' data under their control. However, such collaboration has its advantages as well as disadvantages, the most crucial one being the protection of data privacy and security. It is a well-known fact that health information is among the most personal data that can be breached which would have severe ethical, legal, and financial repercussions. Since AI models depend on data to be trained then issues to do with data sharing and collaboration of AI models should also be done in secure, transparent, and ethical manners. Some of the solutions that are seen and being implemented in the recent past include data anonymization, differential privacy, and SMPC, but these are still topics of current research.

1.3. Federated Learning: A New Paradigm

The main component of the collaborative health intelligence is FL, a novel approach to ML that allows to train state-of-the-art models without centralizing the data. In conventional ML, data is acquired from different sources and is stored in a central server or database and used for training the model (Rose et al., 2025). However, in many medical cases, data cannot be centralized because of the issues of privacy, legal regulations, or ownership of data. This is solved by FL which allows the learning of models on the devices or systems that are decentralized (such as local hospitals or medical institutions) while only syncing the model updates with a central server instead of the data itself. The advantage of FL in healthcare is that it enables the training of AI models using multiple datasets from various healthcare facilities without sharing patients' information over the network. This approach also makes it possible to respect the patient's privacy while at the same time facilitating the development of the AI models by the various health care providers. This way, patients' data is kept secure while healthcare institutions are able to benefit from the data offered by a larger network. In addition, FL can address the data heterogeneity problem at different institutions, which makes it possible for models to work across different settings, including the differences in patients' demographics, diseases' incidence, and practices among other factors. As evidenced from the above discussion, there are numerous advantages of using FL over traditional machine learning techniques in the health-care sector (Ramesh et al., 2024; Gracious, L. A et al., 2024). First, it enhances privacy and security since no one will be required to disclose any information. Second, it helps to link up institutions with different datasets but cannot share them with each other due to compliance or data protection issues. Lastly, FL can help in creating better and more precise models of medical diagnosis that are based on more sources of information, thus improving the health care industry.

1.4. Objective of the chapter

This chapter focuses on the relationship between the Collaborative Health Intelligence and the Federated Learning in the context of the AI based healthcare. In particular, the chapter will review the state of the art of FL in the healthcare sector, discuss its possible uses and advantages, and explore the issues and implications of using such technologies in the healthcare industry. The survey will begin with the basic definitions of Federated Learning and will then explain how it operates and why this learning approach is valuable in the healthcare industry. It will then go through how Federated Learning is being used in real-world health care situations, including examples of its application. The chapter will also look into the ethical, regulatory and security concerns that arise from the application of FL in healthcare and how they are being managed. Lastly, the chapter will explores a vision of the future of AI in healthcare that will be the focus of the next generation of technologies, namely FL. It will also identify the research & development opportunities and the prospect of Federated Learning to revolutionize the healthcare system and promote the decentralized approach based on the patient's needs.

2. FUNDAMENTALS OF FL

FL is a new and revolutionary approach to ML that allows multiple institutions or devices to train models together while keeping their data private. This section starts with explaining what Federated Learning is, how it works, how data privacy is ensured in FL, and some of the issues and limitations of FL in the healthcare domain.

2.1. Overview of FL

FL is a type of ML whereby several clients including the hospitals, medical devices or other research facilities can train a common model without sharing their data(Wen et al 2023). In each client, the local model is trained on the client's data and only the changes to the trained model (such as model parameters or gradients) are transmitted to a central server. In this way, the server collects these updates and enhances the global model. This process is repeated iteratively, and each time each client refines the model while at the same time being able to maintain ownership of its data. It is for this reason that the key principle of FL is the decentralization of data. This is unlike the conventional machine learning, which entails data collection from multiple sources, storage in a central database and then feeding it to the model for training from the database. In Federated Learning, however, data does not move from one place to the other but remains at its original place. The following are the benefits of this approach. First, it enhances data privacy and security since less sensitive information is disclosed. Second, it minimizes the need for huge transfer of data which may be recurrent, expensive and time-consuming. Third, it enables multi-institution collaboration which enhances the applications of AI models since different data sources are used. Relative to centralized ML, FL has several unique advantages. Centralized models are prone to privacy and regulatory issues since they aggregate data from various sources, a factor that is a significant concern when it comes to the collection and management of health records due to the legal guidelines. On the other hand, FL keeps data local and this helps in minimizing risks that are associated with invasion of data privacy and non-adherence to the set privacy standards(Banabilah et al 2022).

Figure 1. Federated Learning

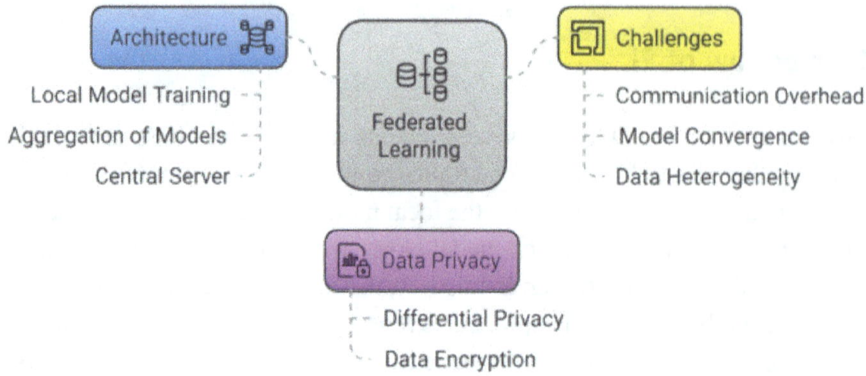

2.2. Architecture and Framework

FL works under a specific architecture that includes local model training, aggregation of models and a central server. It is important to have a clear understanding of the architecture to gain an insight on how the technology operates & how it can be implemented in actual healthcare practice. The process of FL also starts with local model training. Every client, for instance, a hospital or a medical device, trains a model on its own data that only it has access to. This is usually a standard machine learning or deep learning process where the weights of the model are trained using the client's data. After the model is trained locally, it computes the gradients with respect to the parameters of the model based on the loss function used during training. In local training, the client transmits only the model updates which can be weights or gradients to a central server. This server is to receive the updates that have been done on all the clients by the other servers. There is an approach called Federated Averaging (FedAvg), in which the server sums the updates of the clients & updates the global model parameters with the obtained sum. The server does not receive any raw data from any client and it does not store or process this data in any way therefore it is secure. This process goes on in cycles where the clients perform localized updates to the model and then send the updated model to the central server. This continues until the model finds a good solution that generalizes well across the different data sources, even though the author does not have direct access to individual data set. FL models are generally supposed to be extensible, portable and capable of serving a large number of clients. This decentralized architecture is important in the healthcare environment where the data can be scattered across different institutions with different systems and structures. Federated Learning enables data to remain local but contribute to a global model, this means that it is possible to train a model on different data collected from different parts of the world hence improving the healthcare AI systems.

2.3. Data Privacy and Security

One of the most serious issues in managing healthcare data is protection of the patient's data and adherence to the requirements of the law. FL addresses these concerns in several ways, employing various techniques to protect the privacy of the patients and their health information. Currently, one of the common techniques employed to achieve privacy in Federated Learning is differential privacy. This strategy involves making the client's updates noisy and unpredictable so that it cannot be deduced from the aggregated update. Differential privacy makes sure that the information that each client provides does not contain details of specific patients, and even if the adversary tries to reconstruct the model updates, they cannot do so. Differential privacy adds noise to the model gradients to ensure that no individual's data is identifiable or reconstructable from the final model. Besides differential privacy, data encryption is also adopted to secure the updates of the model during the communication. Encryption makes it possible that even if the updates captured during the communication between clients & the central server the data cannot be read without the decryption key. The various techniques such as homomorphic encryption enable the central server to perform computations on the encrypted model updates so that there is no time when the actual data is exposed in an unencrypted manner. There are also issues of security of the collaborative process in Federated Learning apart from data security. It is therefore important for the updates received from each client to be authentic and not containing any viruses. Methods like secure aggregation are used in order to avoid a situation where the attacker introduces wrong updates to the global model. This makes the model more resilient and guarantees that the concept of collaborative learning is not contaminated by any negative influences. However, the security of FL in the context of healthcare is still an open issue. Since the healthcare data is gaining value, there is an increased vulnerability of the decentralized systems to attacks. Therefore, there is a constant emergence of new approaches for data protection, defence against adversarial attacks, and identification of outliers.

2.4. Challenges and Limitations

On the same note, FL has its pros and cons that need to be considered when implemented, particularly in sensitive sectors such as healthcare. There are several issues that have been identified as critical in the design of the system and among the most important is communication overhead. There is always the need for the clients to send their model updates to the central server, which can be a burden in large networks or if the updates are large in size. This can be a major issue in health care systems where an institution may not afford to make use of broadband connections or where the cost of communication is a factor. This problem is currently being addressed through the use of other effective communication methods like model compression and frequency reduction. Another challenge is model convergence. In FL, the training of the model occurs in a decentralized fashion and each client has a subset of the data. This can result in non-convergence of the global model as the local models obtained from training on different data distributions may be contradictory. To overcome these challenges, there is a need to use better aggregation techniques and optimization algorithms to enhance convergence of the global model when dealing with diverse and possibly imbalanced data. The last problem is data heterogeneity which is one of the major challenges in FL especially in the healthcare sector. The data in various institutions may differ greatly in terms of its quality, format, and distribution. For instance, different hospitals may have different policies on data acquisition of the patients, and therefore the data collected may not be uniform. Such heterogeneity can hamper the generalization capabilities of the model and can lead to more erroneous results. In order to address data heterogeneity, there is a need to use algorithms that are able to handle the data and make the global model learn from the data that is available.

3. FL IN HEALTHCARE

FL has a great potential to change the healthcare sector as it allows for the collaborative learning process without sharing the data(Antunes et al 2022). In the context of health care, FL allows the creation of enduring, general models, trained with data from multiple institutions without the need to centralize the information, which can be highly sensitive(Nguyen et al 2022). This section describes the various types of the source of healthcare data that can be used for FL, the potential uses of FL, and several case studies of FL's application.

Figure 2. Federated Learning in Healthcare

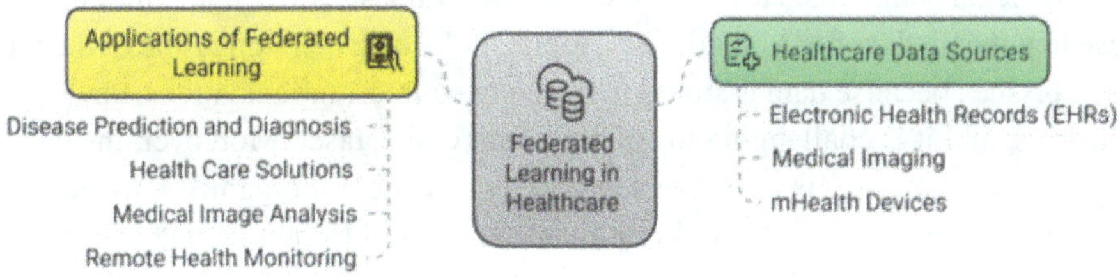
Applications of Federated Learning
Disease Prediction and Diagnosis
Health Care Solutions
Medical Image Analysis
Remote Health Monitoring
Federated Learning in Healthcare
Healthcare Data Sources
Electronic Health Records (EHRs)
Medical Imaging
mHealth Devices

3.1. Healthcare Data Sources

The first and most crucial to any AI health care model is the input data used in training the model. In the case of FL, there are certain types of healthcare data which can be used, which are as follows with the challenges associated with them: EHRs are considered as one of the most valuable sources of health care data. EHRs consist of medical history, diagnosis, treatment plan, laboratory results, and prescription history of a patient. They play an important role in analysis of the patient's health status and as a useful tool in health prognosis. However, EHRs pose certain challenges to the development of AI models, including variation in the data quality, data in completeness, and data format in different hospitals or healthcare providers. Moreover, EHR data can be fraught with bias because its collection may be based on certain medical practices, patients' characteristics, or institutional procedures, which makes it problematic to extend it to other populations. Medical Imaging is another important data type especially when it comes to diagnosing or tracking a disease through techniques such as MRI, CT scans and X-ray. The convolutional neural networks have widely been used in image analysis including detecting of cancer, identification of abnormality and in observations during surgery. Medical imaging data is usually large and of high resolution and therefore poses problems in terms of transmission in Federated Learning systems. In addition, medical imaging data is diverse across different institutions, different imaging modalities, different protocols and different labelling, which can be a challenge when developing the model. It's measured from mHealth devices such as blood pressure meters, glucometer, fitness trackers and others. These devices offer constant data on the signs of the patients such as heart rate, movement, and sleep, which can be useful for managing conditions such as diabetes or cardiovascular diseases. Nevertheless, the data collected by the sensors is noisy, sparse, and a lot of times inconsistent and hence needs to be cleaned before it can be used in the Federated Learning models. Moreover, many of these wearables produce personal data, the privacy of which is an issue that has to be addressed using proper transmission and storage solutions to meet the legal standards. However, there are several issues when it comes to using these healthcare data for AI model development. Data dispersion is one of the most crucial issues because data is stored in different sources, organizations, devices, or platforms, and it is challenging to collect it into one dataset. Moreover, the data in the healthcare industry is also diverse as even two different organizations can store and manage their data in the different formats, using different language or having different standards. Lastly, data privacy and security remain an issue that should be dealt with at all times. Since patient information is highly confidential, models have to be developed in a way that would allow the learners to learn from each other without compromising the privacy of the patient information.

3.2. Applications of FL in Healthcare

FL is a promising solution to many of the issues in healthcare since it allows model training across multiple institutions while keeping data local. The following is a list of some of the most effective ush of Federated Learning in the health sector. Disease Prediction and Diagnosis: FL is most appropriate in the disease prediction and diagnoses of diseases given large and diverse datasets. For instance, in the field of oncology, FL can contribute to the development of models for cancer diagnosis based on medical imaging data including MRI, CT scans from several hospitals. Likewise, in cardiovascular diseases, FL can be applied to build models that can interpret patients' information from various areas, enhancing the prognosis of heart diseases and their potential impacts. FL models can also use information from EHRs, sensor data and lab results to enhance the accuracy of the prediction. This way, with the training of these models across many institutions, the healthcare providers can develop AI systems that can generalize well across patient populations. Health Care Solutions: The application of Federated Learning involves creating AI models that come up with treatment plans tailored for particular patients and taking into consideration their medical history, genetic structure, and other factors. For instance, a model on data collected from a set of different health facilities can prescribe procedures to patients who have cancer based on genotypes, the type of cancer, and the rate of cure of various treatments. Likewise, FL can be used to develop individualized treatment plans for patients with chronic diseases such as diabetes that have to do with adjusting insulin doses based on data collected by wearable devices and the patient's history. This makes FL ensure that the recommendations given are a wider variety of medical practices and patients' data which will be accurate. Medical Image Analysis: The application of AI in medical image analysis is one of the oldest and most established uses of the technology, and Federated Learning is making a great impact in this field. Since FL can obtain data from different hospitals and medical centers, it can be used to train models to recognize diseases from X-rays, MRI, CT scans & other imaging techniques such as tumors, fractures, or infections. Thus, through FL, the medical image models can use a wider range of imaging data and improve the generalization of imaging technology and patients. For example, when developing a Federated Learning model on MRI scans obtained from one hospital and another, the results produced are much more generalized than those of a model developed with one hospital data alone. Remote Health Monitoring: The use of wearable devices and mobile applications in the management of health has made remote health monitoring one of the most important fields in the healthcare sector. Wearable objects including smartwatches, glucose monitors and heart rate sensors produce massive data on now health statistics. This makes it possible for these devices to participate in the training of these AI models without necessarily sharing any sensitive information. Thus, FL can be used in creating models for diagnosis, such as heart disease or chronic diseases like diabetes, by constantly monitoring data from sensors. Furthermore, with the FL models, the healthcare providers are able to monitor the condition of the patients from a distance, make the necessary changes to the treatments as and when needed and all these are done while respecting the privacy of the patients(Bashir et al 2023).

4. ETHICAL CONSIDERATIONS AND REGULATORY CHALLENGES

This section focuses on the ethical and regulatory issues arising from the increased application of FL in the healthcare industry. These have to be resolved to avoid misapplication of artificial intelligence in medical facilities in a way that is legally and ethically wrong. Some of the ethical issues covered in this section include ethical issues of using AI in healthcare, regulatory issues on data protection and AI applications, and the need to establish trust and transparency in the use of FL in medical systems.

4.1. Ethical Concerns in AI-Driven Medical Care

AI models in healthcare, especially those developed through Federated Learning can help in diagnosis, treatment, and general patient care. However, the use of AI in making decisions related to the patient's health has a number of ethical issues that must be discussed to ensure that every patient will benefit from the AI applications and no patient will be harmed by the technology.

Ethical Issues in AI in the Healthcare System: The use of AI in the healthcare sector is not without its drawbacks, and one of them includes bias in the AI models.

Machine learning models, including FL models, are trained on historical data and may contain the same bias that is contained in the healthcare system. For instance, a model trained on data from one ethnic group, for example, white patients, will not be as effective when applied to patients from a different ethnic group such as the blacks. This bias can result in wrong diagnosis, different treatment prescriptions or differential treatment and health outcome which only worsens the inequalities in health. Reducing bias entails using diverse data during training, as well as periodically checking for model performance disparity across diverse patient populations. It is crucial to make sure that the data used in Federated Learning is as diverse and extensive as possible to accommodate all patients and provide equal quality of healthcare. Accountability and Decision-Making in AI Systems: Another ethical issue in AI in the healthcare domain is accountability of the medical decisions made by the AI system. Some AI models especially Federated Learning models create a black box environment where the rationale for the decision made by the model is not easily understandable by the physicians or the patient. The problem with this is that it is challenging to explain how the model came up with a certain recommendation or diagnosis, which is a cause for concern when it comes to assigning blame in the event of an error. It is therefore important that ethical principles and clear protocols should be set down to avoid lack of accountability and to safeguard patient's rights. For similar reasons, the use of explainable AI methods, including interpretable models or post-hoc explanations, in Federated Learning models could enhance its accountability as the process of the decision-making becomes more transparent to the clinicians. Some of the ethical concerns of utilising sensitive health data for training AI models include patient privacy and consent. Health data is sensitive information, and using it for the training of the AI is questionable as it poses risks when patients are not aware of how their data is being used or if their consent was not sought. In some cases, patients may not comprehend the rights of their data being used in an AI system, especially when such systems are trained across different institutions in a FL setting. To address these issues, healthcare organisations must ensure that the patient gives consent to his/her data to be used in the mentioned ways, the use of the data and the parties who will have access to the data and the risks involved in the use of the data. In addition, the privacy-preserving methods of FL like differential privacy and encryption can reduce the potential risks of the data sharing by protecting the patient data and making them anonymous during the training process. However, it is still important to monitor the practices continuously and ensure that ethical practices are followed.

Figure 3. Ethical Considerations and Regulatory Challenges

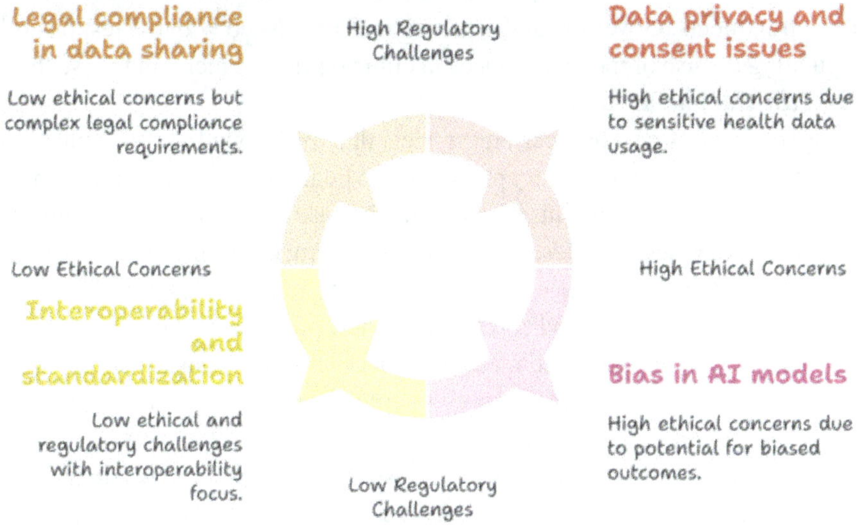

4.2. Regulatory and Legal Challenges

Over time, as Federated Learning is being implemented widely in the healthcare sector, it will encounter different regulatory and legal issues. These frameworks are aimed at safeguarding the patient, maintaining the confidentiality of patients' data and offering a check on the appropriate uses of AI solutions in the practice of medicine. However, the characteristics of Federated Learning are fundamentally different from most of the existing learning models, and thus there are certain regulatory issues that arise in its context. Legal Compliance Issues in Sharing Data: In the context of sharing data, the legal frameworks are very stringent in the healthcare industry due to patient confidentiality. The nature of Federated learning that keeps the patient data local and never has to be sent to a central server. However, the process of collecting updates from various institutions has introduced some new issues concerning these laws. For instance, although the model updates that are shared in FL are not patient data, they can contain patterns or information that can be used to identify patients under certain conditions. This means that regulatory bodies will have to set standards to address the issue of data protection of users in Federated Learning systems as the current laws are not sufficient to guide the implementation of Federated Learning. This might entail establishing fresh guidelines pertaining to Decentralized AI, guaranteeing that FL adequately considers patients privacy, yet allows for data sharing within and across establishments. Legal Restrictions on the Use of AI in the Medical Field: AI in the medical field is still restricted due to legal restrictions in order to protect the health of patients and the efficiency of medical treatments. Governmental organizations are tasked with the responsibility of regulating the use of medical devices in clinical practice including those that are run by artificial intelligence.

Diagnostic tools or other learning models that are applied in the medical field must go through a lot of regulatory procedures to guarantee the safety, effectiveness, and reliability of the model. This is especially the case in a distributed system where the models are trained in different institutions, this makes it difficult to monitor or assess the general performance of the system. The regulators will have to ensure safety measures, disclosure and continuous review process to address the risks that are associated with the AI based medical devices. This is because heterogeneity of systems across the different institutions is a crucial issue that affects the implementation of Federated Learning for healthcare. Some of the challenges encountered when implementing Federated Learning network is the different IT structures, data formats, and standards that are used in healthcare institutions. For instance, the data collected from different hospitals may be formatted or named differently and therefore the model updates cannot be aggregated easily. Currently, there is no standard way of implementing FL and thus regulators and standards organizations need to set common frameworks and standards. This also involves establishing such things as data exchange modes or specifications, communication protocols, means of model assessment to enable harmonized interdisciplinary research. Interoperability and standardization are key to getting the most out of FL in healthcare and to be able to deploy models developed across multiple institutions.

4.3. Trust and Transparency

In order to successfully incorporate Federated Learning in healthcare, two main factors are the need to foster trust and to be transparent. To ensure patient trust, healthcare workers, and regulatory authorities, it is crucial that they are sure that the AI models are used ethically and for the benefit of the patients. The Role of Trust in Collaborative Medical AI: In the healthcare industry, trust is one of the key aspects that people place their trust in doctors and other healthcare facilities. To introduce AI-driven systems based on FL in the healthcare sector, the providers have to be assured that the models are reliable, secure, and relevant to practice. Likewise, patients have to be assured that their data is not misused and that the AI systems will not compromise the quality of care provided to them. Lack of trust on the side of both the health care professionals and the patients will make it hard for them to take AI technologies into practice. Transparency in the mechanism of operation of Federated Learning systems, measures put in place to secure patient data, and the outcome of the AI decisions made. This means that there needs to be cooperation between health care organizations, AI specialists, and other authorities to build the trust of all the parties involved. The following are the elements that must be considered to avoid the misuse of AI models in healthcare: The model must include transparency in the decisions made by the model and the outcomes of the model. Since the implications of such decisions entail crucial issues, for example, the diagnoses or treatment advice, healthcare practitioners and patients should know how the models come to their conclusions. This is especially true in FL where the model is trained across different institutions and therefore the process is even more complicated. It is critical that Federated Learning models should be made interpretable and explainable. It also involves creating ways through which the clinicians can be able to comprehend the rationale that the AI models use to come up with their suggestions and also making the models accountable. It also refers to the patient's right to know how the information about them is being used, how decisions are made, and measures taken to ensure the information is not disclosed to the third party. Transparent systems help to maintain ethical values of artificial intelligence in healthcare because it creates responsibility for the results and aligns the objective with the patient's needs.

5. FUTURE DIRECTIONS

There are many promising developments in FL for health care in the future decades, as AI methods keep on emergently, IoMT technologies are being advanced and an emergence in focus to personalized and predictive medicine is being noticed. As AI continues to be applied in the health care sector, FL presents a solution to health care model development that is cooperative and protects patient's information. This section looks into the future of FL in healthcare in terms of improvement in the FL techniques, the incorporation of IoMT and the move to personalized and predictive healthcare, as well as collaboration across disciplines.

5.1. Advancements in Federated Learning Techniques

There is high potential for FL in healthcare, the efficiency and effectiveness of the technique is expected to increase as new algorithms and techniques are being developed. While FL has been applied to various medical applications, there are still existing issues and challenges that researchers are trying to improve upon to expand the capabilities of FL methods. Federated Optimization is among the fields that are currently witnessing the emergence of new algorithms. Optimization is a key component of FL since it involves making updates based on the data collected from other institutions. However, there are some problems related to the structure of FL: high communication overhead for the aggregation of the model updates, non-convergence of the models, and the heterogeneity of the local data. There are studies on achieving the model federate optimization in which the communication cost is significantly reduced and the model convergence rate is enhanced. For example, some recent approaches such as Federated Averaging or FedAvg has been proposed to tackle these challenges but more researches are required to improve it in order to handle more complex & large health care datasets. Another trend is the integration of Federated Learning with other paradigms of AI: From this perspective, it is possible to identify new trends that have recently started to appear in the literature. For instance, transfer learning is being considered as the practice of using models trained in a centralized manner and then fine-tuned for decentralized data. This can go a long way in decreasing the amount of data and computations needed for each local model training, thus making it possible to implement FL in areas with limited resources like rural or underfunded hospitals. It is also about the possibility of integrating FL with reinforcement learning or even active learning or meta-learning to seek for more flexibility and intelligence of models in healthcare system, which would learn with the increase of experiences or data and achieve better results automatically. Thus, the future of Federated Learning in healthcare will be more efficient and scalable, making it easier to develop more accurate and collaborative models that still protect privacy.

5.2. Integration With IoMT

IoMT refers to a burgeoning network of advanced connective technology medical devices & sensors that monitor patients' health information. Some examples include wearables such as fitness trackers, smartwatches, glucose monitor and blood pressure monitor that engage the patient in a continuous flow of patient data. The combination of FL and IoMT is a promising solution for the future of healthcare since it will improve the level of care and make decision-making more efficient. FL and IoMT: The combination of FL with IoMT devices offers a significant advantage in the healthcare system since it is capable of collecting, analyzing, and updating the models instantly. IoMT devices produce a large volume of real-time data that can be used to track the patient's condition at any given time. This will enable the use of this data without compromising the privacy of patients, since the data is retained on local devices or hospitals while the model's updates are sent to and received in a privacy-preserving manner. This creates an opportunity to offer patient-centered healthcare that interferes with the patient's needs in real-time instead of relying on the traditional paper-based medical records. For example, a wearable device may record the patient's heart rate and periodically provide it to the FL model. It will be able to use these updates and other patients' data to enhance its capability of anticipating future cardiovascular events, offer an early alert to the clinicians, and enable them to intervene earlier. Conducting an IoMT of such Chronic conditions as diabetes or ailments like asthma could relay real-time data to refine models for recommending changes in the medication dosage or alteration of lifestyles. However, dynamic model updates are important in addressing dynamic nature of patient health especially in cases of acute diseases or illnesses. FL and IoMT also allow a model to update from new data as it is received and include it in its decision-making process to make sure that the treatment recommendations are based on the most current patient data. With the growth of FL in conjunction with IoMT, the healthcare system will evolve to a more data-oriented, adaptive, and patient-specific one that adapts to the needs of a patient in real-time.

5.3. Personalized and Predictive Medicine

Another great benefit of FL in healthcare is the aspect of precision medicine & predictive medicine. Personalized medicine is the approach to the medical practice that is based on the individual patient's genetic characteristics, his or her lifestyle, and the disease state. While preventive medicine aims at preventing diseases and illness, predictive medicine employs models to predict the future health conditions of an individual. Precision Medicine: The use of FL in building precision medicine models is possible because many institutions can train a single model jointly without sharing patients' data. These models can take into account such factors as the patient's genetics and medical history, lifestyle and environment in order to determine the most suitable treatment option for the patient. This way, the Federated Learning accumulates data from various populations and prevents the models from being trained in a way that would only suit one group of patients, and thus, it is more universal.

Likewise, Federated Learning can be applied to develop a treatment plan for chronic diseases like diabetes or hypertension, based on the data received from wearable sensors and previous patient's records. Another interesting application of FL in the field of predictive medicine is the use of FL to predict disease outbreaks or health trends from cooperative data sets. FL models can accurately identify potential symptoms of an epidemic like the flu or COVID in different institutions and regions by using data from various healthcare facilities. These predictive models can be used in the following ways: The early interventions can be made, the resources are allocated, and decisions can be made at the national or global level by the public health organizations. In the future, Federated Learning could help to build models for the identification of the spread of the infected diseases, even help to predict the amount of the necessary healthcare resources, and even long-term health prognosis of the patient with the help of many sources of the health-related data.

5.4. Cross-Disciplinary Collaboration

With the current development of FL in healthcare, there will be a need for the integration of different stakeholders. Due to the nature of FL, the need to adopt privacy-preserving technologies, the diverse nature of the healthcare domain that involves AI researchers, healthcare providers, policy makers as well as data security experts. The major problem of the FL in healthcare is the lack of an environment that would unite AI researchers, clinicians, and policy-makers. Academic researchers are needed for the creation of new algorithms and enhancement of the current models of FL, and clinical practitioners provide valuable information on the use of FL in practice. While, policymakers are supposed to guarantee the ethical, lawful, and health effective application of these technologies. Besides, improved innovation, cross-disciplinary collaboration will be also required for the solutions of the regulatory issues related to data sharing, privacy, and integration of FL systems into the current healthcare systems. It is also important for the creation of best practices and policies that would enable the safe, efficient, and fair integration of AI in the provision of health care. Guidelines for the sustainable, ethical, and efficient use of AI: In order to get the best out of FL in healthcare, there are need to have frameworks that will help in the process. These frameworks should ensure that FL models are used in a way that is sustainable, which also means that the use of FL models is conducted in a fair and ethical manner. This also entails policies for data management, patient's consent, model explanation, and framework to monitor the impact of AI decision-making. Furthermore, frameworks need to address the issues of the FL system's flexibility to be introduced into various healthcare facilities, ranging from the small clinics in rural areas to large city hospitals. For FL systems to reap the most benefits from collaborative learning, it is imperative that they are made interoperable across the different institutions and across different regions.

6. CONCLUSION

The use of FL in healthcare is a novel area that could be considered as the future of AI in the field of medicine. Due to its decentralized & privacy-preserving nature, FL offers the healthcare institutions a unique chance to improve patients' outcomes through collaborative model training without compromising the data confidentiality. This piece of technology has the potential to revolutionalise different aspects of health care right from treatment planning and diagnosis to disease prognosis using large distributed health data without invasion of patient privacy. FL in healthcare has multiple advantages that include, data privacy, collaboration intelligence, and model effectiveness. It allows hospitals and clinics, as well as research institutions, to train AI models on the local data without transferring patient information to third parties, which is prohibited by the legal laws. Finally, FL can help achieve fair healthcare due to the fact that it enables the use of data from various patient groups to be included in the model, thus eliminating bias. However, there are several issues that should be discussed with regard to this approach. Firstly, it is communication overhead, secondly, data heterogeneity, thirdly, model convergence difficulties, and finally, the integration of FL with current health systems. However, the issue of the bias of these mostly machine algorithms, responsibility for avoiding bias in resource allocations and decisions made using these systems, and data subjects' ability to consent to their data use will not be out of debate. It is quite evident that Federated Learning is set to define the future of AI in healthcare. With advancing AI models and more interconnection between healthcare organizations, FL could bring about precisely optimized treatments that fit the patient's exact details in terms of their health history at the present data and more. With the help of IoMT and predictive modeling, FL can still go a long way in improving the preventive care and early diagnosis of diseases in patient with chronic diseases. In the future, FL will continue to revolutionize the area of collaborative health intelligence to enhance medical research as well as the public health response and treatment of patients. Thus, overcoming current difficulties, AI in healthcare has a great future and can change the approach to patient care for the better in all aspects, making healthcare more efficient, safe, and accessible for everyone.

REFERENCES

Antunes, R. S., André da Costa, C., Küderle, A., Yari, I. A., & Eskofier, B. (2022). Federated learning for healthcare: Systematic review and architecture proposal. [TIST]. *ACM Transactions on Intelligent Systems and Technology*, *13*(4), 1–23. DOI: 10.1145/3501813

Banabilah, S., Aloqaily, M., Alsayed, E., Malik, N., & Jararweh, Y. (2022). Federated learning review: Fundamentals, enabling technologies, and future applications. *Information Processing & Management*, *59*(6), 103061. DOI: 10.1016/j.ipm.2022.103061

Bashir, A. K., Victor, N., Bhattacharya, S., Huynh-The, T., Chengoden, R., Yenduri, G., Maddikunta, P. K. R., Pham, Q.-V., Gadekallu, T. R., & Liyanage, M. (2023). Federated learning for the healthcare metaverse: Concepts, applications, challenges, and future directions. *IEEE Internet of Things Journal*, *10*(24), 21873–21891. DOI: 10.1109/JIOT.2023.3304790

Boopathi, S., & Khang, A. (2023). AI-integrated technology for a secure and ethical healthcare ecosystem. In *AI and IoT-Based Technologies for Precision Medicine* (pp. 36–59). IGI Global. DOI: 10.4018/979-8-3693-0876-9.ch003

Gopi, B., Kokila, M. S., Bibin, C. V., Sasikala, D., Howard, E., & Boopathi, S. (2024). Distributed Technologies Using AI/ML Techniques for Healthcare Applications. In *Social Innovations in Education, Environment, and Healthcare* (pp. 375-396). IGI Global.

Gracious, L. A., Pajila, P. B., Johncy, G., Anish, T. P., & Prasanth, K. (2024, March). Towards Precision Oncology: A Study of Machine Learning Models for Breast Cancer Prediction. In *2024 10th International Conference on Advanced Computing and Communication Systems (ICACCS)* (Vol. 1, pp. 1938-1943). IEEE. DOI: 10.1109/ICACCS60874.2024.10717246

Indu, V. T., Elumalai, M., & Gracious, L. A. (2026). Optimization Algorithms for Machine Learning Model Enhancement in Healthcare. In *AI Model Design and Data Management for Disease Prediction* (pp. 159–192). IGI Global Scientific Publishing.

Keerthika, K., Kannan, M., & Khang, A. (2023). Medical data analytics: Roles, challenges, and analytical tools. In *AI and IoT-Based Technologies for Precision Medicine* (pp. 1–15). IGI Global. DOI: 10.4018/979-8-3693-0876-9.ch001

Khang, A. (Ed.). (2023). *AI and IoT-based technologies for precision medicine*. IGI Global. DOI: 10.4018/979-8-3693-0876-9

Mangairkarasi, S., Ramana, T. V., Vaishnavi, R., Agalya, S., Sathya, V., & Subramanian, R. S. (2025). Advancing Healthcare Through Artificial Intelligence: Applications, Challenges, and Future Directions. In *Responsible AI for Digital Health and Medical Analytics* (pp. 113-134). IGI Global Scientific Publishing.

Nguyen, D. C., Pham, Q. V., Pathirana, P. N., Ding, M., Seneviratne, A., Lin, Z., Dobre, O., & Hwang, W. J. (2022). Federated learning for smart healthcare: A survey. *ACM Computing Surveys*, *55*(3), 1–37. DOI: 10.1145/3501296

Ramesh, P., Bhargavi, V. S., Shiney, S. A., Dinesh, M. G., & Nalini, M. (2024, October). Exploring the Transformative Impact of Machine Learning in Healthcare: Applications, Challenges, and Future Directions. In *2024 2nd International Conference on Self Sustainable Artificial Intelligence Systems (ICSSAS)* (pp. 620-627). IEEE.

Rose, R. M., Varun, C. M., Sivasakthi, K., Kennady, R., & Lekha, D. (2025, May). Leveraging AI and IoT Data for Predictive Modelling and Preventive Healthcare. In *2025 Third International Conference on Augmented Intelligence and Sustainable Systems (ICAISS)* (pp. 628-633). IEEE. DOI: 10.1109/ICAISS61471.2025.11041733

Saraswat, D., Bhattacharya, P., Verma, A., Prasad, V. K., Tanwar, S., Sharma, G., Bokoro, P. N., & Sharma, R. (2022). Explainable AI for healthcare 5.0: Opportunities and challenges. *IEEE Access : Practical Innovations, Open Solutions*, *10*, 84486–84517. DOI: 10.1109/ACCESS.2022.3197671

Wen, J., Zhang, Z., Lan, Y., Cui, Z., Cai, J., & Zhang, W. (2023). A survey on federated learning: Challenges and applications. *International Journal of Machine Learning and Cybernetics*, *14*(2), 513–535. DOI: 10.1007/s13042-022-01647-y PMID: 36407495

Chapter 5
Collaborative Health Intelligence:
Federated Learning and the Future of AI in Medicine

Nancy Soni
Amity Institute of Biotechnology, India

Asomi Chowdhury
Amity Institute of Biotechnology, India

Hina Bansal
https://orcid.org/0000-0003-1683-1581
Amity University, Noida, India

ABSTRACT

Federated Learning empowers hospitals and research centres to train AI models collaboratively without sharing patient records. It is the decentralized alternative in which AI models can be trained across multiple healthcare organizations. The patient data is stored securely at multiple parties rather than being shared in raw data. FL makes it possible to share learned knowledge while still adhering to strict data-specific privacy regulations. This chapter provides a comprehensive overview of FL's foundational principles, architecture, and challenges. It highlights the various ways FL can assist with data protection for patients and research participants, decentralized data governance, enhance security, and scale FL across hospitals and research institutions. It gives insights on FL implementation in healthcare practice, including radiology with NVIDIA Clara, AI-driven rare disease diagnosis,

DOI: 10.4018/979-8-3373-3306-9.ch005

COVID response solutions, and wearable health monitoring trackers. Additionally, it discusses possible combinations of FL and blockchain systems, edge AI, IoT in a medical context.

1. INTRODUCTION

Current opportunities for disease diagnosis, personalized medicine, and medical research have been made possible through the rapid growth of artificial intelligence (AI) in the health sector. Yet, because the conventional model of AI depends on centralized data gathering, patient confidentiality, data security, and regulatory compliance, these become big issues. Thanks to logistical, ethical, and regulatory hurdles, research institutions and hospitals tend to reside in silos of data, which hamper collaborative innovation. AI frameworks are now capable of learning from dispersed data repositories without direct sharing of data because of Federated Learning (FL), an innovative process. Federated learning is a paradigm revolution in machine learning whereby models are being trained on several devices or institutions without moving raw data out of its domicile. The technology is GDPR, HIPAA, and other privacy regulation-compliant, and thus, it is especially revolutionizing healthcare. Through enabling collaborative intelligence (Yurdem et al., 2024). This chapter explores the foundations, applications, and future potential of federated learning in medicine.

In summary, this introduction highlights the transformative potential of technology on communication, presents the challenges of centralized data management, and proposes federated learning as a possible, privacy-preserving means to tap into collective benefits while remaining compliant with the regulatory requirements around medical data.

2. FUNDAMENTALS OF FEDERATED LEARNING

Federated Learning (FL) is a learning framework for collaborative model training on distributed data sources with no sacrifice of data privacy. In this section, the essential principles, architecture models, and relative strengths behind FL systems are critically examined.

2.1 Workflow and Core Principles

Federated Learning (FL) is a decentralized learning approach where multiple models are jointly trained on respective devices or servers with local dataset samples without shared data. The approach distinguishes itself from regular centralized learning in that data does not have to be central to a specific server before learning. Figure 1 represents the overview of Federated Learning (FL). A central server maintains a global model, while multiple clients (e.g., hospitals) train local models on their private data. The global model is updated by aggregating local model parameters without sharing raw data, preserving privacy.

The fundamental concept of FL is global model aggregation and local model training. In typical federated practice, a client (such as a hospital, smartphone, or diagnostic device) privately trains a model on local data. Model parameters (such as weights or gradients) are uploaded to a central server, and the server aggregates them to produce an updated global model. The updated model is broadcast to all the clients for training in the next iteration.

This iterative process allows for collaborative learning with data always retained in the source, ensuring privacy and data protection laws like HIPAA and GDPR are implemented. A federated learning workflow typically includes a series of critical activities:

- **Client Selection**: A subset of the clients is selected in each round.
- **Model Distribution**: The global model is distributed to chosen customers.
- **Local Training**: Every client is trained on its local data.
- **Model Upload**: Customers upload updated model parameters to the master server.
- **Aggregation**: The server aggregates (typically using FedAvg) safely to create a new global model (Panda et al., 2025).

Federated Learning (FL) is a collaborative model training framework in which distributed data sources work together without having to share the data, protecting privacy.

To sum up, FL allows elegant collaborative model training without ever having to share the data, all the while preserving privacy by keeping data on the devices locally and aggregating model updates. In a decentralized fashion, the workflow consists of client selection, model distribution, local training, secure upload of model parameters, and safe aggregation of model parameters. This decentralized workflow is inherently compliant with privacy and data protection legislation. Therefore, it is especially useful for healthcare organizations that want to collaborate and build models together while not sharing patient data.

Figure 1. Schematic overview of Federated Learning (FL).

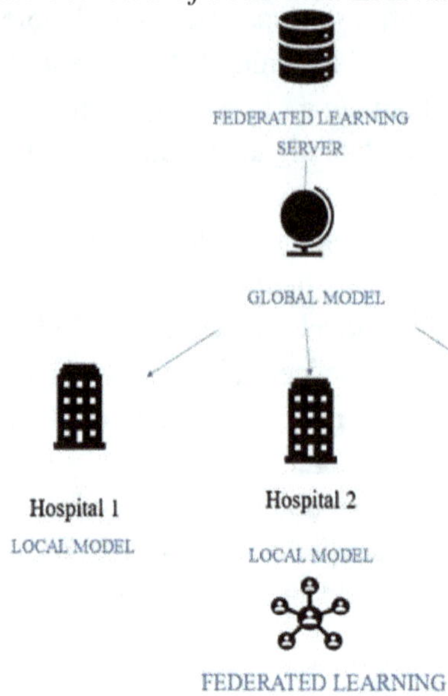

2.3 Essential Components and Architecture Frameworks

Federated learning depends on a range of interdependent architectural elements and communication protocols to ensure robust, high-performance, and trustworthy model training across distributed systems.

A. Essential Elements

- Clients (Edge Devices/Nodes) are the data owners that train the local model. One of quite a diverse array of data owners, they can be tools such as wearables, mobile phones, hospitals, etc. Each client has potentially a different distribution of data, known as non-IID (non-independent and identically distributed) data.
- Federated Server - the central coordination server that orchestrates the training rounds and aggregates the models. It facilitates client selection and updates to the model and ensures efficient communication (Zhang et al., 2023).

B. Key Features

- The privacy layer includes secure aggregation, differential privacy, and cryptographic verification.

- Model management encompasses version control, federated hyperparameter tuning, and cross-site validation.
- Transformations in Healthcare: integration of DICOM/HL7, adherence to regulatory standards, and modules for clinical concept mapping.

C. Execution Frameworks

- TensorFlow Federated (TFF) serves as a robust FL solution for medical imaging and clinical AI.
- OpenFL: Tailored specifically for medical research in imaging.
- FATE: An enterprise-level platform focused on pharmaceutical and population health analytics (Oh & Nadkarni, 2023).
- PySyft (OpenMined): For EHR and clinical trials with GDPR-compliant privacy features.
- NVIDIA FLARE: Advanced framework for 3D imaging and multi-site training with HIPAA-aligned architecture.

The architecture in this federated learning process combines heterogeneous client devices and a central coordination server in order to enable secure, privacy-preserving collaborative training. It balances and manages the models while enabling common healthcare data standards and compliance with regulations. Dedicated execution frameworks provide scalable, robust solutions optimized for a number of different medical research and clinical applications. Table 1 shows a comparative summary of federated learning frameworks and their capabilities for privacy-preserving healthcare applications. This table highlights privacy mechanisms, data compatibility, medical relevance, and compliance-supporting features of each platform.

Table 1. A comparative summary of federated learning frameworks and their capabilities for privacy-preserving healthcare applications.

Framework	Developer	Privacy Features	Healthcare Use Cases	Data Type Support	Regulatory Compliance Tools
TensorFlow Federated	Google	Differential privacy, secure aggregation	Medical imaging, clinical predictions	DICOM, structured clinical	HIPAA audit logging
PySyft	OpenMined	SMPC, homomorphic encryption	Clinical trials, EHR analysis	Tabular, time-series	GDPR compliance modules
FATE	Linux Foundation	Vertical FL, federated transfer learning	Drug discovery, population health	Multi-modal (images, omics)	IRB approval tracking

continued on following page

Table 1. Continued

Framework	Developer	Privacy Features	Healthcare Use Cases	Data Type Support	Regulatory Compliance Tools
OpenFL	Intel/NVIDIA	Medical imaging optimizations	Radiology, pathology AI	DICOM, whole-slide images	De-identification tools
NVIDIA FLARE	NVIDIA	Federated analytics, 3D imaging	Multi-institutional training,diagnostics	3D medical images (e.g., CT, MRI)	HIPAA-aligned architecture, audit logs

2.4 Federated Learning vs. Traditional AI

While traditional AI methods rely on centralized data collection and processing, federated learning decentralizes model training to prioritize data privacy, control, and compliance. The table below compares both paradigms across critical dimensions in the healthcare domain (Zhou et al., 2024).

Table 2 highlights the key differences between Federated Learning (FL) and traditional centralized AI approaches across various criteria, including data handling, privacy, compliance, training efficiency, and use case suitability. It illustrates how FL offers enhanced privacy and scalability, making it well-suited for sensitive domains like healthcare.

In contrast to centralized AI, where raw data must be aggregated, federated learning trains models on devices locally, so sensitive information stays private while enhancing compliance on using restricted data. This offers a broader and more scalable type of AI better suited for sensitive healthcare applications, where patient data protection and accessibility are equally important.

Table 2. Differences between Federated Learning (FL) and traditional centralized AI approaches

Criteria	Federated Learning	Traditional AI
Data Location	Remains at the source (client-side)	Centralized server
Privacy Risk	Low –raw data is never shared	High –data is transmitted and stored
Regulatory Compliance	Easier to comply with HIPAA/GDPR	Risk of non-compliance due to aggregation.
Training Efficiency	Lower –due to network latency and heterogeneity	Higher –centralized, optimized hardware
Data Quality Management	Complex – data heterogeneity and imbalance	Easier – data can be pre-processed uniformly.

continued on following page

Table 2. Continued

Criteria	Federated Learning	Traditional AI
Scalability	High – enables global, distributed training	Moderate – limited by data acquisition
Use Case Suitability	Ideal for sensitive, siloed data (e.g., hospitals)	Suitable for general non-sensitive datasets

3. SIGNIFICANCE OF FEDERATED LEARNING IN HEALTHCARE

Healthcare systems today are producing more sensitive patient data than ever before: this includes electronic health records (EHR), imaging diagnostics, genomics, and wearables. However, the use of this extensive patient data to support artificial intelligence (AI) is complicated due to ethical, legal, and technical issues. In recent years, Federated Learning (FL) has become a new way of collaborating around model training, needing access to the model rather than data. FL is important to healthcare because it helps improve data privacy, helps break down institutional barriers, and encourages worldwide academic collaboration on AI research (Kumar & Singla, 2021).

3.1 Improving Data Security and Privacy

Federated learning has significant privacy-preserving features that are attractive to the medical community. FL protects the raw patient data that remains secured by the healthcare organizations. With traditional machine learning, data is co-located for training, which can have limitations with patient privacy and the use of data analytics. With FL, the model parameters or weights and gradients are sent to the central server for aggregation. By doing this, there is a reduced risk of misuse, mishandling, interception, or even wrongful access of patient data.

From a regulatory perspective, FL aligns with international data protection laws, like the Health Insurance Portability and Accountability Act (HIPAA) in the United States or the General Data Protection Regulation (GDPR) in Europe. These regulations prohibit the unrestricted sharing of personally identifiable health information across borders or entities, which FL inherently addresses by eliminating the need to transmit such data in the first place (Al-Huthaifi et al., 2023).

Furthermore, privacy-enhancing technologies can be applied to FL to add additional layers of security: Differential privacy adds noise to the model updates, the reverse engineering of patient intelligence from the shared parameters. Secure Multiparty

Computation (SMPC) ensures that during the aggregation, the server cannot see user contributions. Homomorphic encryption enables computations to be conducted with encrypted data, enabling security to be maintained while conducting the computations. Thus, in FL, security is reframed so that learning occurs collaboratively, but custodianship of data remains custodial for each healthcare institution-- that is entirely necessary in a modern medical ecosystem (Cui et al., 2021).

To summarize, federated learning is a new approach to privacy-preserving data analysis for healthcare that allows for model training to happen in partnership and without transferring sensitive patient records to a central server. By transferring only model parameters and not raw datasets, FL lowers the potential impact of data breaches, uses/misuses, and unauthorized access. FL is also easily aligned with a variety of the world's privacy laws, including HIPAA and GDPR. The use of advanced privacy-enhancing techniques, such as differential privacy, secure multiparty computation, and homomorphic encryption, can further improve security capabilities. Federated learning covers the use of data as well as protecting an institution's ability to control data, along with the potential for large-scale medical collaborations that are safe.

3.2 Breaking Data Silos in Medicine

Worldwide, healthcare systems are highly fragmented and possess enormous systems of data silos among hospitals, research organizations, and diagnostic laboratories. These silos profoundly obstruct the development of robust and generalized AI models. No single institution typically has sufficient heterogenous datasets to access the complete continuum of disease etiology, patient populations, and clinical practice.

Federated learning occurs in the environment of disseminated data holders, enabling data owners to engage in model training without ceding data control. For example, a cardiology model, trained using FL technology, utilizes echocardiogram data from hospitals on different continents, which may include urban hospitals in Europe, rural clinics in Asia, and community hospitals in North America, all without data movement or storage to a central server. By having data from a variety of hospitals, the degree of generalizability and clinical reliability of the model is exponentially greater. Academic institutions, medical centre's, private hospitals, and health systems can deploy AI tools in various patient and demographic backgrounds.

Furthermore, FL presents a tactical answer to institutional resistance to sharing data. Many healthcare organizations are wary of collaboration for competitive reasons or reasons of intellectual property, and they often cite non-interoperability as a hurdle. FL avoids these barriers and produces a collaborative model without data exposure, thus creating trust between groups and encouraging equity in AI advancement (Reilly et al., 2023).

In conclusion, federated learning tackles perhaps one of health care's most perfidious and obstinate barriers: the fragmentation of medical data between institutions and geographies. By allowing hospitals, labs, and research facilities to collaboratively build models and report findings without sharing the underlying datasets, FL maintains privacy and increases the quality of the models through engagement with the greatest volume and variability of data possible. This yields better generalization, greater confidence that the clinical findings won't be denied by institutional intermediaries with proprietary competition issues, and builds trust between organizations and ultimately across the medical community, while simultaneously improving medical AI fairness and equity.

3.3 Enabling Global Collaboration Without Data Sharing

In the time of pandemics, global disease surveillance, and international clinical research, the importance of global collaboration on delegated AI projects is more crucial than ever. Ethical and legal frameworks for the use of patient data, conversely, differ from country to country, making it not only infeasible to gather data in a central repository but also -in certain cases -impossible to do so based on local law!

Federated learning allows for a natural and seamless method of collaborating globally, whereby institutions are able to train and/or work together on a federated AI model while still obeying local data governance laws. Federated learning becomes particularly relevant in multinational clinical trials where the data is not legally allowed to leave the country of origin. Global health research where institutions in developing countries could contribute to model training without compromising national sovereignty and cross-border epidemic surveillance where early-warning systems rely on timely and real-time data from distant and geographically varying institutions (Sprenkamp et al., 2024).

In addition, FL actively promotes inclusiveness in AI model development. Traditionally, AI models are built using datasets from higher-income countries with better digitally supported infrastructures. Federated learning enables underrepresented countries with value-added data that is not translatable to other contexts to participate in AI model training.

Building AI models in this way avoids bias towards higher-income countries and recognizes the legitimacy of underrepresented countries' contributions. The inclusion of national health data into AI training is of value and significance in all parts of the world.

This functionality is especially revolutionary for diseases that have geographic identity or genetic identity; for example:

- Tuberculosis and malaria in sub-Saharan Africa
- Cardiometabolic diseases in South Asia
- Liver and gastric cancers in East Asia

FL represents a return to investigating new AI models unrestricted by data privacy and ownership while offering global institutions equal participation in model building, thereby advancing the healthcare AI ecosystem in a more collaborative, inclusive, and ethically sound manner (Treloar, 2014).

In conclusion, federated learning represents a pathway to global collaboration in medical research, as it removes both regulatory and ethical barriers to the transnational exchange of data. It provides an avenue for medical institutions globally, regardless of technological readiness and financial capacity, to securely contribute to model development and persist with national data sovereignty. This approach enables reduced bias, which is prevalent when only relying on high-income region-predominated datasets for training models. By offering a method for geographically and genetically specific disease data to be included, FL is a practice to encourage socially equitable, ethically supervised, and globally pertinent healthcare innovation.

4. HEALTHCARE APPLICATIONS

There is increasing recognition of Federated Learning (FL) as a potential disruptor in healthcare, which enables artificial intelligence models to be built on different data sources while protecting patients' data privacy and complying with strict health laws. FL has multiple potential use cases, including diagnostic imaging, clinical decision support systems (CDSS), electronic health record (EHR) analytics, genomics, remote patient monitoring, wearable health technologies, and drug discovery. FL allows institutions to work together while preserving the raw data in a logical, legal, ethical, and technical way. Better models can be developed using distributed methods to build robust models that are unbiased and generalizable because we are enabling model training using different datasets from different sites with different populations and health profiles.

FL may allow multiple radiology departments from different hospitals to collaborate on training deep learning models for objectives such as detecting tumors, fractures, or lesions from diagnostic images, including X-rays, MRIs, and CT scans. For instance, if an FL model is trained on chest X-rays from institutions across Asia, Europe, and North America, it will generalize better compared to a model trained in isolation, which would reduce bias in the model and increase diagnostic performance when applied across populations. Similarly, FL shows great potential in histopathology, whereby high-resolution pathology slides can be used to perform cancer detection while guaranteeing that sensitive patient data never leaves the host institution (Chaddad et al., 2023).

In the area of clinical decision support, FL expands physician ability to forecast patient outcomes, recommend personalized treatments, and alert clinicians to significant adverse events. Models that have been trained via federated networks incorporate the organizational knowledge of multiple care providers, improving the accuracy of predictions for critical conditions such as sepsis, acute kidney injury, and cardiovascular disease. By nature, decision-making in clinical practice occurs in real-time and therefore lends itself exceptionally well to FL, as it enables models to be continually updated across distributed clinical environments without breaking data governance policies.

The advancement of FL in the analysis of electronic health records (EHR) is also noteworthy. In centralized approaches, there are often fears of the implications related to patient privacy and data security. However, FL permits researchers and health care companies to analyze data sourced from EHRs across hospitals and health systems while not exposing identifiable patient information. Discoveries from EHR data are invaluable to restock estimates of disease trends and support epidemiological studies and public health intervention planning.

FL underpins pandemic preparedness and response. During global health emergencies, like COVID-19, FL has offered many avenues for model specification for early detection, triage, and treatment optimization without necessitating the aggregation of patient data that may be limited by national or institutional policies. Consequently, naturally, FL is now viewed as an integral part of the global digital health infrastructure (Wang et al., 2023). Figure 2 outlines the key themes in the application of Federated Learning (FL) in healthcare.

In summary, FL holds the promise of broad impact across healthcare at a time when institutions can collaborate on the development of sophisticated models across diverse datasets while securing patients' privacy, meeting stringent regulations, and operating in compliance with existing privacy best practices. Its uses encompass diagnostic imaging, clinical decision support, EHR analytics, genomics, remote monitoring, and pandemic readiness while generating more accurate, lower-bias, and generalizable models. By enabling a higher level of trust among institutions and allowing them to collaborate globally without the risk of exposing their raw data, FL builds trust between institutions, supports the collaborative approach, and enables the generation of robust, scalable, and ethically rigorous AI solutions to modern healthcare issues.

Figure 2. Application of Federated Learning (FL) in Healthcare

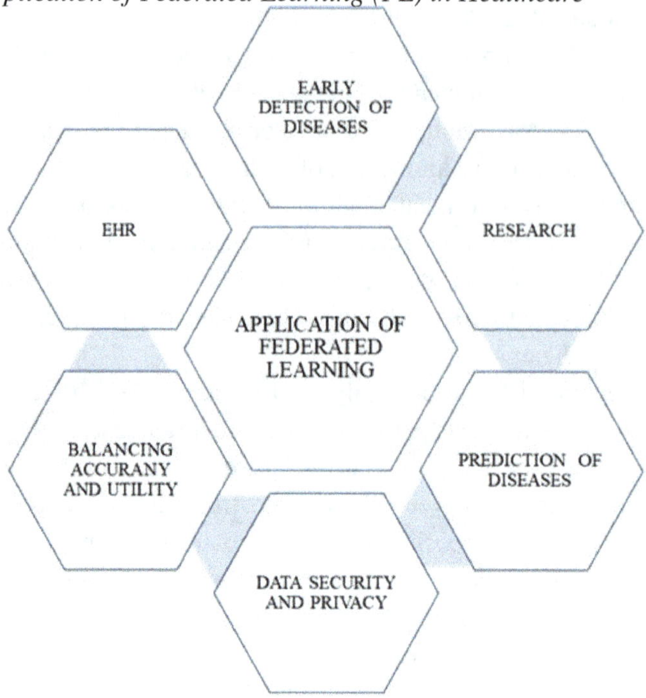

5. ADVANTAGES OF FEDERATED LEARNING IN HEALTHCARE

Federated Learning (FL) expands upon the current state of the art in healthcare to address important challenges concerning privacy, ownership of data, and ethical AI. High-stakes healthcare often involves sensitive patient data (and in extreme circumstances, health systems have been forced to change practical procedures/policies to avoid liability issues), such that traditional machine learning and other forms of centralized approaches involve individually linked data repositories, resulting in adverse patient privacy risks. These risks also place the system (or steward of the data) in a position of legal liability. FL maintains the data in local environments, where the data is under the stewardship of the local healthcare provider, and thus, there is potential for reduced privacy risk, increased trust in the application of AI, and shared accountability in unique systems of local healthcare. Many of the standards that govern patient privacy, ethics, and data ownership -like the General Data Protection Regulation (GDPR) in Europe and the Health Insurance Portability and Accountability Act (HIPAA) in the United States -exist to protect patients' rights and maintain the confidentiality of health information (e.g., protect patient data). Thus, FL is a natural mechanism to develop ethical ways of administering data in research and in practice, provide a normative standard of privacy for model development, and enable robust collaborations and applied research without sacrificing patient trust, institutional violations, or any issues of contractual compliance/legal liabilities.

FL represents an important paradigm shift toward equitable, safe, and interoperable health AI ecosystems (Bogdanova et al., 2020). It is a transformative shift in healthcare AI that solves significant issues of privacy, ownership of data, and ethical compliance. By keeping the data in its environment of origin, it protects legal liability, maintains patient trust, and promotes fairness and interoperability to allow healthcare players to collaborate. This basic premise allows AI innovation to occur safely, in compliance with laws and at scale, following international regulations on data protection.

5.1 Enhanced Data Privacy and Security

The key strength of federated learning (FL) is that it is thoughtfully designed with privacy & security in mind. When using FL, the raw data never leaves the source institutions and will help eliminate many risks for the constraints that data loss, data breaches, and data compliance can pose for centralized machine learning models. Instead of sending identifiable personal health information, approximate model updates or gradients are sent to a central aggregator to improve the model. These updates can also benefit from various security technology features, such as differential privacy (statistical noise added to the data) and secure multiparty computation (SMPC, where computations occur without exposing the data that anyone is using) (Jebreel et al., 2022).

Furthermore, FL also supports homomorphic encryption (computations on encrypted data) and federated analysis (descriptive statistics to produce, without restrictions, industry-standard summary statistics about data using aggregations without losing the privacy of the data). All of these innovations are essential for the healthcare space, where datasets can contain some of these attributes: genetic data, clinical notes, diagnostic images, and patient history.

By using FL, healthcare institutions can confidently engage in collaborative AI research and model development while complying with locally dictated/protective data laws and international governing laws such as HIPAA, GDPR, and the Indian PDP Bill. This privacy-protective architecture enhances patient trust, which is vital for scalable adoption of digital health technology. Furthermore, privacy by design encourages AI innovation and advancement without ethical dilemmas regarding exposing and/or centralizing personal health data, providing a secure, trustworthy environment for shared data in medicine (Gu et al., 2023).

In conclusion, FL's privacy-by-design architecture guarantees that sensitive patient data is stored and never leaves the originating institution, limiting risk from breaches, unauthorized access, and violations of regulations. Through the exchange of only model parameters along with robust protections such as differential privacy, secure multiparty computation, and homomorphic encryption, FL allows AI applications in healthcare that are compliant, secure, and trustworthy, while preserving the utility of varied medical datasets.

5.2 Decentralized Data Control and Ownership of Data

Federated Learning (FL) shifts the data governance approach of allowing regulatory organizations to have full authority and ownership over datasets through the different phases of the machine learning cycle. There are regulatory and legal barriers in the healthcare data space because they are critical, strategic, sensitive, and regulated. FL provides hospitals, research institutions, and clinics opportunities to jointly develop artificial intelligence (AI) models without losing custody of data, which is a major disadvantage in this area. With FL, decentralized, distributed AI lowers the cost and risk of data sovereignty, compliance, and intellectual property concerns; limits potential breach risk of an organization's data; and reduces infrastructural cost of a centralized architecture that may require massive datasets in healthcare. The importance of stakeholder confidence and trust to allow for ethically grounded and patient-centric AI development cannot be overstated, because most institutions may not even want to share raw data due to competitive, legal, or cultural reasons. FL enables cooperation with trust institutions which can receive information and contribute to the collective information without providing their data to the wider organization (Wang et al., 2018).

Additionally, FL enables cross-border and inter-organization collaborations that had typically been restricted within the boundaries of privacy laws and regional data privacy laws. For example, healthcare providers in different countries can now collaboratively train diagnostic models that are compliant with numerous national laws, including GDPR in Europe, HIPAA in the United States, and data localization laws in countries like India and China.

Decentralized control over data also encourages data equity. Smaller agencies such as rural hospitals, under-resourced clinics, or new care centers generally have valuable local data that include diverse patient populations and are often excluded from large AI initiatives simply due to a lack of localized capacity or fear of sharing data. FL provides these groups with the opportunity to be involved in global research and access cutting-edge AI tools, improving, in turn, health equity and minimizing systemic bias in AI training. Moreover, FL enables a sustainable use of data in which institutions do not have to replicate or duplicate data storage, which is cumbersome and costly. FL also minimizes the attack surface for cyber threats by maintaining the data demand locally while including an audit trail for all data exchanges at the same time.

However, FL gives institutions complete custody and control of their data while developing AI in collaboration. This decentralized structure lowers compliance risk, allows for cross-border partnerships strictly within legal limits, enhances equity to allow smaller or under-resourced providers to participate, takes care of a competitive, legal, and cultural interest in developing those models, builds trust, promotes data sovereignty, and supports equitable model development for the benefit of more health care settings.

5.3 Growing AI in Hospitals and Beyond

Artificial Intelligence (AI) is now being integrated into hospitals and other health care systems with the hope of transforming how health care is delivered through better diagnosis, better operational efficiencies, and individualized treatment. "AI" is used to refer to a growing list of applications, as well as a range of individual applications as they are woven more tightly into clinical workflows. While many applications of AI are in radiology, pathology, surgery, and patient monitoring, hospitals are also considering how to utilize AI for operational efficiencies such as predicting patient admissions, assessing hospital resources, or optimizing workflows. As AI continues to penetrate hospital settings, it is also reshaping health care delivery remotely and in the community setting. Wearable technology and home-based monitoring equipment are generating vast amounts of ongoing health information that can be translated through federated learning (FL)—a process that builds collaborative intelligent models without sacrificing the data privacy of the participants. This means different stakeholders can all leverage their ownership of the data to act on insights for earlier disease detection and personalized care in the community, and not just in the traditional clinical care environments (Jiang et al., 2017). Enabling infrastructure - made up of 5G networks, edge computing, and interoperable data platforms to allow real-time analytics and decision-making over a distributed care ecosystem - will support the continued evolution of AI through ongoing validation, clinician trust, and equitable access to support responsible and inclusive development.

To sum up, AI is evolving from a hospital-based system to a connected, intelligent health ecosystem. Federated learning will be essential to this evolution, as it will facilitate privacy with security. As trust and infrastructure and policy change, AI will evolve in ways that redefine health and healthcare beyond clinical walls and within clinical walls (Rieke et al., 2020).

5.4 Enabling Cooperation Without Data Transfers

Inter-institutional collaboration in contemporary healthcare is essential for constructing robust and generalizable artificial intelligence (AI) models. Privacy laws, the control of data ownership, and institutional silos for data sharing, however, can serve as impediments to centralized data sharing. In this context, federated learning (FL) provides a paradigm shift in cooperation where raw data does not need to flow between institutions. Instead, AI models are trained in hospital and/or clinic and/or wearable device environments, with model updates being shared without sharing raw data. Encrypted model updates, for example, gradients or weights, are shared with a central aggregator. FL allows data sovereignty of data while collaborating on the overall knowledge derived from multiple data generators. This model offers a distributed approach for newer collaborative forms of medical AI, especially in respect to more sensitive areas of medical care, such as electronic health records (EHRs), imaging data, or real-time biosensor data. In these cases, federated learning preserves data at the organization of origin while providing a cooperative route toward model development innovation while simultaneously complying with relevant privacy regulations (such as GDPR and HIPAA). Federated learning approaches also reduce the risk of data exposure and reduce complex anonymization processes that can diminish data utility. And also provide security during model training and aggregation.

These technologies provide an infrastructure of privacy - preserving intelligence (PPI), whereby several organizations can co-develop predictive models for diagnostic, treatment planning, or disease outbreak prediction or forecasting, without the need to transfer patient - level data from each organization more than necessary (Yang et al., 2019).

To summarize, federated learning is the next frontier for collaborative medical AI. As a collective technical infrastructure, it allows for the alignment of ethics, law, and operations for healthcare stakeholders in an environment where collaboration can occur at scale, while assuring privacy, confidentiality, and trust of all patients' data.

6. CHALLENGES

There is considerable potential for collaborative health intelligence and federated learning (FL) to transform health care, but several barriers may limit the ability to scale these types of operations. These challenges range from technical, ethical, and regulatory to infrastructural challenges that represent significant obstacles or impediments to realizing the innovation potential that AI-enabled health services have to offer.

1. Data Heterogeneity and Quality Variation

One of the principal challenges of working in the federated learning environment is that health data collected may not be IID (independently and identically distributed) across hospitals, clinics, or networks of wearable devices. Given the difference between hospitals and clinics as well as differences in protocols, hardware, or demographic populations, there are variances in the quality, structure, and completeness of the data collected. This heterogeneity is problematic in terms of slowing convergence of the medical federated learning model, resulting in biased learning in federated learning and generalizability in healthcare contexts [21].

2. Computational and Network Constraints

Federated learning depends on edge computing and, thus, requires sufficient local computing resources to train models. Most edge devices and institutional infrastructures lack the necessary hardware acceleration, energy efficiency, or memory to deal with complex models, particularly in resource-constrained environments. Also, in situations with greater network latency or limited bandwidth, timely synchronization of model updates can become impossible, which slowly optimizes the global model and adversely affects responsiveness in critical care.

3. Privacy, Security, and Adversarial Threats

Federated learning improves on privacy by keeping data local, but it is not without privacy and security risks. For example, a malicious attacker can carry out a gradient leakage attack, a model inversion attack, or a model poisoning attack to reveal patients' sensitive information. Moreover, many privacy and security controls, like differential privacy, secure multiparty computation, and homomorphic encryption, which may be needed in federated learning systems, add to computational costs and increase system complexity (Mendieta et al., 2022).

4. Interoperability & Standardization

The interoperability of the participants' nodes of federated healthcare networks is restricted by inconsistent standardization of data schemas, ontologies, and communication protocols. Incorporating data from diverse data sources becomes increasingly complex, particularly when the healthcare organizations already rely on different contexts, technologies, and uses for data. Standardization is being pursued for healthcare data interoperability; the degree of progress differs both regionally and nationally (e.g., Europe is taking steps towards standardization).

Standardization ultimately poses a challenge for cross-border collaboration around health data (Li et al., 2020).

5. Ethics and Regulatory Challenges

Federated learning presents a fresh constellation of ethical issues around data sovereignty and governance, algorithmic liability, and informed consent, as well as differences in the regulation of data and jurisdiction. There exist issues of overlapping but sometimes conflicting statutory obligations within regulatory frameworks like HIPAA (U.S.), GDPR (EU), and the Data Governance Act. What emerges in terms of restrictions is complex enough to navigate to facilitate global cooperation and collaboration while addressing an environment of regulation, compliance, innovation, and equitable access (Hassani et al., 2024).

6. Model Validation and Clinical Integration

The process of validating federated models across diverse healthcare systems is complicated by the availability of independent ground truth or standardized tests. The implementation of AIs and their outputs into clinical workflow is more than the accuracy of models; it may also involve (1) development of user-centered interfaces, (2) training of clinical users to use AIs, and (3) modification of workflows or care pathways.

In summary, federated learning in healthcare has a number of limitations: disparate data quality, limited computational infrastructures, privacy and security risks, and the lack of universal standards. In addition, ethical and regulatory challenges also have an impact on cross-border collaboration, while the ability to adopt models in clinical settings is limited by issues related to model validation, workflow inclusion, and user training. Finding tangible ways to overcome these challenges will be vital to developing safe, interoperable, and broadly trusted health AI systems.

7. CASE STUDIES

The case studies show applications in pandemic response, radiology, rare disease research, remote care, and emerging technologies, such as IoT and blockchain. It also provides examples of how federated AI preserves patient privacy, regulates compliance, and allows operational efficiency.

7.1 Radiology Federated Learning: NVIDIA Clara

Nvidia's Clara Federal Learning is a cutting-edge edge computing solution developed specifically for radiology to meet the demand for increased disease detection while protecting patient privacy. Radiology is potentially one of the most data-rich areas of medicine, but the advancement of artificial intelligence (AI) in radiology has been stymied by data privacy regulations, restrictions on data-sharing, and ethical considerations. NVIDIA Clara, a federated learning (FL) platform focusing on healthcare, enables contributors to develop and share AI models without the sharing of raw medical data. In this initial project, NVIDIA partnered with our launch collaborator, the American College of Radiology (ACR), and several leading hospitals to improve diagnostic models for breast cancer detection through mammography data (Wen & Wen, 2022).

The FL project included more than 20 institutions, all of which kept their data in their facilities while contributing to the overall model. Through Clara FL, the hospitals were able to train their AI models locally on-site and shared only encrypted model parameter updates to a central server. The model contributions were modeled locally, so full ingestion of patient data was maintained while enabling large-scale generalization of the model. In total, more than 33,000 mammograms were used from across the sites in this, one of the largest multi-institutional FL projects in medical imaging. The outcome was promising: the federated model showed better sensitivity and specificity compared to most site-based models, and it also showed robustness to differences across imaging devices, patient populations, and patterns of clinical imaging practice. Most importantly, smaller hospitals - which often do not have enough data to train a reliable AI model on their own - were able to access and contribute to a high-performance collaborative model (Johnson, 2020).

In conclusion, this case study illustrates how federated learning can combine heterogeneous and geographically dispersed radiology data securely. By assisting 20-plus institutions to train a breast cancer detection model on 33,000 mammograms without sharing proprietary data, NVIDIA Clara enhanced detection sensitivity for breast cancer and improved access/institutional generalizability to detection algorithms for married hospitals and did so in a manner that preserves site privacy and establishes data silos while promoting equity in AI use for healthcare.

7.2 Rare Disease Joint Research

Rare diseases present remarkable challenges to researchers and clinicians, particularly because of their small population sizes, diagnostic complexities, and the challenge of finding advanced medical expertise. So, data adequate for training an AI model cannot be acquired at one institution with sufficient data to be effective.

Federated learning (FL) has been used to support collaboration between multiple institutions in their work diagnosing and researching rare diseases, specifically in radiology and neurology. An excellent real-world application of FL in rare disease research is the Federated Tumour Segmentation (FeTS) project for glioblastoma, a rare, aggressive brain cancer. The FeTS project engaged 71 institutions from 6 continents, and the FL extension was used to train an AI model for the research project from a dataset of 25,256 MRI scans of 6,314 patients (Pati et al., 2022). In this instance, each institution trained a model locally and shared only encrypted weight updates to preserve privacy and compliance. The federated model made substantial improvements in tumor boundary identification. A 33% increase in surgically delineable tumor definition and a 23% increase in tumor extent were observed, compared to models trained on public data. Using federated learning improved diagnostic performance and stayed compliant with data protection regulations such as HIPAA and GDPR.

In summary, this case would show an early pathway to transformative federated learning in rare disease evaluation. Federated learning enables less resource-rich institutions to collectively create, improve, and access a high-performing generalizable AI model while still ensuring compliance with privacy regulations. The FeTS glioblastoma project exemplifies the value of FL in rare disease research, providing 71 institutions on six continents the opportunity to jointly train on over 25,000 MRI scans while maintaining data sovereignty. The federated model showed significant improvements in tumor boundary detection, demonstrating FL's potential in overcoming data scarcity and regulatory limitations in niche medical spaces.

7.3 AI and Federated Learning in COVID-19 Response

The COVID-19 pandemic illustrated a need for fast, efficient, accurate, and scalable decision-support tools in healthcare. Conventional artificial intelligence (AI) approaches often faced considerable challenges because of privacy regulations and operational complexities in assembling sensitive patient data across institutions. Federated learning (FL) offered a new solution, as it allowed the opportunity to collaboratively build models with data without sharing or centrally aggregating raw data, which is especially important during a public health crisis (Dayan et al., 2021). An inspiring example of FL was the EXAM (Electronic Medical Record Chest X-ray AI Model) project with institutions around the world that incorporated data from over 16,000 cases. The purpose of this project was to build an AI model that could predict the future oxygen needs of symptomatic COVID-19 patients, which we developed using information from vital signs, lab work, and chest X-rays. Each institution trained its model locally using its data, and the only information shared with the central server was model updates concerning patient privacy and regulations, such as HIPAA and GDPR.

The federated EXAM model achieved an average area under the curve (AUC) greater than 0.92 when predicting clinical outcomes at 24 and 72 hours after presentation in the emergency room. The federated model had a 16% improvement in average AUC and a 38% improvement in generalizability across unharmonized datasets from different continents when compared to models trained with data from individual sites only. Furthermore, for the prediction of mechanical ventilation or death at 24 hours at the largest independent test site, sensitivity was 0.950, and specificity was 0.882. These results elucidate how FL can accelerate privacy-preserving data science collaborations and provide robust models that generalize across heterogeneous healthcare settings. FL enabled learning from multi-source and multi-modality data, e.g., chest radiographs paired with electronic health records, and protects PHI without unreasonably burdening the data harmonization process at a critical and urgent time in a diverse COVID-19 response (Ridley, 2021).

In conclusion, the EXAM project demonstrates the importance of federated learning (FL) in emergency healthcare and exemplifies a global collaborative effort to accurately anticipate the oxygen requirement of patients with COVID-19 while using multimodal data, spanning a cohort of greater than 16,000 cases. The federated model not only demonstrated more accuracy but also explicitly provided improved generalizability compared with any single-site model. These outcomes illustrate the potential of privacy-preserving, large-scale AI development for projects that must adhere to urgent timelines and, in many cases, heterogeneous clinical scenarios.

7.4 Remote Care Wearable Devices

The rapid evolution of wearable health monitoring devices - including smartwatches, biosensors, and mobile health applications -has opened up tremendous possibilities in the field of remote patient care. These devices provide some form of data, such as heart rate variability, blood pressure, oxygen saturation, sleep quality, and more. These devices provide the ability to offer continuous monitoring of many aspects of our lives, using real-time physiological data. The issue of scaling the privacy, security, and ethical shortcomings when dealing with sensitive data that can be used for predictive analytics is significantly intensified. To circumvent these issues, Kakao Healthcare has launched a large-scale federated learning (FL) project in collaboration with 16 large hospitals in South Korea, focused on developing predictive healthcare models using data from wearable devices and electronic medical records (EMRs) to follow data protection regulations. Conceptually, the data is secured within each hospital in their respective cloud environment, and it was simply model updates (gradients and weights) that were encrypted, and pooling processes back to a central server greatly reduced the privacy risks (Kakao Healthcare, n.d.).

An example of this federated system is the creation of a breast cancer recurrence prediction model. In this example, the federated model predicted breast cancer recurrence probability by analyzing 25,000 patient records - even wrist biometrics data in real time from wearables. The performance of the federated model achieved an unprecedented predictive accuracy of 0.8482 within an accuracy range of 0.6397 to 0.8362 for previous attempts using traditional models. The external validation cohort also performed extremely well, achieving an area under the curve population of 0.7769 and demonstrating the ability of this type of model to generalize across heterogeneous populations. Importantly, beyond predictive accuracy, this approach greatly saved significant time for data analysis in a federated model with traditional models, eliminating the requirement for identifiable data sharing (from 2 years to 4 months).

In summary, this case study illustrates the exciting possibilities of federated learning within remote healthcare. By enabling real-time, privacy-preserving training of AI models across existing distributed networks, this case sets a foundation for an equitable, collaborative, and scalable health intelligence approach (Lee et al., 2025). Kakao Healthcare's FL initiative that leverages both wearable and EMR data from 16 hospitals shows how distributed AI can leverage community data for accurate and privacy-compliant predictive models for events such as breast cancer recurrence. The project reduced model development time substantially while providing good generalization potentials across populations -evidence of FL's robustness and scalability across real-time remote health monitoring.

7.5 New Tech: IoT, Blockchain, Edge AI

The conjunction of the Internet of Things (IoT), blockchain technology, and edge Artificial Intelligence (AI) is becoming a transformative paradigm in collaborative health intelligence, particularly through the context of federated learning (FL). Collectively, these technologies resolve some significant barriers to conducting good health and well -being collaborative work, including issues of healthcare data privacy, latency, scalability, and trust, allowing for powerful, real-time clinical decision support systems. An interesting real-world example is the blockchain-augmented edge AIoT platform for secure and streamlined health data management and analysis. IoT devices—wearable implantable sensors -continuously monitor real-time physiological data for the patient. Instead of sending raw data to a centralized server, edge AI performs analysis on IoT devices at the edge to minimize latency locally, thus minimizing access to raw data.

The platform's security model is powered by blockchain technology using a sharding, proof-of-authority (PoA) consent framework, which allows for the management and auditing of all transactions, including updates to AI models and recordings of clinical decisions. This method provides an immutable, transparent, and tamper-proof data provenance and also protects patient privacy. The blockchain also provides lifecycle management of personalized AI models (AI adaptors) for managing traceability and version control, which are requirements of clinical accountability. One mechanism in action was the network of hospitals that came together to utilize this platform to support the provision of remote monitoring and diagnostics for chronic conditions, including cardiovascular diseases and diabetes. The architecture of the platform allowed these hospitals to collaboratively train federated AI models using individuals' locally held and processed data from wearables, sharing encrypted model updates through the blockchain network. This enabled the scalability of AI-driven diagnostic approaches involving multiple institutions with a variety of data sources. Operational results showed improved memory efficiency, which can be attributed to sharding, resulting in a halved time of accessing data. The system also allowed for real-time analytics that enabled acute care and remote patient management that adhered to rigid standards of data privacy, including HIPAA and GDPR (Jun, 2025).

This case study exemplified the synergistic relationship of IoT, blockchain, edge AI, and federated learning to resolve various barriers to implementing AI in health care environments while establishing a framework for scalable, secure, and privacy-preserving collaborative intelligence and paving the way for future smart health environments and innovations in precision medicine.

In summary, this example demonstrates how combining FL with IoT, blockchain, and edge AI tackles security, transparency, and latency challenges in distributed healthcare. A blockchain-augmented AIoT platform enabled real-time, privacy-preserving diagnostics for chronic diseases across several hospitals and evidenced the value of converging emerging technologies for scalable and compliant collaborative intelligence.

7.8 Lessons from Practice: Insights

The integration of federated learning (FL) in the healthcare industry, while exciting, has revealed some important lessons learned from actual real-world initiatives across institutions. These lessons highlight the potential for change as well as the complexity of implementing AI-driven collaborative health intelligence at scale.

A good example of this is the Swarm Learning initiative by Hewlett-Packard Enterprise (HPE), which was applied during the initial phase of COVID-19. In this distributed learning environment, multiple academic hospitals (with sites in Germany, the Netherlands, and the USA) worked to create a predictive AI model for COVID-19 infection (severity and triage). Each institution contributed their model locally to a global model without exchanging raw patient data. Each of the original contributing sites trained the model locally and sent model parameters in an encrypted format to a shared, blockchain-coordinated global model. Then the global model converged in a fraction of the time we initially expected, while adhering to strict data privacy frameworks, including GDPR and HIPAA (Pinto-Coelho, 2023).

Learnings from Practice -There were a few overall learnings from 'real-world' implementations of federated learning (FL):

- Interoperability is crucial: Differences in electronic health record systems and in data formats reduce the interface utility to FL. More standard ontologies like OMOP and FHIR would support data harmonization.
- Strong governance enables collaboration: Strong legal frameworks in advance, a role in stakeholder engagement, and commitment to developing trust in advance all serve to enable collaboration on the project.
- Data diversity enhances model robustness: In previous FL implementations there is perceived potential for models to improve generalization and fairness because they are trained on federated and heterogeneous data, such as best practices utilized in initial FL implementations conducted in different areas of Canada.
- Scalable decentralized infrastructures are key: In the FL context, edge computing and cloud-native tools offer low-latency model updating capabilities while keeping sensitive data on the device or in safe data environments.
- Clinician representation is important to support adoption: Engagement with clinicians is also equally important for their engagement, explainability, and usability of the AI when engaging clinicians on how they can trust the AI and building the appropriate workflows that ideally would be a smooth integration.

In summary, real-world implementations show that for FL to be effective, there are many factors. a) interoperability b) good governance frameworks c) breadth and representativeness of data d) a scalable decentralized infrastructure e) clinical buy-in. Considered together, these lessons illuminate that technical implementations cannot exist out of the trust framework and community stakeholder engagement or standardized processes through which such technologies can be continuously adopted.

8. AI-DRIVEN MEDICAL CARE IN THE FUTURE

Artificial Intelligence (AI) is anticipated to profoundly influence national healthcare systems and markets worldwide through 2030. From diagnostics to treatment, research, and streamlining healthcare workflows, AI will have pervasive impacts across some, if not all, aspects of healthcare. For example, AI systems will ingest and analyze vast amounts of information—electronic health records, medical imaging, and genomic information, for example—to find clinical patterns, inform early diagnosis, and facilitate preemptive intervention. This will allow for very individualized care that incorporates a patient's specific genetics, lifestyle, and medical history. Table 3 gives an overview of artificial intelligence (AI) areas of applications in healthcare and their major functional properties, measurable outcomes, and real-world applications.

Moreover, AI will democratize healthcare further through telemedicine, virtual consultations, and distance monitoring of patients. Intelligent virtual assistants and chatbots will empower patients to participate in triage with prompts to schedule appointments and initial clinical advice. Wearable technology will facilitate real-time continuous health monitoring. Non-local or non-native patients will have access to AI-enabled telehealth platforms and multilingual planning tools, which would mitigate geographic and language

Transformational Uses

- Precision Diagnostics (Insilico Medicine, n.d.)
- Predictive and Preventive Care
- Drug Discovery Simplification (Blanchard, 2025)
- Contactless Care and Telemedicine
- Surgical Robotics (Baucas et al., 2023)

Table 3. Applications of AI in healthcare and their major functional properties, measurable outcomes, and real-world applications.

AI Application Area	Key Functional Capabilities	Quantifiable Impacts	Real-World Examples	Healthcare Outcome Improvements
Precision Diagnostics	AI-based imaging analysis (MRI, CT, retinal scans); pattern recognition in clinical data	- Up to 95% diagnostic accuracy- 10% reduction in diagnostic errors	Zebra Medical Vision	Faster, more accurate diagnosis; reduced clinician workload
Predictive & Preventive Care	Early detection using EHRs, wearables, and genomic data; risk stratification for chronic diseases	- Prediction of conditions years in advance Real-time anomaly alerts	Apple Watch detecting atrial fibrillation	Enables early intervention; reduces long-term disease burden
Drug Discovery Acceleration	Generative AI in target identification, molecular modelling, and trial design	- Reduction in drug development time from 10 years to 2–3 years Cost reduced from ~$2.6B to a fraction	Insilco Medicine (fibrosis candidate in 46 days)	Speeds up access to new treatments; lowers R&D costs
Remote Monitoring & Telemedicine	AI-integrated wearables and remote patient monitoring (RPM); telehealth consultation platforms	- 38% reduction in hospital readmissions- Over $200B annual savings	RPM systems; virtual care in rural communities	Improves access, supports chronic care management, and lowers systemic costs.
Surgical Robotics	AI-assisted robotic systems for precision, motion scaling, and intraoperative guidance	- 35% fewer surgical complications-20% reduction in hospital stay duration	Da Vinci Surgical System	Enhanced surgical safety; reduced recovery time

8.1 Integrating AI with Emerging Technologies

The future of AI healthcare will depend on how it leverages next-generation technologies, including blockchain, the Internet of Things (IoT), 5G/6G networks, and quantum computing. The symbiosis of these technologies presents groundbreaking use cases. To illustrate, the future AI researching and developing on blockchain will allow for stopping the tracing of federated learning, as well as automatically optimizing smart contracts patented by AI amending insurance claims. And IoT devices (wearables/implants) will continuously stream health events to Edge AI models to reduce latency and improve timely responses (Hassani et al., 2024). Next-generation low-latency networks (5G, 6G) will support use cases like telesurgery and remote diagnostics, while quantum computing will speed drug discovery by simulating molecular biology. Table 4 represents hypothetical integrations of technologies, with related examples for actual use in healthcare.

In summary, the integration of AI with blockchain, IoT, 5G/6G, and quantum computing will fundamentally transform healthcare. Blockchain provides secure and auditable federated learning; IoT devices leverage Edge AI for real-time awareness of information in the smart hospital; advanced networks enable remote diagnostic or telesurgical services; and quantum computing can accelerate drug discovery. Collectively, these technologies can provide scalable, secure, and transformative solutions for healthcare.

Table 4. Hypothetical integrations of technologies, with related examples for actual use in healthcare:

Technology	Integration with AI	Healthcare Use Case
Blockchain	Secures health records and ensures auditability of AI decisions and federated learning	AI-enhanced smart contracts for claims, decentralized patient data ledgers
IoT / Edge AI	Real-time AI processing of sensor data minimizes latency and protects privacy.	Continuous glucose monitoring, AI in surgical robots (e.g., NVIDIA Clara Holoscan)
5G/6G Networks	Enables ultra-low latency AI applications	Telesurgery, AR-based remote diagnostics (e.g., 5G Smart Hospital in South Korea)
Quantum Computing	Accelerates AI model training, enhances complex simulations	AI-driven drug discovery and disease pathway analysis (e.g., IBM Quantum initiatives)

8.2 Trust in AI for Medicine

In order for Artificial Intelligence (AI) systems to be appropriated in medicine, trust must be built first. While AI technologies promise enormous opportunities before us - from automating diagnostics to making personalized treatment recommendations - embedding AI into clinical workflows also requires considerations of transparency, fairness, accountability, reliability, and ethical governance. Trust becomes paramount when AI is integrated into complex collaborative health intelligence ecosystems that involve multiple organizations and utilize federated learning and/or utilize sensitive personal patient data directly from devices and sensors, social media, EMR, and others. A significant part of developing that trust is explainability, or the AI system's ability to provide an explanation of how its predictions were drawn that is interpretable and acceptable for clinical users and patients alike. Many modern AI models—particularly deep neural networks—are perceived too often as “black boxes,” compared to statistical tools developed in the past. When employing a federated learning approach, researchers may be further limited in their ability to produce interpretable models because of a decentralized model-training process (“An expert hybrid federated learning,” 2025). A significant factor is the robustness and reliability of medical AI models. If a medical AI model performs robustly across different populations, imaging modalities, and sensor types, then it can be reliably used in parallel clinical environments. The federated paradigm helps with reliability and robustness because most federated systems will likely exhibit data heterogeneity, as the participating nodes (e.g., a hospital system or wearable device) will be experiencing varying levels of demographic, environmental, and technical heterogeneity. Federated learning improves perception of trustworthiness because it maintains the integrity of the local context, avoiding central bias; however, a validation process still needs to be seen across all nodes in order to make sure all nodes are delivering the appropriate standards of fairness and reduce the chance of misdiagnosis or treatment errors given the standard distribution processes.

Regarding privacy and data safety, this too is more likely to be a means to provide trust in proceeding with an AI project. Whether it is the patients and families or the providers, they will be more likely to engage with AI if they think their sensitive data will not be compromised. Federated learning has an advantage here because the raw data will always stay local, and only the encrypted model parameters are shared. When this is combined with differential privacy, secure multiparty computation, or blockchain-based audit trails, the enterprise should match or exceed regulatory and ethical standards, increasing the trust of the public and providers (Barth, 2023).

In conclusion, trust in AI for medicine is not a purely technical problem; trust is multidimensional for transparency, equity, security, and human-centered design. Federated learning, as a form of collaborative health intelligence, provides a fascinating structure to build this trust and align data privacy. Figure 3 shows the five pillars of trust in medical AI—explainability, fairness, privacy and security, reliability, and human-AI collaboration - are adjacent to the concept of federated learning. Together, these pillars ensure a secure, transparent, and fair AI system in medical care.

Figure 3. The five pillars of trust in medical AI—explainability, fairness, privacy and security, and reliability.

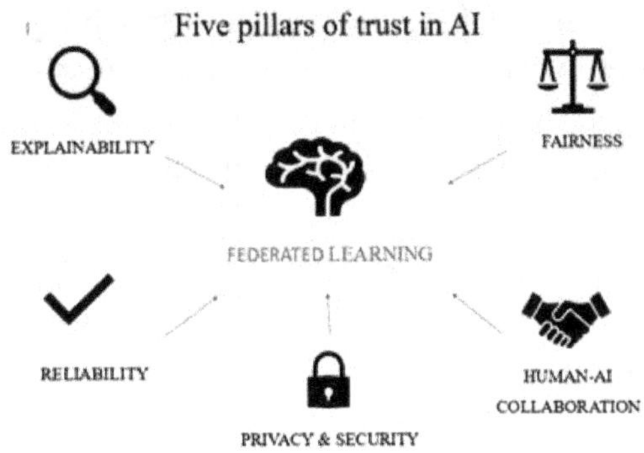

8.3 AI Care Policy and Global Cooperation

With artificial intelligence (AI) becoming more integrated into healthcare delivery, diagnostics, and public health surveillance, now is the time to begin developing comprehensive policy related to AI care and to think about the role of global cooperation. AI systems, especially those that use collaborative intelligence -such as federated learning -operate outside of institutional and national contexts. To implement AI safely and sustainably in a range of healthcare applications, attention must also be paid to creating aligned regulations, policies, and ethical frameworks that collectively contribute to equitable, secure, and responsible AI implementations.

AI care policy means the set of legal, ethical, and operational guidance for the design, implementation, and evaluation of AI in health systems (European Commission, 2025). The decentralizing structure of federated learning has unique policy challenges and possibilities; while federated learning ultimately creates a privacy-preserving approach by keeping data local, it also requires a new paradigm for governance of machine learning models, data sovereignty, and trust among institutions in different jurisdictions. This ecosystem is built on worldwide cooperation. WHO, OECD, and GPAI projects are building frameworks for medical AI systems focusing on fairness, safety, and interoperability. For example, the WHO Guidance on Ethics and Governance of AI for Health identifies the need to develop inclusive governance mechanisms, transparency and accountability in model development, and alignment with rights frameworks for global health. We are also beginning to see the movement towards AI certification and auditing, with potentially the same level of scrutiny that we see with clinical trials, coming from jurisdictions that are managing at -scale digital health (e.g., the EU, Canada, South Korea, and Singapore). Since federated learning is decentralized, we can work within the regulations associated with data and protection based on the different regions (i.e., General Data Protection Regulation (EU) and Health Insurance Portability and Accountability Act (U.S.A.)). In order to capitalize on the opportunities with federated learning, we will need global standards, interoperable data formats, and ethical frameworks that help us operationalize these possibilities and that cannot be formed in silos (European Commission, 2025).

COVID-19 and other recent crises have brought back to the forefront the imperative toward collaborative systems for making rapid diagnoses, tracking outbreaks, or other types of health interventions. In summary, the future of AI in medicine, and in particular federated learning contexts, will be driven not just by technological advancement but by global alignment on policies, ethics, and collaboration. Agendas that champion inclusive, adaptive, and future-oriented AI care policies based on global consensus and human-centeredness will be necessary to make collaborative health intelligence equitable and responsible for the global community (Regulatory Affairs Professionals Society, n.d.).

In essence, the meaningful adoption of AI in healthcare, including approaches like federated learning, requires a globally coordinated strategy that aligns policy, ethics, and interoperability standards. Addressing issues of fairness, safety, transparency, and legal compliance (such as, GDPR and HIPAA) is already the focus of international efforts led by bodies like the WHO and OECD. Ultimately, the future of collaborative health intelligence will depend as much on robust global governance in these areas as on continued technological advancements.

9. LIMITATIONS OF USING FEDERATED LEARNING

Federated Learning (FL) represents a paradigm shift that allows the authors to harness the power of collaborative artificial intelligence without sacrificing patient privacy. There are key limitations that become apparent during its real-life application within the health care domain, which must be resolved before any feasible and widely adopted health care applications of FL can be developed.

1. Data Heterogeneity and Quality Differences

FL models will need to deal with datasets from many different hospitals and clinics, as well as clinical devices. These providers will have several variations based on differences in demographics, clinical protocols, equipment characteristics, and record-keeping practices. This level of non-uniformity is often referred to as non-IID (independent and identically distributed) data and can hinder model convergence, introduce bias, or reduce accuracy when applied to a new population of patients.

2. Computational and Network Constraints

FL relies fundamentally on the local processing power for training models, which is then fed back to the server for aggregates to happen before updates are assumed. FL is likely to provide a smoother update path than centralized AI systems. However, many healthcare organizations, especially those in low-resource contexts, do not have high-performance hardware, a consistent energy supply, or reliable bandwidth to perform this efficiently.

3. Privacy and Security Issues

While FL doesn't involve the sharing of information directly, there are still threats to privacy and security in the form of adversaries threatening to triangulate models with the intent to attack them. Some threats include gradient leakage, model inversion attacks, and model poisoning attacks, which are some examples of adversarial threats. To counter adversarial threats, techniques such as differential privacy, secure multiparty computation, and homomorphic encryption can expand on FL but incur some efficiency and complexity in exchange for low add-ons to privacy or security.

4. Gaps in interoperability and standardization

The lack of standardized data schemas, ontologies, and communication protocols means that it is problematic to integrate environments, and interoperability problems are compounded into collaboration across borders because of variations in privacy regulation, data formats, and technical systems.

5. Ethical, Legal, and Regulatory Complexity

Multiple overlapping (and occasionally contradictory) regulatory frameworks such as HIPAA, GDPR, and national data localization laws present an enormous challenge. Algorithmic liability, patient consent, and data governance remain unsettled questions that raise issues of fairness, transparency, and accountability in federated healthcare AI.

6. Validate Models and Integrate Clinically.

Validation of federated models is difficult to achieve in practice because there is no standard evaluation metric or ground truth dataset to evaluate with. Also, the clinical integration of these models requires careful usability evaluation, clinician training, and often redesign of the paradigms used to work with models that can delay implementation.

Concluding, Federated learning presents a fascinating opportunity for privacy-preserving collaborative artificial intelligence (AI) in the field of medicine, while recognizing that there are many technical, infrastructural, security, and governance hurdles that need to be addressed. For federated learning to transition from an idea to an aspect of the global health AI environment will require continuous collaborative efforts and shared insights across disciplines, including clinicians, technologists, policymakers, and government officials.

10. CONCLUSIONS

Deductive reasoning suggests that Federated Learning (FL) represents a paradigm shift in healthcare artificial intelligence (AI), as it offers a comprehensive approach to addressing the persistent issues of data privacy, data security, and compliance with regulations. FL enables collaborative model training without a centralized data repository, which allows patient information to remain within institutional borders. Data aggregation does not occur, and, as a result, AI models that are accurate and generalizable can be created. FL's decentralized methods provide additional AI model accuracy, encompassing various institutions and geographically dispersed locations. With an increased accuracy of AI models and adherence to HIPAA, along with GDPR, stakeholders comprising healthcare providers, researchers, and patients can trust such frameworks.

The applications of FL in medicine are very broad and changing. In addition to aiding in image diagnosis, CLARA enables cooperation between various institutions and thus aids in cross-institutional applications by training on heterogeneous datasets and increasing the robustness of the model to varying populations, as demonstrated by NVIDIA Clara's federated mammography analysis. Other areas where FL has aided are furthering research in rare diseases, aiding in the response to pandemics such as the EXAM model for COVID-19, and monitoring patients through wearables. Other supplements to FL, such as integrating blockchain technology, edge computing, and the Internet of Medical Things (IoMT), allow for an increase in the scope of application of real - time, secure, scalable, AI - powered healthcare technologies.

Regardless, FL's full potential is still far from being realized due to several obstacles. The limitations of data diversity, computational resources, system threats, and cross-system collaboration are some notable challenges. Moreover, ethical scrutiny involving fairness and access, algorithm transparency, bias minimization, and equal opportunities also needs to be considered. Forming unified policies alongside set compliance governance structures will aid in the responsible widespread use and adoption of FL.

In the scope of AI technology in medicine, FL is believed to lower restrictions on international borders while addressing bias in AI models, allowing near-universal access to advanced diagnostics and personalized treatments. With a shift towards a privacy-respecting, patient-led, integrated healthcare framework, FL will act as a collaborative health intelligence backbone. Its growth will be reliant on multi-domain planning as well as flexible but strong institutional policy models combined with focused, responsible AI use and ethical principles.

In conclusion, federated learning is a paradigm shift in the development and application of healthcare AI that balances innovation with privacy, security, and equity. It is not just a technical breakthrough. In order to fully realize its potential in influencing the direction of medicine, the journey has only just begun, and its success will depend on ongoing cooperation between technologists, clinicians, legislators, and patients.

11. REFERENCES

Al-Huthaifi, R., Li, T., Huang, W., Gu, J., & Li, C. (2023). Federated learning in smart cities: Privacy and security survey. *Information Sciences*, *632*, 833–857. DOI: 10.1016/j.ins.2023.03.033

Barth, S. (2023, April 14). AI in healthcare. *ForeSee Medical*. https://www.foreseemed.com/artificial-intelligence-in-healthcare

Baucas, M., Spachos, P., & Plataniotis, K. (2023). Federated learning and blockchain-enabled fog-IoT platform for wearables in predictive healthcare. *arXiv*. https://arxiv.org/abs/2301.04511

Blanchard, S. (2025, May 13). Inside the cutting-edge NHS wards where robots assist surgeons – turning major ops into day cases. *The Scottish Sun*. https://www.thescottishsun.co.uk/health/14781345/million-pound-machine-keyhole-surgery-health-operations/

Bogdanova, A., Attoh-Okine, N., & Sakurai, T. (2020). Risk and advantages of federated learning for health care data collaboration. *ASCE-ASME Journal of Risk and Uncertainty in Engineering Systems. Part A, Civil Engineering*, *6*(3), 04020027. Advance online publication. DOI: 10.1061/AJRUA6.0001078

Chaddad, A., Wu, Y., & Desrosiers, C. (2023). Federated learning for healthcare applications. *IEEE Internet of Things Journal*, *11*(5), 7339–7358. DOI: 10.1109/JIOT.2023.3325822

Cui, L., Qu, Y., Xie, G., Zeng, D., Li, R., Shen, S., & Yu, S. (2021). Security and privacy-enhanced federated learning for anomaly detection in IoT infrastructures. *IEEE Transactions on Industrial Informatics*, *18*(5), 3492–3500. DOI: 10.1109/TII.2021.3107783

Dayan, I., Roth, H. R., Zhong, A., Harouni, A., Gentili, A., Abidin, A. Z., Liu, A., Costa, A. B., Wood, B. J., Tsai, C., Wang, C., Hsu, C., Lee, C. K., Ruan, P., Xu, D., Wu, D., Huang, E., Kitamura, F. C., Lacey, G., & Li, Q. (2021). Federated learning for predicting clinical outcomes in patients with COVID-19. *Nature Medicine*, *27*(10), 1735–1743. DOI: 10.1038/s41591-021-01506-3 PMID: 34526699

European Commission. (2025, March 28). Artificial intelligence in healthcare. *Public Health*. https://health.ec.europa.eu/ehealth-digital-health-and-care/artificial-intelligence-healthcare_en

Gu, X., Sabrina, F., Fan, Z., & Sohail, S. (2023). A review of privacy enhancement methods for federated learning in healthcare systems. *International Journal of Environmental Research and Public Health, 20*(15), 6539. Advance online publication. DOI: 10.3390/ijerph20156539 PMID: 37569079

Hassani, H., Huang, X., & Silva, E. S. (2024). Trustworthy federated learning: Privacy, security, and beyond. *arXiv*. https://arxiv.org/html/2411.01583

Hassani, H., Silva, E. S., & Al Kaabi, A. M. (2024). Federated learning, ethics, and the double black box problem in medical AI. *arXiv*. https://arxiv.org/html/2504.20656v1

Insilico Medicine. (n.d.). IPF – Phase 1. https://insilico.com/blog/ipf-phase1

Jebreel, N. M., Domingo-Ferrer, J., Blanco-Justicia, A., & Sánchez, D. (2022). Enhanced security and privacy via fragmented federated learning. *IEEE Transactions on Neural Networks and Learning Systems, 35*(5), 6703–6717. DOI: 10.1109/TNNLS.2022.3212627 PMID: 36260588

Jiang, F., Jiang, Y., Zhi, H., Dong, Y., Li, H., Ma, S., Wang, Y., Dong, Q., Shen, H., & Wang, Y. (2017). Artificial intelligence in healthcare: Past, present and future. *Stroke and Vascular Neurology, 2*(4), 230–243. DOI: 10.1136/svn-2017-000101 PMID: 29507784

Johnson, K. (2020, April 16). Health care organizations use NVIDIA's Clara federated learning to improve mammogram analysis AI. *VentureBeat*. https://venturebeat.com/ai/healthcare-organizations-use-nvidias-clara-federated-learning-to-improve-mammogram-analysis-ai/

Jun, M. (2025). Platform framework for blockchain-enhanced healthcare AIoT systems. *Frontiers in Communications and Networks, 6*, 1538965. Advance online publication. DOI: 10.3389/frcmn.2025.1538965

Jun, M. (2025). Platform framework for blockchain-enhanced healthcare AIoT systems. *Frontiers in Communications and Networks, 6*, 1538965. Advance online publication. DOI: 10.3389/frcmn.2025.1538965

Kakao Healthcare. (n.d.). Kakao Healthcare to link data platform with 17 major hospitals. *Pulse*. https://pulse.mk.co.kr/news/english/11290677

Kumar, Y., & Singla, R. (2021). Federated learning systems for healthcare: Perspective and recent progress. In *Studies in computational intelligence* (pp. 141–156). Springer., DOI: 10.1007/978-3-030-70604-3_6

Lee, T., Shiau, J., Chen, C., Yun, W., Wuu, C., Huang, Y., Yeh, S., Chen, H., & Chao, P. (2025). A machine learning model for predicting breast cancer recurrence and supporting personalized treatment decisions through comprehensive feature selection and explainable ensemble learning. *Cancer Management and Research, 17*, 917–932. DOI: 10.2147/CMAR.S514693 PMID: 40357238

Li, T., Sahu, A. K., Talwalkar, A., & Smith, V. (2020). Federated learning: Challenges, methods, and future directions. *IEEE Signal Processing Magazine*, *37*(3), 50–60. DOI: 10.1109/MSP.2020.2975749

Mendieta, M., Yang, T., Wang, P., Lee, M., Ding, Z., & Chen, C. (2022). Local learning matters: Rethinking data heterogeneity in federated learning. In *Proceedings of the IEEE/CVF Conference on Computer Vision and Pattern Recognition* (pp. 8387–8396). CVPR., https://openaccess.thecvf.com/content/CVPR2022/html/Mendieta_Local_Learning_Matters_Rethinking_Data_Heterogeneity_in_Federated_Learning_CVPR_2022_paper.html DOI: 10.1109/CVPR52688.2022.00821

Oh, W., & Nadkarni, G. N. (2023). Federated learning in health care using structured medical data. *Advances in Kidney Disease and Health*, *30*(1), 4–16. DOI: 10.1053/j.akdh.2022.11.007 PMID: 36723280

Panda, S., Dubey, R., Jena, B., Pareek, V., Tsai, L., & Saxena, S. (2025). Federated learning frameworks in smart e-healthcare: A systematic literature review with bias evaluation. *Applied Soft Computing*, *171*, 112747. Advance online publication. DOI: 10.1016/j.asoc.2025.112747

Pati, S., Baid, U., Edwards, B., Sheller, M., Wang, S., Reina, G. A., Foley, P., Gruzdev, A., Karkada, D., Davatzikos, C., Sako, C., Ghodasara, S., Bilello, M., Mohan, S., Vollmuth, P., Brugnara, G., Preetha, C. J., Sahm, F., Maier-Hein, K., & Bakas, S. (2022). Federated learning enables big data for rare cancer boundary detection. *Nature Communications*, *13*(1), 7346. Advance online publication. DOI: 10.1038/s41467-022-33407-5 PMID: 36470898

Pinto-Coelho, L. (2023). How artificial intelligence is shaping medical imaging technology: A survey of innovations and applications. *Bioengineering (Basel, Switzerland)*, *10*(12), 1435. Advance online publication. DOI: 10.3390/bioengineering10121435 PMID: 38136026

Regulatory Affairs Professionals Society. (n.d.). The global regulatory landscape for AI/ML-enabled medical devices. *RAPS*. https://www.raps.org/News-and-Articles/News-Articles/2024/9/The-global-regulatory-landscape-for-AI-ML-enabled

Reilly, J. B., Kim, J. G., Cooney, R., DeWaters, A. L., Holmboe, E. S., Mazotti, L., & Gonzalo, J. D. (2023). Breaking down silos between medical education and health systems: Creating an integrated multilevel data model to advance the systems-based practice competency. *Academic Medicine*, *99*(2), 146–152. DOI: 10.1097/ACM.0000000000005294 PMID: 37289829

Ridley, E. L. (2021, September 16). Strength in numbers: Federated learning boosts AI for COVID-19. *AuntMinnie*. https://www.auntminnie.com/clinical-news/digital-x-ray/article/15629249/strength-in-numbers-federated-learning-boosts-ai-for-covid-19

Rieke, N., Hancox, J., Li, W., Milletari, F., Roth, H. R., Albarqouni, S., Bakas, S., Galtier, M. N., Landman, B. A., Maier-Hein, K., Ourselin, S., Sheller, M., Summers, R. M., Trask, A., Xu, D., Baust, M., & Cardoso, M. J. (2020). The future of digital health with federated learning. *NPJ Digital Medicine*, *3*(1), 119. Advance online publication. DOI: 10.1038/s41746-020-00323-1 PMID: 33015372

Sprenkamp, K., Fernández, J. D., Eckhardt, S., & Zavolokina, L. (2024). Overcoming intergovernmental data sharing challenges with federated learning. *Data & Policy*, *6*, e19. Advance online publication. DOI: 10.1017/dap.2024.19

Treloar, A. (2014). The Research Data Alliance: Globally co-ordinated action against barriers to data publishing and sharing. *Learned Publishing*, *27*(5), 9–13. DOI: 10.1087/20140503

Wang, S., Zhang, Y., & Zhang, Y. (2018). A blockchain-based framework for data sharing with fine-grained access control in decentralized storage systems. *IEEE Access : Practical Innovations, Open Solutions*, *6*, 38437–38450. DOI: 10.1109/ACCESS.2018.2851611

Wang, T., Du, Y., Gong, Y., Choo, K.-K. R., & Guo, Y. (2023). Applications of federated learning in mobile health: Scoping review. *Journal of Medical Internet Research*, *25*, e43006. Advance online publication. DOI: 10.2196/43006 PMID: 37126398

Wen, Y., & Wen, Y. (2022, September 2). Federated learning powered by NVIDIA Clara. *NVIDIA Technical Blog*. https://developer.nvidia.com/blog/federated-learning-clara/

Yang, Q., Liu, Y., Chen, T., & Tong, Y. (2019). Federated machine learning. *ACM Transactions on Intelligent Systems and Technology*, *10*(2), 12. Advance online publication. DOI: 10.1145/3298981

Yurdem, B., Kuzlu, M., Gullu, M. K., Catak, F. O., & Tabassum, M. (2024). Federated learning: Overview, strategies, applications, tools and future directions. *Heliyon*, *10*(19), e38137. Advance online publication. DOI: 10.1016/j.heliyon.2024.e38137 PMID: 39391509

Zhang, F., Shuai, Z., Kuang, K., Wu, F., Zhuang, Y., & Xiao, J. (2023). Unified fair federated learning for digital healthcare. *Patterns (New York, N.Y.)*, *5*(1), 100907. Advance online publication. DOI: 10.1016/j.patter.2023.100907 PMID: 38264718

Zhou, T., Lin, Z., Zhang, J., & Tsang, D. H. (2024). Understanding and improving model averaging in federated learning on heterogeneous data. *IEEE Transactions on Mobile Computing*, *23*(12), 12131–12145. DOI: 10.1109/TMC.2024.3406554

Chapter 6
Enabling Decentralized Clinical Insights:
Federated Learning in Smart Healthcare Systems

Sonam Gupta
https://orcid.org/0000-0002-4323-6991
Ajay Kumar Garg Engineering College, Ghaziabad, India

Pradeep Gupta
Ajay Kumar Garg Engineering College, Ghaziabad, India

Lipika Goel
Sridevi Women's Engineering College, Hyderabad, India

Sachin Jain
https://orcid.org/0000-0002-2948-7858
Ajay Kumar Garg Engineering College, Ghaziabad, India

ABSTRACT

Healthcare AI has federated learning as a transformational approach in which clinical research can be conducted collaboratively and in patient privacy is preserved. This chapter considers federated learning and how it enables healthcare institutions to learn from sensitive data without centralizing it and without access to that data. It consists of the technological architecture, companding local computational resources, secure communication channels, and model aggregation servers, each with a suitable algorithm for dealing with data heterogeneity between institutions. Its integration with existing healthcare infrastructure (IoMT devices, EHR systems) ensures operational efficiency thus being integrated into the existing

DOI: 10.4018/979-8-3373-3306-9.ch006

system. By balancing innovation with privacy, federated learning is positioned as a cornerstone technology for the development of the personalized medicine — which with technology giants as the players the only type in which patient privacy can be respected while taking advantage of the collective clinical wisdom.

1. INTRODUCTION

Today, healthcare institutions generate enormous clinical data daily on the basis of thousands of such outlets using the digital transformation of healthcare. Rich datasets are continuously being produced by the electronic health records (EHRs), medical imaging repositories, genomic database, and wearable devices and there is great opportunity for improving patient care, advancing medical research, optimizing healthcare operation (Rajkomar et al., 2018). Although such data abundance stands in contradiction with the need for aggregating these distributed datasets to drive medical breakthroughs, the sensitive nature of healthcare information and the strict privacy regulations are generally inconsistent with the use of conventional data pooling approaches (Price & Cohen, 2019).

Federated learning is a revolutionary paradigm in artificial intelligence that allows to carry out collaborative model training across institutions without having to share patients' data. Federated learning, as a way of distributed machine learning with an emphasis on preservation of privacy, was first proposed by McMahan et al. (2017) at Google, and the method has been quickly adopted by the community. Interestingly, this approach holds promise to alleviate this tension in healthcare so specifically (Rieke et al., 2020). Federated learning keeps data where it originates and achieves the statistical power of multi-institutional collaboration by allowing models to train locally at each institution if, and only if, validated by a central authority.

Further, rare disease research is burdened by small sample sizes at any one institution making for lack of statistical significance and model generalizability (Rajkomar et al., 2019). As in population health initiatives, models that more reflect healthcare disparities and clinical practices across geographical regions and health systems are preferred if they are diverse in demographic representation.

Further, it is scrutinized the regulatory frameworks and the ethical considerations including how federated learning deals with HIPAA and GDPR, and broader problems of the algorithmic transparency, fairness, and accountability. Organizational structures and policies to sustain federated learning ecosystems in healthcare are outlined for the governance section under the task, incentive models, the stakeholder engagement strategies, and the collaborative frameworks.

We then stretch our necks towards the future of federated learning in healthcare, anticipating its performance in emerging research in directions, stressing advanced technological changes and evolving healthcare delivery models that will append a shape to the evolution. We hold a dual perspective throughout this chapter: on the one hand, technological complexity of federated systems is taken into account; on the other hand, the human dimensions of healthcare delivery are acknowledged; in both cases, patient outcomes, clinical decisions, and access to healthcare are to be considered the ultimate measures of success.

2. TECHNICAL FOUNDATIONS OF FEDERATED LEARNING IN HEALTHCARE

2.1 Federated Learning Architecture

The idea of federated learning consists of a distributed machine learning approach that allows collection of multiple parties to collaboratively train their respective learning algorithms for the same task without such underlying data being exchanged (McMahan et al., 2017). The typical use case of this architecture in healthcare contexts considers three major components: local nodes representing individual healthcare providers or institutions, a federated server that coordinates the learning process and aggregates model updates, and communication channels of secure type among these entities (Kaissis et al., 2020).

In standard federated learning protocol, an iterative process goes on as follows (Li et al., 2020): (1) The federated server initializes a global model and sends it to the participating nodes, (2) then nodes train the model on their local data, (3) the resulting model updates (not local data) are sent to the federated server, (4) The server aggregates the updates to refine the global model. (5) And the improved global model is rehashed to the participants for the next iteration of training. It keeps on evolving until the model converges or meets predetermined performance metrics. The architecture is as shown in figure 1.

There are several healthcare implementations that come with several architectural variants. The predominant approach in institutional healthcare, cross-silo federated learning, involves a relatively small number of organizations at a hierarchy that have substantial resources (computational and data) to contribute to the federation (Kairouz et al., 2021). Such organizations may include hospitals, research institutions, health care systems, and many others. On the other hand, cross device federated learning involves large number of edge devices that have limited computational capacity, ranging from wearables and mobile health applications in use by single patients (Rieke et al., 2020).

Different policies govern the coordination mechanisms in federated learning. It includes centralized federations, where there is one orchestrating entity that does the aggregation and distribution of a model, and decentralized, where runners do not rely on a central authority (Boughorbel et al., 2019). Based on blockchain, implementations in decentralized governance of healthcare federations are promising frameworks that form transparent and immutable record of model updates and participant's contributions (Nguyen et al., 2021).

Figure 1. Federated Learning Architecture in Healthcare

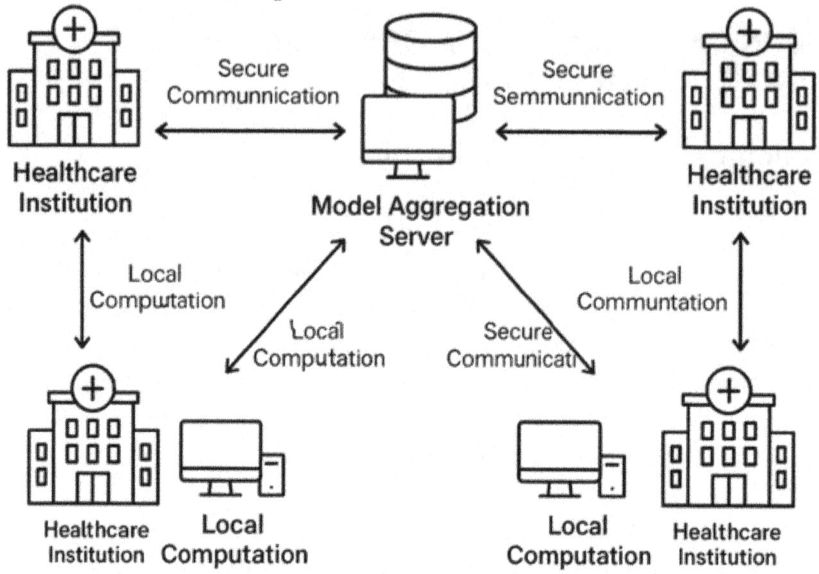

2.2 Federated Learning Algorithms

Several of the federated optimization algorithms have been adapted or developed specifically to healthcare applications. However, Federated Averaging (FedAvg) as introduced by McMahan, et al. (2017) is the fundamental type of implementation, where weighted averaging of local model updates, based on each institution's dataset size. Yet healthcare data presents special challenges requiring the invention of the algorithm.

Statistical heterogeneity, particularly due to data heterogeneity—the divergence of a patient populations, diagnostic practice and recording standard across institution—increases model's statistical heterogeneity, which compromises model's performance (Kairouz et al., 2021). This challenge has led schools and institutions to develop personalized federated learning algorithms that allow them to keep pieces of the model tailored to their patient populations, and benefit from the sharing of collaborative insights (Kulkarni et al., 2020). For example, FedProx (Li et al., 2020) and SCAFFOLD (Karimireddy et al., 2020) address statistical heterogeneity by limiting the local updates to be within a constrained space or correcting the client drift.

In the classification tasks of rare diagnosis, federated focal loss and federated re-weighting have been proved to be more effective in handling the imbalanced data for data distributions common in healthcare, where rare conditions may need additional representation only when looked in multiple institutions. (Chen et al., 2021) Moreover, it has been shown that federated transfer learning approaches are promising for when there are some limited labeled data and knowledge from data rich participants can be used to help others with smaller data sets.

Continual federated learning frameworks based on sequential learning paradigms have been developed to enable models to adapt over the course of clinical practice and diseases patterns.

2.3 Privacy and Security Mechanisms

The first motivation for federated learning in healthcare is privacy preservation. Then beyond the intrinsic privacy value of being able to contain data within the data center footprint, other schemes add further resistance to potential inference exploitation (Kaissis et al., 2020). Differential privacy adds calibrated noise around the model updates to make sure the presence or absence of any single patient record is not deducible from the shared model (Dwork & Roth, 2014). In healthcare implementations, privacy budget has restrictions for both patient protection and model utility and especially for the rare conditions where small samples make privacy-utility tradeoffs harder (Yale et al., 2019).

Secure aggregation protocols allow federated servers to maintain anonymity and compute an aggregated model update that is consistent with each contributory without knowing each contributor's (Bonawitz et al., 2017). In the healthcare settings, PATE (Private aggregation of teacher ensembles) (Papernot et al., 2018) has also shown effectiveness by aggregating predictions of several locally trained models instead of sharing the model parameters.

Those defense mechanisms against adversarial attacks are particularly necessary to ensure the integrity of the federated learning process. In Byzantine robust aggregation algorithms, compromised participants are detected and shielded against potential attempts to poison the model through malicious contributions from which harmful biases or backdoors could be introduced (Li et al., 2019). Particularly important in clinical decision support applications in which model recommendations directly impact patient care are these protections.

Commonly, standard cryptographic protocols, such as TLS (Transport Layer Security), coupled with healthcare specific, but compliant with standard clinical systems, authentication mechanisms are typically used for communication between participating nodes and federated servers (Rieke et al., 2020). Some implementations leverage secure hardware enclaves like Intel SGX or ARM TrustZone for the implementation of isolated execution environments for model training that protects the model training where data is stored from privileged adversaries within participating institutions (Mo & Haddadi, 2019).

3. IMPLEMENTATION CONSIDERATIONS FOR HEALTHCARE ORGANIZATIONS

3.1 Technical Infrastructure Requirements

Deep learning in medical imaging requires substantial GPU resources at participating sites (Sheller et al., 2020). It must assessed whether existing infrastructure is able to serve local model training in a way that doesn't interfere with clinical operations (e.g. requiring dedicated computational resources or a solution based on the cloud for model training) (Roth et al., 2020).

However, even with federated learning which greatly decreases the data transmission, the model parameters can be large payloads (esp. for the complex neural network used in the imaging applications, Xu et al., 2021). Timely model update necessitates that organizations must have sufficient network capabilities to support the timely updates, and thus must design for a tradeoff between communication overhead and network capabilities without a sacrifice to model performance.

Integration system is a key barrier to clinical environments where interoperability among the disparate health information systems persists. Due to this, federated learning implementations need to interface with electronic health records, picture archiving and communication systems (PACS), laboratory information systems, and other clinical data repositories (Rajkomar et al., 2018). Because inputs to federated training workflows often require extraction of, transformation and normalization of data from different heterogeneous systems, middleware solutions are often necessary to form input data (Kaissis et al., 2020).

Therefore, due to its promising edge computing architectures, model training and inference can be performed at local nodes around data source locations, easing reliance on central computing resources (Silva et al., 2019). If they are federating learning, organizations should take into consideration how to integrate IoMT (Internet of Medical Things) devices, point of care diagnostics, and other distributed data sources that reside at the edge in their federated ecosystem (Nguyen et al., 2021).

3.2 Data Standardization and Interoperability

The main challenge in federated learning for the healthcare domain is data heterogeneity, since data structures, coding systems, and documentations practices afford variations and we cannot train the model across institutions (Rieke et al., 2020). On the semantic level, foundational reference points are supplied by standard medical terminologies such as SNOMED CT, LOINC, ICD-10 or RxNorm, however, due to implementation variations and legacy systems as well as the implementation of FHIR, proper harmonisation work is typically needed (Lehne et al., 2019).

Federated learning in organizations is more practical for CDMs, which standardize the representations of data across the participating sites. Such models as OMOP (Observational Medical Outcomes Partnership), PCORnet, i2b2, etc. provide structured frameworks for transforming individuated clinical data into formats that are appropriate for federated analysis (Garza et al., 2016). Typically these CDMs would include data schemas alongside with rules that transform the data and processes that validate that the data is semantically consistent across sites.

In the context of federated healthcare environment, Fast Healthcare Interoperability Resources (FHIR) has been emerging as a key standard for interoperability (Ayaz et al., 2021). FHIR's RESTful API architecture and resource approach supports standardized data access pattern through which these workflows can be integrated. In the context of federated learning, those organizations should consider the possibility of integrating Federated Health Interoperability Resources (FHIR) discovery and implementation in their interoperability strategy and possibly even supporting distributed analytics based on FHIR specific frameworks.

To decrease the variability in data that could otherwise hamper the federated model's performance (Liu et al., 2020), it is possible to develop consistent annotation guidelines and quality control processes, as well as utilize text normalization pipelines with natural language processing pipelines.

3.3 Workflow Integration and Clinical Validation

For federated learning integration into clinical workflows to be successful, the user experience, operational processes as well as validation measures have to be carefully taken into account. In order for federated analyses to be initiated by clinicians and researchers, without heavy reliance on technical expertise in distributed machine learning, the interfaces need to be designed by organizations (Rajkomar et al., 2019). The interfaces for these collection modules should be on par with existing clinical systems in terms of additional workload, but maximize utility.

Challenges in model validation in federated setting are different from the centralized approaches. Therefore, robust validation framework must be deployed in the organizations to assess the model performance which is not only on local test data, but it also must rely on federated groups to validate the generalizablility between sites without data centralization.

Implementation of workflow will be greatly constrained by regulatory issues, especially in the case of federated models, for their intended use as clinical decision support. Organizations have to navigate multifarious approval pathways that could involve institutional review groups, data governance committees, and external regulatory bodies (such as FDA's Software as a Medical Device (SaMD) framework) (Gerke et al., 2020). Federated approaches involve specific regulatory challenges associated with distributed development and validation that warrant documentation of training procedures across the sites involved.

Feedback mechanisms over the continuous monitoring of model performance are essential in keeping model performance in dynamic clinical environments'. Kaissis et al. (2020) states that organizations need to put in place systems that track the drift of the model, detect drop in performance, and foster the model retraining when needed.

3.4 Real-World Deployment Challenges

Implementing federated learning (FL) in healthcare settings involves several practical barriers beyond the core technical considerations. These challenges must be addressed for successful, sustainable deployment.

1. Infrastructure Costs
    - **Barrier:**
        - o High-performance computing (HPC) resources such as GPUs, secure network infrastructure, and data storage solutions are essential for FL.
        - o Smaller healthcare institutions often lack the budget to procure and maintain these systems.
    - **Strategies:**
        - o Adopt **cloud-based FL platforms** to reduce on-site hardware investment.
        - o Implement **edge computing** for local model training to lower central server demands.
        - o Explore **public-private partnerships** for shared infrastructure costs.
2. Staff Training and Expertise
    - **Barrier:**
        - o FL requires specialized technical, clinical, and compliance expertise.

- o Lack of trained personnel can slow deployment and introduce operational risks.
- **Strategies:**
  - o Provide **cross-disciplinary training** for IT teams, clinicians, and compliance officers.
  - o Use **user-friendly FL frameworks** (e.g., OpenFL, NVIDIA Clara) to lower the technical entry barrier.
  - o Include FL modules in continuing medical education (CME) programs for clinicians.

3. Legal Liability and Risk Management
   - **Barrier:**
     - o Errors in FL-driven predictions could result in patient harm, raising liability concerns.
     - o Jurisdictional differences in legal frameworks complicate multi-institution collaborations.
   - **Strategies:**
     - o Define **clear governance agreements** outlining responsibilities and accountability.
     - o Use **regulatory sandboxes** to test FL models under controlled conditions.
     - o Obtain **appropriate insurance coverage** for AI-assisted decision-making tools.
4. Integration with Existing Systems
   - **Barrier:**
     - o FL must work seamlessly with existing Electronic Health Records (EHR) systems, PACS, and laboratory information systems.
     - o Variations in interoperability standards cause delays and technical complexity.
   - **Strategies:**
     - o Use **FHIR-based APIs** for standardized data exchange.
     - o Employ **middleware solutions** to harmonize data flows between legacy systems and FL platforms.
     - o Plan integration during early project stages to avoid costly post-deployment fixes.

4. CLINICAL APPLICATIONS AND USE CASES

The various applications of Federated Learning in Healthcare is as shown in figure 2.

4.1 Medical Imaging Analysis

Medical imaging is one of the most successful application areas where federated learning is adopted in healthcare as a result of high data dimensionality, intensively computationally expensive requirements, and privacy sensitivities (Sheller et al., 2020). We have found that particularly useful in radiology where image acquisition protocols, equipment specifications, interpretation practices are widely different across institutions which prohibits traditional centralized models.

Figure 2. Applications of Federated Learning in Healthcare

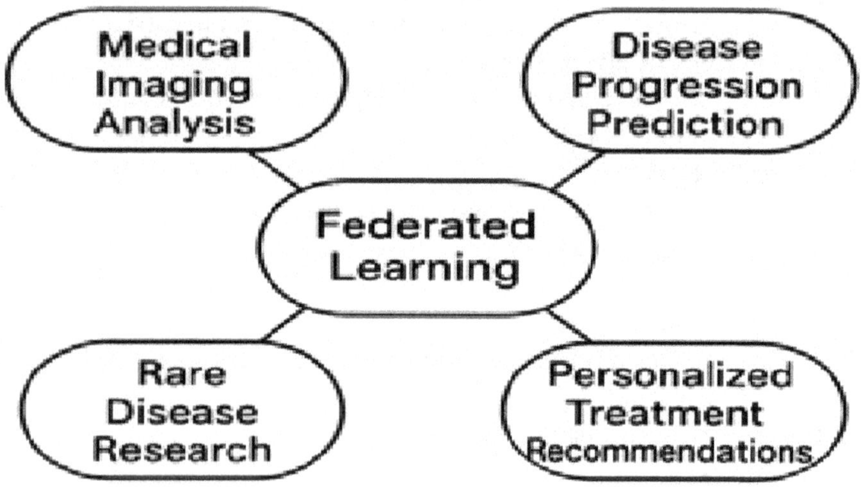

Radiology demonstrates how federated learning can be useful in particular, brain tumor segmentation. To demonstrate federated learning for the scenario of multi-institutional collaborations on delineating tumors without image sharing (potentially identifiable patient images) we used the BraTS (Brain Tumor Segmentation) challenge dataset (Sheller et al., 2020). Federated models are studied to be able to achieve the same performance as centralized approaches while preserving patient privacy, with special motivation on techniques dealing with statistical heterogeneity between two institutions (Li et al., 2019).

Some of the federated learning applications have been leveraged in histopathology towards developing cancer detection and classification models across different institutions using different staining protocols and scanner specifications (Lu et al., 2022). Whole slide images have high pixel level detail, both advantages and challenges for federated approaches, transfer learning techniques and domain adaptation methods are used to handle within and between site variability in tissue preparation and imaging (Poirot et al., 2019).

Similarly, federated learning has also been demonstrated in molecular imaging tasks that include PETCT for cancer staging and treatment response assessment (Xu et al., 2021). Such applications are especially sensitive to multiinstitutional collaboration, since individual centers have limited sample sizes and difficult variability in imaging protocols.

4.2 Predictive Modeling for Clinical Outcomes

Another large application domain is pulmonary related chest Xray analysis. Federated learning has enabled the accelerated design of such models when operating across international boundaries without having to send sensitive patient data. They also provided privacy benefits, as well as a more generalizable model that was able to leverage diverse populations and imaging equipment through the federated approach.

4.3 Predictive Modeling for Clinical Outcomes

Cancer treatment response prediction is just an example of how federated learning can progress towards a singular, personalized medicine without localizing the private data at a central party (Kaissis et al., 2021).

Federated learning is an approach which addresses specific challenges of rare disease diagnosis and management. Historically rare disease research has faced statistical power limitations due to the fact that there are limited patient populations at any one institution (Rajkomar et al., 2019). Collaboration across multiple centers that care for these rare conditions through federated approaches of model development is possible without transferring potentially identifiable patient information.

Federated learning is used to make pharmacogenomic applications to predict medication responses from genetic variants and clinical characteristics, among others (Denny et al., 2010). Among these have been implementations where the healthcare delivery organizations work with research institutions to combine clinical outcome data with genomic information to build prediction models that guide selective meditation without centralized sensitive genetic data.

In the case of a VERTIGO project, the project showed how federated learning can improve coronary artery disease risk prediction by learning from data throughout multiple European healthcare systems that incorporates regional risk factors and outcomes variations in risks in a manner which does not move patient data across national boundaries (Passerat-Palmbach et al., 2020).

4.4 Case Studies: Real-World Federated Learning Deployments in Healthcare

Case Study 1: MELLODDY Project – Privacy-Preserving Drug Discovery

The **MELLODDY (Machine Learning Ledger Orchestration for Drug Discovery)** project demonstrates the large-scale application of federated learning in the pharmaceutical sector. It involves **10 major pharmaceutical companies**, academic partners, and technology providers collaborating to build AI models without sharing proprietary data.

- **Objective:** Predict molecular bioactivity and drug-target interactions using diverse datasets without exposing sensitive intellectual property.
- **Approach:**
  - o Used **cross-silo federated learning** to train models across proprietary datasets.
  - o Implemented secure aggregation and homomorphic encryption to ensure data confidentiality.
  - o Utilized blockchain-based orchestration for transparent model update tracking.
- **Outcome:** Improved model accuracy compared to single-institution models, while maintaining **full compliance with IP protection and privacy requirements**.
- **Relevance to Healthcare:** Although designed for drug discovery, MELLODDY's privacy-preserving model training principles can be adapted to clinical data scenarios such as genomic analysis and rare disease research.

Case Study 2: NVIDIA Clara – Federated Learning for Medical Imaging

NVIDIA Clara is an AI application framework that supports federated learning for healthcare providers. It has been deployed in multiple hospitals to collaboratively train medical imaging AI models without moving patient data.

- **Objective:** Enhance AI-based diagnostic imaging models (e.g., radiology, pathology) across institutions with heterogeneous datasets.
- **Approach:**
  - o Leveraged **Clara Federated Learning SDK** to connect hospitals' local GPU infrastructure.
  - o Applied secure communication protocols and differential privacy mechanisms.
  - o Integrated with existing PACS and radiology workflow systems to minimize disruption.

- **Outcome:** Models trained with Clara achieved **higher generalization performance** across diverse imaging protocols compared to models trained on local data only.
- **Relevance to Healthcare:** Clara's approach proves the feasibility of **multi-institutional AI development in regulated medical environments** while preserving patient confidentiality.

5. POPULATION HEALTH AND EPIDEMIOLOGICAL RESEARCH

To meet the requirements of preserving the privacy of individuals while monitoring infectious disease patterns in disease surveillance networks, federated learning has been used to enable disease surveillance data to be shared in an enclave. Early detection of outbreaks and atypical disease patterns is possible through these systems by analyzing trends in a number of healthcare systems without transferring information about identifiable patients between institutions.

6. CHALLENGES AND LIMITATIONS

6.1 Data Heterogeneity and Quality Issues

Data heterogeneity is one of the most significant challenges in healthcare federated learning. It includes differences in documentation practices, coding systems, and clinical workflows across institutions (Rieke et al., 2020). However, a different terminology systems, unique codes, and documentation templates create semantic barriers in the use of federated learning in healthcare systems (Lehne et al. 2019). There are yet another set of major challenges, especially the variation in the data completeness due to the discrepancies in documentary thoroughness, availability of diagnostic testing, and practice of follow up that lead to systematic variation in data availability across institutions (Beam et al., 2020).

Healthcare organizations broadly vary in how they assure the data quality and use different validation rules, completeness requirements, and correction workflows to affect the data reliability (Johnson et al, 2016). Quality variations of these federated learning implementations need to be considered and these implementations may have to perform some local preprocessing to try to identify and solve any quality problems prior to model training to stem the propagation of bad patterns into the global model. Data Variations in Federated Learning has the various challenges described in Figure. 3.

Figure 3. Challenges of Data Variations in Federated Learning

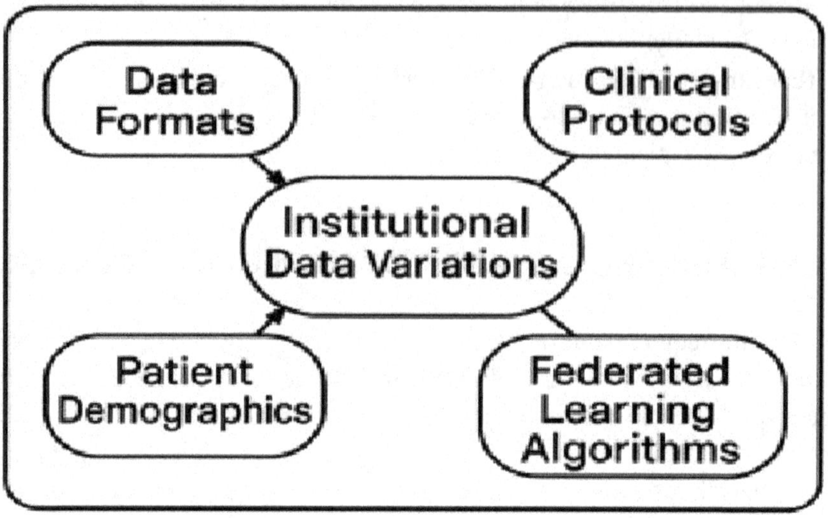

6.2 Statistical Challenges in Distributed Learning

Fundamental to federated optimization are statistical heterogeneity across institutions. However, if not dealt with underlying data distribution, especially if patient populations and the clinical patterns are non-IID (Independent and Identically Distributed) across the participating sites, model convergence and generalizability may be compromised using certain algorithms (Li et al., 2020). And healthcare is especially challenged today because patient demographics, disease prevalence, and practice patterns all change greatly from institution to institution. For example, catastrophic forgetting can occur when sequential updates disproportionately put emphasis on more recent data or on one particular institution from among the many institutions we support, which causes decreased performance on previously learned tasks or populations (Kairouz et al., 2021). To address this mismatch, it is necessary to carefully design mechanisms for aggregating across multiple and diverse patients as well as regularisation approaches that maintain knowledge across different populations of patients for different applications and clinical scenarios. In addition, the imbalance in participation across federated participants can introduce further statistical challenges, either from skewed dataset sizes, which can lead the global models to be towards the patterns present in larger contributors (Kairouz et al., 2021).

Challenges in the outlier detection and robustness in federated settings are more complicated than centralized ones. When you have no direct access to raw data, finding anomalous patterns or contributing values that might erroneously affect the model requires special techniques (Li et al. 2019) on making model updates instead of individual observations. Byzantine-robust aggregation methods solve these problems by identifying and neutralizing potentially harmful contributions, but doing so may unintentionally discard valuable information for patients served by institutions with properly exclusive patient populations.

In federated settings, model evaluation is a concern that needs to be carefully addressed: performance metrics and the appropriate validation methods. Since in distributed environments the data cannot be pooled centrally, traditional cross validation approaches have to be adapted, resulting in techniques like federated validation, leave one institution out testing, and model agnostic meta analysis of local performance metrics.

Computational and Communication Efficiency

However, substantial computational demands are detrimental to the federated learning adoption in the resource limited healthcare environments. Affordable GPU resources are often needed for deep learning models to be used in applications such as medical imaging analysis, but such resources might not be available at all potential participating institutions (Sheller et al., 2020). The disparity in these computations can result in participation inequalities in which less resource endowed organizations such as those that serve the populations that are underrepresented, cannot contribute to, or derive meaningful learning from, federated learning initiatives.

The second challenge is communication overhead, which is especially challenging for models with many parameters: millions can be common (Kairouz et al., 2021). However, in federated learning, the model updates still constitute a significant network payloads despite taking orders of magnitude less than centralized approaches. In organizations with limited bandwidth or unstable connections training cycles can be long and participation success is undermined due to communication failures.

Healthcare organizations are increasingly attentive to the energy consumption considerations in their attempts at sustainability. Due to the computational intensity of model training especially in deep learning approaches, there is a conflict with institutional sustainability goals (Xu et al., 2021).

Standard federated learning protocols impose synchronization requirements that present operational difficulty in healthcare environments that are intermittent in computational resources (Kairouz et al., 2021). In order to accommodate irregular participation patterns, asynchronous federated learning approaches are a promising alternative that allows institutions to contribute when resources are available without slowing down the whole training process.

In the healthcare delivery organization where computational infrastructure is primarily used for patient care activities (Rieke et al., 2020), federated learning resource allocation needs to carefully solved with clinical operational needs. For federated learning to be used in practice, organizations need resource management strategies for training activities that do not undermine time sensitive clinical applications, possibly through scheduling policies that limit intensive training to off the peak hours.

7. PRIVACY AND SECURITY VULNERABILITIES

Federated learning's privacy provable against central approaches comes with a tradeoff—many potential vulnerabilities must also be studied and avoided when applying federated learning in the healthcare domain. One important problem related to inference attacks is that adversaries can recover training data or extra sensitive information from model updates (Kaissis et al., 2020). Therefore, it would be possible for these attacks to compromise the patient privacy even without direct access to the underlying data, and defensive mechanisms are necessary such as differential privacy which prevents leaking information through model parameters.

Healthcare contexts show some particular concerns for membership inference attacks in which simple participation to a set of cohorts of diseases can reveal personal information (Shokri et al., 2017). Similar to the model inversion attacks, model inversion attacks aim to reconstruct representative examples of training data categories from model parameters so they can be used to recover sensitive information that includes facial characteristics from medical imaging models or clinical patterns from diagnostic models (Fredrikson et al., 2015). Healthcare application based on biometric data as well as rare cases with distinctive characteristics are especially feared with these attacks.

However, backdoor and poisoning attacks threaten model integrity since the malicious participants aim to control global model behavior by injecting specially crafted inputs when local training (Bagdasaryan et al., 2020). Such attacks could be dangerous, for instance, in the healthcare context where they would introduce dangerous diagnostic or treatment recommendations in a specific population of patients, and therefore robust federation protocols with anomaly detection and contribution verification mechanisms are required.

However, secure aggregation protocols (Bonawitz et al., 2017) which ensure privacy by preventing the coordinating server from seeing the full set of updates, may introduce vulnerabilities if cryptographic implementation of the secure aggregation protocol contains flaws in the protocol and/or1 key management practices are insufficient. To prevent privacy compromises, implementation of these techniques in the healthcare organizations requires cryptographic soundness and key governance.

8. REGULATORY FRAMEWORKS AND ETHICAL CONSIDERATIONS

8.1 Privacy Regulations and Compliance

Healthcare FL implementations face a number of complex and jurisdiction dependent regulatory landscapes in terms of institution type and/or data category. In the United States, HIPAA (Health Insurance Portability and Accountability Act) is the primary regulatory body that sets out how protected health information (Cohen & Mello, 2018) can be used and the manner in which electronic protected health information (Cohen & Mello, 2018) should be secured. Generally, federated learning approaches adhere to HIPAA's minimum necessary principle by keeping raw data local, but there is a lot of care that must be taken in implement to consider whether model parameters or their gradients could contain protected health information that needs additional safeguards.

For European institutions, federated learning must comply with the **General Data Protection Regulation (GDPR)**. While FL supports GDPR's data minimization principle, additional requirements apply:

- **Transparency** in how the model operates.
- **Purpose limitation** to ensure data is used only for agreed objectives.
- **Right to explanation** for complex AI model decisions.

As this is the case, organizations must also be conscientious to document how federated learning meets these regulatory requirements, possibly including algorithmic impact assessments which assess potential privacy risk (Price & Cohen, 2019)..

In addition to these, there are other international and regional regulations which add to the compliance considerations for the global federated learning initiatives. Special requirements for cross-border federated learning implementations introduced by China Personal Information Protection Law (PIPL), Japan Act on the Protection of Personal Information (APPI), and Brazil General Law of Personal Data Protection (LGPD) apply (Gerke et al., 2020). These overlapping regulatory frameworks themselves must govern organizations that are part of an international federation, which may have to roll out jurisdiction-specific safeguards in a federated architecture.

There are special considerations for federated learning implementations in academic and research context based on research regulations. Cohen and Mello (2018) mention that the requirements for IRB oversight are different in the case when analyses are federated and they involve human subjects research with or without testing specific hypotheses for model development. There are a few institutions that developed the specialized IRB protocols for federated learning which consider its characteristics of privacy preserving and provide enough ethical oversight. With the emergence of AI specific regulations that affect federated learning implementations potentially used for clinical decision support, these regulations are having increasing effect on federated learning. In his work on the FDA's proposed regulatory framework for AI/ML based Software as a Medical Device (SaMD), Gerke et al. (2020) has introduced considerations that would impact federated implementations differently than traditional centralized approaches (Gerke et al., 2020).

8.2 Ethical Frameworks for Collaborative AI

Thoughtful implementation of federated learning in healthcare goes beyond ethical regulatory compliance, designing acceding values into the federated learning itself. Federated model training is a foundational consideration requiring organizations to decide whether the standard clinical consent forms are sufficient to cover federated model training or if consent for development of an AI was required (Rajkomar et al., 2018). To address the issue of inequity, some institutions have implemented a tiered consent models whereby patients consent to various extent and categories in the AI development activities. Given that in federated settings, model training spans across diverse patient populations and different health settings, algorithmic fairness and health equity considerations become highly applicable. Therefore, federated fairness evaluation mechanisms such as (Rajkomar et al., 2018) can be implemented allowing organizations to detect and compensate for potential biases that may further exacerbate healthcare disparities without centralized storage of sensitive attributes. A first consideration for these mechanisms should be obtaining both representation bias and label bias, the latter being systematic differences in documentation of clinicals.

Once again, when it comes to model development across multiple institutions with disparate levels of interpretability requirements like in the federated healthcare settings, transparency and explainability present significant challenges (Doshi-Velez & Kim, 2017). Given the need for clinician and patient understanding of model behavior, federated explainability may be the way to balance the complexity added by privacy preserving techniques.

Questions related to how value produced in federated learning should be distributed between the institutions that contribute, patients, and the broader society are answered in benefit sharing frameworks (Price & Cohen, 2019). When substantial variations are present in participation, in data volume, quality, diversity, the issue is to manage the allocation of intellectual property, financial returns, and recognition, within federated initiatives. When instances of federations are spanning institutions with different resources and capabilities, these considerations are intimately related to cases of algorithmic colonialism and exploitation.

In federated environments, accountability mechanisms need to be distributed model development and deployment (Rieke et al. 2020). This means that organizations should spell out who is responsible for monitoring model performance, investigating adverse events, and update across the federation. This should cover both technical components as well as governance structures defining what institutional roles and responsibilities are binding.

9. GOVERNANCE MODELS FOR FEDERATED LEARNING

To successfully implement federated learning for healthcare, we need strong governance structures which have been implemented to respond to technical and organizational issues. Common governance approaches for cross-institutional federated learning are modeled in consortium models which defines formal criteria for membership, participation expectations and decision making processes (Passerat-Palmbach et al. 2020). Such consortia tend to include both data contribution agreements, intellectual property frameworks and publication policies which balance out institutional interests against collective goals.

Questions of data stewardship, data quality and acceptable use are handled by data governance frameworks about federated learning (Rieke et al., 2020). These federation processes have also lead to organizations participating in federations building common data quality metrics, harmonization processes, and validation processes, amongst other things, in order to enforce the minimum standards for federated training on local datasets. Potentially, the federated profiling may entail techniques whose evaluations are not centralized, such as those pertaining to dataset characteristics.

Conflict resolution mechanisms are an important part of governance in federated environments where there will be times when institutional priorities diverge (Rajkomar et al., 2018). To reduce disagreements within the organization, on what should be the federation direction, what is the model development priority, and what will be the model implementation approach, clear processes for resolving the issues should be created. This may be tiered escalation pathways where technical discussions would lead to leadership engagement only on a case by case basis.

Longer term viability of federated learning initiatives is the area addressed by sustainability models. To sustain the ongoing technical maintenance, governance, and model update activity, organizations need to think about how the activity will be funded or the initial enthusiasm will wane (Rieke et al., 2020). Successful federations transfer from a project model funded by grants, to an operational model, integrated with clinical or research workflow, so that resource allocation is supported by value generation.

10. FUTURE DIRECTIONS AND EMERGING TRENDS

10.1 Technological Advancements

However, some of the current limitations in federated learning in healthcare now have solution counterparts in a few technological trends, while new possibilities are presented. In vertical federated learning (features partitioned, not samples), complementary data sources, including clinical record, genomic sequence and social determinants (Yang et al., 2019), can be combined in novel ways. Holistic patient modeling is made possible while concerns about privacy are addressed, such that diverse data categories are not required to be centralized.

Since transfer learning in healthcare settings has limited labeled data, federated transfer learning approaches like transferring the knowledge across institutions and tasks while preserving software and privacy safeguards (Liu et al., 2020). These methods enable information from any institution with smaller datasets to be leveraged by those that possess more data without direct sharing of the data, thereby diminishing healthcare disparities between resource deficient and resource rich communities.

A new paradigm for optimizing clinical decision support systems across multiple institutions without a central repository of patient trajectories is what federated reinforcement learning is. They allow for the development of collaboration among efforts to develop treatment recommendation systems that learn from disparate clinical practices and patient outcomes, while keeping sensitive treatment sequences within its originating institution. Federated reinforcement learning can be applied to applications in domains of sepsis management, medication dosing and ventilator weaning amongst others to aid in clinical decision making.

With edge AI integration to federated learning, the model that learns and infers gets closer to the point of generating data, and this reduces latency and communication requirements (Silva et al., 2019). This integration can support healthcare domain applications for real time monitoring devices, Point of Care diagnostics as well as mobile health apps.

10.2 Multimodal and Integrative Approaches

Temporal modeling in federated healthcare contexts, one of the recent developments in temporal modeling, features longitudinal patient care and therefore allows pattern recognition across patient's complex clinical trajectories without the centralization of the patient's sensitive medical histories (Huang et al., 2020). The temporal pattern recognition can be applied to chronic disease management, post-operative monitoring and treatment response prediction in a variety of patient populations, thus transforming problems posed in them.

The domain of clinical text federated natural language processing is a growing application domain, that enables extracting insights from the narrative documentation while these are being protected by privacy safeguards (Liu et al., 2020). Techniques including federated pretraining, domain adaptation and vocabulary harmonization handle the challenges in institutional language distribution, documents templates and abbreviations usage. Extracting structured as opposed to unstructured insights from unstructured clinical narratives has the potential to be applied to clinical phenotyping, adverse event detection, and care quality assessment across institutions.

Federated meta learning learn how to learn in a variety of healthcare environments and it is emerging paradigm for developing models fast adapt to new clinical contexts at low cost of training (Li et al., 2020). In particular, these approaches are highly complementary when there are limited exemplar data at a single institution, and when these few exemplars represent rare diseases.

10.3 Organizational and Economic Models

Innovative organizational and economic models for sustainable implementation of federated learning in healthcare are needed that will align incentives amongst participating institutions. In value based federation models, accepting participation is conditioned on the quality improvements and cost reductions that can be achieved through improved clinical decision support, which directly lead to ongoing contribution with financial incentives (Rieke et al., 2020). The models commonly use federalized learning as a way to attain quality metrics and outcome improvements within these existing value based payment frameworks.

Federated learning implementations that span academic, industry, and healthcare delivery organizations have emerged as promising environmental frameworks of public-private partnerships (Federated learning advocacy person to person, 2020). Intellectual property frameworks of such partnerships allow the balancing of commercial interest and public health benefits for the set ups that would allow sustainable collaboration while guaranteeing equitable access to innovations derived from these partnerships. An example of this approach is the MELLODDY consortium, consisting of pharmaceutical companies as well as academic institutions and dedicated technology providers in order to perform federated drug discovery research.

Governance models adopted by open federated learning communities are based on those of open-source software development and facilitate the establishment of open transparent contribution mechanisms, shared model repositories, and collaborative development processes (Roth et al., 2020). These communities democratize federated learning capabilities that normally require enormous technical infrastructure or expertise, and provide smaller institutions a way to participate in model development without extreme technical or scientific expertise from the start. Technically, there are such projects as OpenFL and PySyft, which offer easy to use frameworks for federated implementation.

Federated healthcare AI can be tested in regulatory sandboxes with controlled environments to minimize the uncertainty of regulatory interventions and make it approached with appropriate oversight (Gerke et al., 2020). In response, organizations can set up these programs, having collaboration between a healthcare institution and its regulatory body to establish those programs so that specifically during programs federated learning can be done with modified compliance requirements in exchange of increased transparency and monitoring. Such technology innovation acceleration techniques harness the strengths of these approaches in guaranteeing both patient privacy and safety.

10.4 Integration with Emerging Healthcare Delivery Models

By their nature federated learning fits well within emerging healthcare delivery models based around decentralization, coordination and patient centrist ideas. Federated learning is implemented in accountable care organizations (ACOs) and integrated delivery networks more often in an effort to foster care coordination and quality improvement within institutional boundaries (Brisimi et al., 2018).

The COVID-19 pandemic accelerated telehealth expansion and, along with it, has opened new possibilities and new hurdles for federated learning. Large amounts of data are generated with virtual care platforms distributed over large areas with often unconventional boundaries and alternative privacy concerns. Collaborative model development across telehealth networks is facilitated by federated approaches which ensure data segregation among participating providers and technology platforms, but still allow for collaborative model development amongst participating providers as if it was performed by a fabricated single provider.

Federated learning is an emerging concept that merges learning health system frameworks which leverage federated learning as a tool for continuous quality improvement and generation of evidence without compromising privacy (Rajkomar et al., 2018). By these implementations, healthcare systems can learn about routine care delivery without infringing on appropriate boundaries between clinical operations and research activities. Knowledge generation and dissemination of knowledge is enabled over distributed care environments by federal approaches that respect the institutional autonomy and patient privacy.

Federated learning has emerged as a mechanism to enable collaborative model development across resource settings without the extraction of data from vulnerable populations as world wide initiatives for global health equity have started (Rieke et al., 2020). Resultantly, healthcare institutions from low and middle income countries are facilitated to engage equitably in AI development by sharing their special clinical wisdoms as well as laying claim to their data sovereignty. Such approaches meet the concerns with algorithmic colonialism in global health AI, by ensuring that the models thus generated are beneficial to the contributing populations.

11. IMPLEMENTATION ROADMAP FOR HEALTHCARE ORGANIZATIONS

11.1 Strategic Planning and Stakeholder Engagement

Since federated learning is repurposing training data and enlisting data from multiple locations, one should start with comprehensive strategic planning in order to decide about center/boundary ownership, choose clear objectives, find appropriate uses cases, and align with other institutional priorities. This planning process should evaluate the clinical, operational and research applications, weight factors like dataset characteristics, collaboration opportunities, technical feasibility and potential impact (Rieke et al., 2020). Given that federated approaches tend to only make sense where there is a clear advantage relative to the alternatives of both local and centralized approaches, organizations should prioritize use cases involving sensitive data that cannot be pooled, as well as applications which get significant benefit from being multi-institutional.

Therefore, stakeholder engagement has emerged as a critical success factor for the implementation of federated learning across different perspectives of an organization (Rajkomar et al., 2018). Domain expertise in the use case selection, feature identification and validation of model is available with clinical leaders, technical teams evaluate infrastructure needs and approaches of implementation, legal and law compliance concerned to handle regulatory requirements and executive leadership to make sure that the strategic focus and resource allocation are aligned.

In terms of federated learning planning, patient and community engagement should be included (Price & Cohen, 2019), especially for applications that may pose an ethics concern or that act on vulnerable populations. For example, mechanisms such as patient advisory boards, community consultations and open communication of federated learning activities and security measures should be considered by organizations. In addition to addressing ethical considerations, these engagement approaches involve 'diverse' perspectives on the use case priorities and outcome measures that enhance implementation.

The risks and mitigation planning for federated implementations should consider special challenges such as technical failures, inequality of participants' involvement, privacy risks, and regulatory uncertainties (Kaissis et al., 2020). Therefore, organizations should develop contingency plans in such a case when a participant withdrew, the model performance degrades or the Regulatory requirements evolve. As the federated implementation completes more maturation and new risks appear, these assessments should be reissued periodically.

11.2 Technical Implementation Considerations

First, technical implementation should start with data readiness assessment including availability, quality, and standardization of data across participating institutions for the use cases that have been selected (Lehne et al., 2019). The required data harmonization for effective federated training needs to be identified for organizations, i.e. identifying maps on terminology, feature extraction approaches and quality improvement processes. Typically, these assessments identify institutional differences in documentation practices, diagnostic coding, data completeness, which must be assuaged prior to being put into place.

When selecting federated learning framework, implementation maturity, security features, interoperability with other existing systems and alignment with the use case should be considered (Rieke et al., 2020). There is a variety of established frameworks such as TensorFlow Federated, PySyft, FATE, OpenFL, that organizations can use or custom implementations may be developed if organizations have specialized requirements. All of these factors should be taken into account in choosing this selection: current capabilities, development trajectories, and community support for further maintenance and enhancement of the forecast system.

A crucial technical consideration for implementations of the system supporting direct patient care is the integration with existing clinical systems. The gap between federated learning platforms and electronic health records, imaging systems, laboratory information systems and other clinical repositories is the topic for organizations to develop interfaces for (Rajkomar et al., 2018). Data extraction for training the model and delivery of results to support clinical decisions must be captured in these integrations, and they should fit into existing workflows to avoid disrupting them.

Technological wraps must ensure security at multiple levels (data access controls, communication channels, privacy enhancing technologies relevant to the case and risk profile) (Kaissis et al., 2020). They should use encryption for data at rest and in transit, access logging, secure aggregation protocols, as well as other privacy safeguards, such as differential privacy, as necessary.

11.3 Governance Implementation

Formal structures that span the participating institutions are needed for effective governance implementation, but that do not compromise on maintaining autonomy at participating organizations. The strategic part of these federated steering committees frequently serves to create answers — to whom to be the priority, who to partner with, what to fund, etc. — and thus involves questions of prioritization of use cases, resource allocation, and development of partnerships. According to these committees, they should have executive representation from each of the participating organizations, decision making among institutional interests and collective goals.

Federated implementations are operational governed through technical working groups that answer questions of data standards, model architectures, training protocols, and validation methods (Rieke et al., 2020). Usually, these groups will consist of data scientists, software engineers and clinical informaticists from the participating institutions as well as domain experts to contribute, as there is a need to address implementation challenges and to maintain uniform technical approaches across the federation.

The federation (Rajkomar et al., 2018) establishes standards for the contribution of data; quality assessment, as well as the acceptable use of the data, across the federation. In most cases, they develop common data models, privacy safeguards, quality metrics and contribution expectations that balance federated training with institutional data stewardship responsibility. Often, effective implementations include federated data profiling mechanisms that quantify the degree of dataset differences across participants without bringing together sensitive information into a central repository.

Machines to compliance oversight mechanisms — compliance oversight mechanisms are used to ensure compliance to regulatory requirements, ethical standards, federation policies within the participating institutions (Gerke et al., 2020). They usually involve regular process of auditing, demanding documentation and reporting structures that can show how appropriate safeguards can be used without excessive administrative burden. They oversee effective implementations which standardize documentation of compliance while taking into consideration jurisdiction specific variations.

12. EVALUATION AND CONTINUOUS IMPROVEMENT

Federated learning implementations require the evaluation on a number of technical, clinical, operational efficiency and ethical dimensions. Metrics should be set up in each dimension based on the measurement approach that acknowledges the federated nature of the implementation. These evaluations need to look at both the institutional impacts and the federation-wide outcomes, including instances in which collective benefits will not be the same as the results for the individual.

Part of model performance monitoring should be automated appraisal of statistical performance on individual contributors involved in the model to flag quality-based problems like model drift, widespread differences in mobile performance across subphantoms, or completely unpredicted observations (Kaissis et al., 2020). Such monitoring systems should also have alert mechanism to notify relevant governance bodies when metrics fall beyond acceptable ranges, leading the trigger of investigation and possible intervention.

In order to determine the clinical impact of federated models, it should be evaluated whether it provides the expected improvement in care quality, efficiency, or outcomes when it is implemented in practice (Rajkomar et al., 2018). They may consist of pre/post comparisons or interrupted time series evaluations, or if possible randomized evaluations. Implementations are effective because they take into account that what may be impact for some institutions may not be impact for others because of different patient populations, clinical workflow and implementation approaches.

To assess workflow integration, federated learning capabilities incorporated into clinical operations should be evaluated based on the extent to which they are accepts by users, are efficient in the workflow and sustainable at an operational level (Rieke et al., 2020). When these assessments consist of both quantitative metrics of system utilization and qualitative feedback from clinicians and operational staff, they are typically referred to as these. This feedback is used to implement this in continuous improvement cycles to improve integration.

In participation equity, contribution quality, and governance effectiveness, federation health assessment should cover the collaborative ecosystem (Passerat-Palmbach et al., 2020). However, these assessments tend to be oriented towards factors like participation rates, contribution diversities, decision satisfaction, and such sustainability metrics. These assessments are used effectively to fulfill the stakeholders' goals of defining improvement opportunities in federation structure, incentive models, and governance process for long term viability.

13. CONCLUSION

Federated learning could be considered as a major stride in the healthcare AI because it forms a sophisticated approach to solving the trade off between data driven advancement and privacy preservation. This approach roughly achieves the operational necessity of large rich datasets whilst complying with the ethic and legal requirements imposed on healthcare information by enabling collaborative training of machine learning models in multiple healthcare institutions, keeping those sensitive patient data in siloes within their respective facilities.

Federated learning seems on its way to being a big thing in healthcare, and while multimodal learning, edge computing, special AI hardware have been emerging and will continue to improve capabilities and eliminate barriers to implementation. Governed by a thoughtful set of frameworks and building on sustainable business models, as well as future technological innovations, federated learning provides a way to personalized medicine as well as evidence based healthcare through respecting institutional boundaries, without destroying established boundaries for individual benefits by generating collective knowledge.

REFERENCES

Ayaz, M., Pasha, M. F., Alzahrani, M. Y., Budiarto, R., & Stiawan, D. (2021). The Fast Health Interoperability Resources (FHIR) standard: Systematic literature review of implementations, applications, challenges and opportunities. *JMIR Medical Informatics, 9*(7), e21929. DOI: 10.2196/21929 PMID: 34328424

Bagdasaryan, E., Veit, A., Hua, Y., Estrin, D., & Shmatikov, V. (2020, June). How to backdoor federated learning. In *International conference on artificial intelligence and statistics* (pp. 2938-2948). PMLR.

Beam, A. L., Manrai, A. K., & Ghassemi, M. (2020). Challenges to the reproducibility of machine learning models in health care. *Journal of the American Medical Association, 323*(4), 305–306. DOI: 10.1001/jama.2019.20866 PMID: 31904799

Bonawitz, K., Ivanov, V., Kreuter, B., Marcedone, A., McMahan, H. B., Patel, S., Ramage, D., Segal, A., & Seth, K. (2017). Practical secure aggregation for privacy-preserving machine learning. In *Proceedings of the 2017 ACM SIGSAC Conference on Computer and Communications Security* (pp. 1175-1191). DOI: 10.1145/3133956.3133982

Boughorbel, S., Jarray, F., Venugopal, N., Moosa, S., Elhadi, H., & Makhlouf, M. (2019). Federated uncertainty-aware learning for distributed hospital ehr data. *arXiv preprint arXiv:1910.12191.*

Brisimi, T. S., Chen, R., Mela, T., Olshevsky, A., Paschalidis, I. C., & Shi, W. (2018). Federated learning of predictive models from federated electronic health records. *International Journal of Medical Informatics, 112*, 59–67. DOI: 10.1016/j.ijmedinf.2018.01.007 PMID: 29500022

Chen, Y., Yang, X., Qin, X., Yu, H., Chen, J., & Sun, J. (2021). FedHealth 2: Weighted federated transfer learning via batch normalization for personalized healthcare. In Machine Learning for Healthcare Conference (pp. 1-22).

Cohen, I. G., & Mello, M. M. (2018). HIPAA and protecting health information in the 21st century. *Journal of the American Medical Association, 320*(3), 231–232. DOI: 10.1001/jama.2018.5630 PMID: 29800120

Denny, J. C., Ritchie, M. D., Basford, M. A., Pulley, J. M., Bastarache, L., Brown-Gentry, K., Wang, D., Masys, D. R., Roden, D. M., & Crawford, D. C. (2010). PheWAS: Demonstrating the feasibility of a phenome-wide scan to discover gene–disease associations. *Bioinformatics (Oxford, England), 26*(9), 1205–1210. DOI: 10.1093/bioinformatics/btq126 PMID: 20335276

Doshi-Velez, F., & Kim, B. (2017). Towards a rigorous science of interpretable machine learning. arXiv preprint arXiv:1702.08608.

Dwork, C., & Roth, A. (2014). The algorithmic foundations of differential privacy. *Foundations and Trends in Theoretical Computer Science*, *9*(3-4), 211–407. DOI: 10.1561/0400000042

Fredrikson, M., Jha, S., & Ristenpart, T. (2015). Model inversion attacks that exploit confidence information and basic countermeasures. In *Proceedings of the 22nd ACM SIGSAC Conference on Computer and Communications Security* (pp. 1322-1333). DOI: 10.1145/2810103.2813677

Garza, M., Del Fiol, G., Tenenbaum, J., Walden, A., & Zozus, M. N. (2016). Evaluating common data models for use with a longitudinal community registry. *Journal of Biomedical Informatics*, *64*, 333–341. DOI: 10.1016/j.jbi.2016.10.016 PMID: 27989817

Gerke, S., Minssen, T., & Cohen, G. (2020). Ethical and legal challenges of artificial intelligence-driven healthcare. In *Artificial Intelligence in Healthcare* (pp. 295–336). Academic Press. DOI: 10.1016/B978-0-12-818438-7.00012-5

Huang, L., Yin, Y., Fu, Z., Zhang, S., Deng, H., & Liu, D. (2020). LoAdaBoost: Loss-based AdaBoost federated machine learning with reduced computational complexity on IID and non-IID intensive care data. *PLoS One*, *15*(4), e0230706. DOI: 10.1371/journal.pone.0230706 PMID: 32302316

Johnson, A. E., Pollard, T. J., Shen, L., Lehman, L. W. H., Feng, M., Ghassemi, M., Moody, B., Szolovits, P., Anthony Celi, L., & Mark, R. G. (2016). MIMIC-III, a freely accessible critical care database. *Scientific Data*, *3*(1), 1–9. DOI: 10.1038/sdata.2016.35 PMID: 27219127

Kairouz, P., McMahan, H. B., Avent, B., Bellet, A., Bennis, M., Bhagoji, A. N., ... & Zhao, S. (2021). Advances and open problems in federated learning. *Foundations and trends® in machine learning, 14*(1–2), 1-210.

Kaissis, G., Ziller, A., Passerat-Palmbach, J., Ryffel, T., Usynin, D., Trask, A., Lima, I.Jr, Mancuso, J., Jungmann, F., Steinborn, M.-M., Saleh, A., Makowski, M., Rueckert, D., & Braren, R. (2021). End-to-end privacy preserving deep learning on multi-institutional medical imaging. *Nature Machine Intelligence*, *3*(6), 473–484. DOI: 10.1038/s42256-021-00337-8

Kaissis, G. A., Makowski, M. R., Rückert, D., & Braren, R. F. (2020). Secure, privacy-preserving and federated machine learning in medical imaging. *Nature Machine Intelligence*, *2*(6), 305–311. DOI: 10.1038/s42256-020-0186-1

Karimireddy, S. P., Kale, S., Mohri, M., Reddi, S., Stich, S., & Suresh, A. T. (2020, November). Scaffold: Stochastic controlled averaging for federated learning. In *International conference on machine learning* (pp. 5132-5143). PMLR.

Kulkarni, V., Kulkarni, M., & Pant, A. (2020, July). Survey of personalization techniques for federated learning. In *2020 fourth world conference on smart trends in systems, security and sustainability (WorldS4)* (pp. 794-797). IEEE. DOI: 10.1109/WorldS450073.2020.9210355

Lehne, M., Sass, J., Essenwanger, A., Schepers, J., & Thun, S. (2019). Why digital medicine depends on interoperability. *NPJ Digital Medicine*, *2*(1), 79. DOI: 10.1038/s41746-019-0158-1 PMID: 31453374

Li, T., Sahu, A. K., Talwalkar, A., & Smith, V. (2020). Federated learning: Challenges, methods, and future directions. *IEEE Signal Processing Magazine*, *37*(3), 50–60. DOI: 10.1109/MSP.2020.2975749

Li, T., Sahu, A. K., Zaheer, M., Sanjabi, M., Talwalkar, A., & Smith, V. (2020). Federated optimization in heterogeneous networks. *Proceedings of Machine learning and systems, 2*, 429-450.

Li, X., Gu, Y., Dvornek, N., Staib, L. H., Ventola, P., & Duncan, J. S. (2020). Multi-site fMRI analysis using privacy-preserving federated learning and domain adaptation: ABIDE results. *Medical Image Analysis*, *65*, 101765. DOI: 10.1016/j.media.2020.101765 PMID: 32679533

Li, X., Huang, K., Yang, W., Wang, S., & Zhang, Z. (2019). On the convergence of FedAvg on non-IID data. In *International Conference on Learning Representations.*

Liu, Y., Kang, Y., Xing, C., Chen, T., & Yang, Q. (2020). A secure federated transfer learning framework. *IEEE Intelligent Systems*, *35*(4), 70–82. DOI: 10.1109/MIS.2020.2988525

Lu, M. Y., Chen, R. J., Kong, D., Lipkova, J., Singh, R., Williamson, D. F., Chen, T. Y., & Mahmood, F. (2022). Federated learning for computational pathology on gigapixel whole slide images. *Medical Image Analysis*, *76*, 102298. DOI: 10.1016/j.media.2021.102298 PMID: 34911013

McMahan, B., Moore, E., Ramage, D., Hampson, S., & Arcas, B. A. (2017, April). Communication-efficient learning of deep networks from decentralized data. In *Artificial intelligence and statistics* (pp. 1273–1282). PMLR.

Mo, F., & Haddadi, H. (2019, March). Efficient and private federated learning using tee. In *Proc. EuroSys Conf.,* Dresden, Germany (p. 1).

Nguyen, D. C., Ding, M., Pathirana, P. N., Seneviratne, A., Li, J., & Poor, H. V. (2021). Federated learning for internet of things: A comprehensive survey. *IEEE Communications Surveys and Tutorials*, *23*(3), 1622–1658. DOI: 10.1109/COMST.2021.3075439

Papernot, N., Song, S., Mironov, I., Raghunathan, A., Talwar, K., & Erlingsson, Ú. (2018). Scalable private learning with pate. *arXiv preprint arXiv:1802.08908.*

Passerat-Palmbach, J., Farnan, T., Miller, R., Gross, M. S., Flannery, H. L., & Gleim, B. (2020). A blockchain-orchestrated federated learning architecture for healthcare consortia. *arXiv preprint arXiv:1910.12603.*

Poirot, M. G., Vepakomma, P., Chang, K., Kalpathy-Cramer, J., Gupta, R., & Raskar, R. (2019). Split learning for collaborative deep learning in healthcare. arXiv preprint arXiv:1912.12115.

Price, W. N.II, & Cohen, I. G. (2019). Privacy in the age of medical big data. *Nature Medicine*, *25*(1), 37–43. DOI: 10.1038/s41591-018-0272-7 PMID: 30617331

Rajkomar, A., Dean, J., & Kohane, I. (2019). Machine learning in medicine. *The New England Journal of Medicine*, *380*(14), 1347–1358. DOI: 10.1056/NEJMra1814259 PMID: 30943338

Rajkomar, A., Oren, E., Chen, K., Dai, A. M., Hajaj, N., Hardt, M., Liu, P. J., Liu, X., Marcus, J., Sun, M., Sundberg, P., Yee, H., Zhang, K., Zhang, Y., Flores, G., Duggan, G. E., Irvine, J., Le, Q., Litsch, K., & Dean, J. (2018). Scalable and accurate deep learning with electronic health records. *NPJ Digital Medicine*, *1*(1), 18. DOI: 10.1038/s41746-018-0029-1 PMID: 31304302

Rieke, N., Hancox, J., Li, W., Milletari, F., Roth, H. R., Albarqouni, S., Bakas, S., Galtier, M. N., Landman, B. A., Maier-Hein, K., Ourselin, S., Sheller, M., Summers, R. M., Trask, A., Xu, D., Baust, M., & Cardoso, M. J. (2020). The future of digital health with federated learning. *NPJ Digital Medicine*, *3*(1), 119. DOI: 10.1038/s41746-020-00323-1 PMID: 33015372

Roth, H. R., Chang, K., Singh, P., Neumark, N., Li, W., Gupta, V., & Kalpathy-Cramer, J. (2020, September). Federated learning for breast density classification: A real-world implementation. In *MICCAI Workshop on Domain Adaptation and Representation Transfer* (pp. 181-191). Cham: Springer International Publishing. DOI: 10.1007/978-3-030-60548-3_18

Sheller, M. J., Edwards, B., Reina, G. A., Martin, J., Pati, S., Kotrotsou, A., Milchenko, M., Xu, W., Marcus, D., Colen, R. R., & Bakas, S. (2020). Federated learning in medicine: Facilitating multi-institutional collaborations without sharing patient data. *Scientific Reports*, *10*(1), 12598. DOI: 10.1038/s41598-020-69250-1 PMID: 32724046

Shokri, R., Stronati, M., Song, C., & Shmatikov, V. (2017, May). Membership inference attacks against machine learning models. In *2017 IEEE symposium on security and privacy (SP)* (pp. 3-18). IEEE. DOI: 10.1109/SP.2017.41

Silva, S., Gutman, B. A., Romero, E., Thompson, P. M., Altmann, A., & Lorenzi, M. (2019, April). Federated learning in distributed medical databases: Meta-analysis of large-scale subcortical brain data. In *2019 IEEE 16th international symposium on biomedical imaging (ISBI 2019)* (pp. 270-274). IEEE.

Vepakomma, P., Gupta, O., Swedish, T., & Raskar, R. (2018). Split learning for health: Distributed deep learning without sharing raw patient data. *arXiv preprint arXiv:1812.00564*.

Xu, J., Glicksberg, B. S., Su, C., Walker, P., Bian, J., & Wang, F. (2021). Federated learning for healthcare informatics. *Journal of Healthcare Informatics Research*, *5*(1), 1–19. DOI: 10.1007/s41666-020-00082-4 PMID: 33204939

Yale, A., Dash, S., Dutta, R., Guyon, I., Pavao, A., & Bennett, K. P. (2019, April). Privacy preserving synthetic health data. In *ESANN 2019-European Symposium on Artificial Neural Networks, Computational Intelligence and Machine Learning*.

Yang, Q., Liu, Y., Chen, T., & Tong, Y. (2019). Federated machine learning: Concept and applications. [TIST]. *ACM Transactions on Intelligent Systems and Technology*, *10*(2), 1–19. DOI: 10.1145/3298981

Chapter 7
Enhancing Security and Insight in Federated Learning for AI-Driven Healthcare

Manju M. S.
https://orcid.org/0009-0007-2029-4666
Maulana Azad National Institute of Technology, Bhopal, India

ABSTRACT

This chapter explores the integration of Federated Learning (FL) and Explainable Artificial Intelligence (XAI) in healthcare, emphasizing their potential to revolutionize AI-driven medical solutions while preserving data privacy and building trust. It examines how FL enables collaborative model training across decentralized data sources without sharing sensitive patient information, addressing critical issues of data security and compliance. The chapter also investigates the role of XAI in enhancing interpretability and transparency in federated models, a crucial factor for clinical adoption. Through discussion of local and global explainability, real-world applications, and emerging challenges such as data heterogeneity, communication costs, and algorithmic bias, the chapter provides a comprehensive view of how FL and XAI jointly contribute to more secure, accountable, and effective AI systems in healthcare.

1. INTRODUCTION

Artificial intelligence (AI) has dramatically impacted the field of healthcare and is changing the way diseases are identified, monitored, and treated. The extent

DOI: 10.4018/979-8-3373-3306-9.ch007

of AI-enabled systems ranges from automated image interpretation to predictive modelling of patient outcomes, creating the possibility of more timely, accurate, and cost-effective interventions. The healthcare sector produces extensive amounts of data, such as electronic health records (EHRs), medical imaging, genomic sequences, and readings from wearable devices. AI methods, particularly those based on deep learning, can identify patterns and relations in dataset resources that are often difficult to accomplish using traditional statistical methods or by human clinicians. For example, convolutional neural networks (CNNs) have provided high-quality classification for diabetic retinopathy (Gulshan et al., 2016), breast cancer (Yala et al., 2019), and skin lesions (Esteva et al., 2017), while recurrent models have provided patient risk predictions from sequential EHR data (Choi et al., 2016). All these innovations have resulted in better diagnostic accuracy, earlier disease detection, and personalized treatment recommendations. AI is also instrumental in pandemic response planning, resource allocation, drug discovery, and the management of real-time patient monitoring areas in which speed and scalability matter (Topol, 2019, p. 51).

Figure 1. Centralized AI in Healthcare

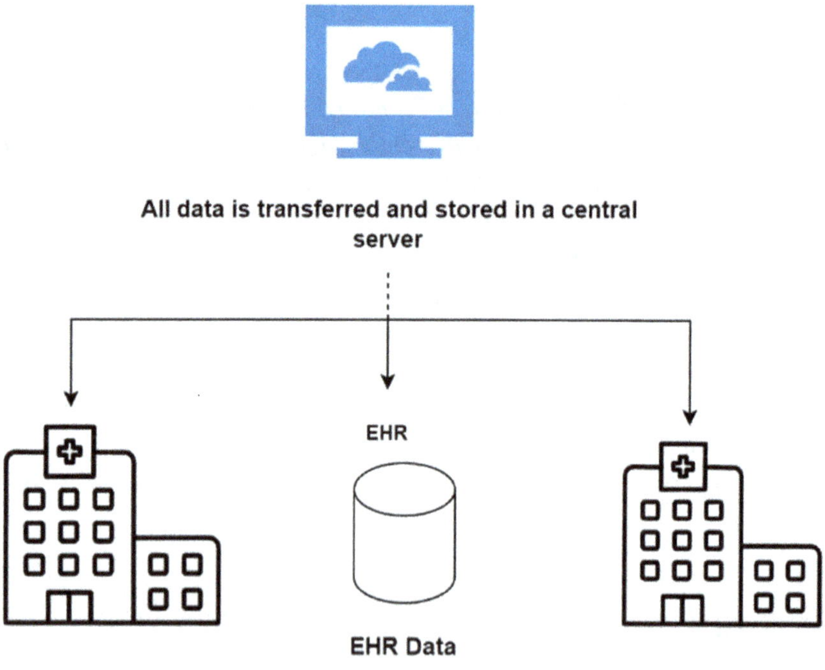

While AI has transformational potential, its clinical implementation is complicated by ethical, legal, and technical barriers, many stemming from centralized models.

Figure 1 illustrates a centralized AI model where EHR data from multiple hospitals is transmitted to and stored on a central server. While this setup allows unified model training and analysis, it raises significant concerns about data privacy, legal compliance, vulnerability to failures, and lack of inclusivity. Protected by laws such as HIPAA (USA) and GDPR (EU), patient data cannot be easily shared without legal and ethical implications (Kaissis et al., 2020). Additionally, centralized AI models represent single points of failure, suffer from algorithmic bias, particularly underrepresented populations (Rajkomar et al., 2018), and are inherently opaque, which makes it difficult for clinicians and patients to trust them. Given these challenges, there is a rising need for AI systems in healthcare that are decentralized, secure, and interpretable. The ideal AI model in healthcare should meet three key criteria:

- Data privacy: Patient data should not leave the institution.
- Model transparency: The system should be interpretable to foster trust.
- Collaborative learning: Knowledge should be aggregated from multiple sources to improve model generalization.

This necessitates a paradigm that supports privacy, inclusivity (allowing smaller hospitals to participate), and trustworthiness. Federated Learning (FL) is one such framework that supports these goals.

Table 1. Comparison with Traditional Centralized Learning

Centralized Learning	Federated Learning
All data is transferred and stored in a central server	Data remains local at each participating institution
High risk of data breaches and privacy violations	Improved privacy and security through data locality
Single point of failure and potential data monopoly	Decentralized architecture minimizes systemic risk
Limited data diversity if participation is low	Inclusion of diverse datasets from multiple institutions

Table 1 compares centralized learning and federated learning, showing a few of the differences in data handling, privacy, system architecture, and data diversity. Centralized learning requires all data to be uploaded, stored, and processed on one central server, which introduces various risks, including data breaches, systemic failure, and privacy breaches. FL increases participant privacy as the data can remain at the site. FL architecture gathers all data together, but a decentralized framework increases privacy and security. Additionally, federated learning has the advantage of more datasets from a range of contributing sources for learning, for better generalization across tasks. This chapter proceeds as follows: Section 2 introduces the foundations of FL in healthcare. Section 3 outlines key security architectures used in FL. Section 4 explores Explainable AI (XAI) techniques in federated settings. Section 5 highlights real-world applications of FL in clinical practice. Section 6 discusses major challenges and research opportunities. Finally, Section 7 concludes with reflections on the future of secure and interpretable AI in healthcare.

2. FEDERATED LEARNING (FL)

Federated Learning, first popularized by Google (McMahan et al., 2017, p. 1273), is a decentralized machine learning (ML) approach that enables multiple parties to collaboratively train a shared model without transferring raw data. Instead, institutions train models locally and send only model updates (like gradients or weights) to a central server, which aggregates them (e.g., via Federated Averaging) and updates a global model. This global model is then redistributed to participants.

Figure 2. Federated Learning in Healthcare

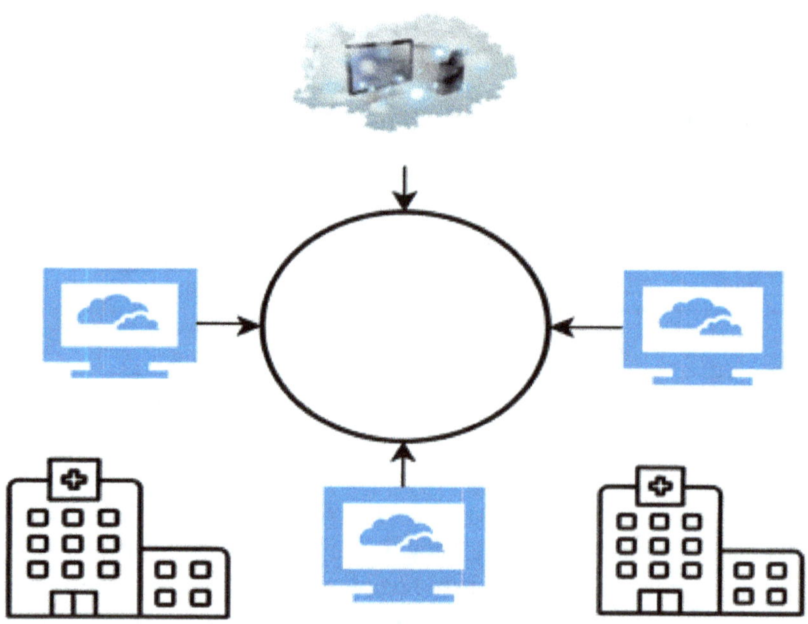

Figure 2 shows there are a number of hospitals, shown as buildings, that each have local computers to train their own machine learning models using their own patient data. Each of these computers shares the updates of the models to an aggregation server, shown as a circular hub, which aggregates the updates and sends back a better global model. The cloud is there to remind you about the role of cloud infrastructure in providing secure communication and supplying centralized aggregation of patient data without ever having sensitive data being shared. FL ensures compliance with data protection laws while enhancing security and maintaining performance. Research shows FL's effectiveness in medical imaging tasks such as brain tumor segmentation (Sheller et al., 2018, 92–93; W. Li et al., 2019) and COVID-19 diagnosis, achieving results comparable to centralized learning. It supports generalization through exposure to diverse data sources and adapts over time via "federated continual learning" (Yang et al., 2024). However, challenges such as communication cost, non-IID data, and model attacks persist and are addressed using techniques like secure multiparty computation, differential privacy, and robust aggregation (Rieke et al., 2020, pp. 2-3). FL operates by training models at each participating site and sharing only model parameters, preserving patient data privacy. It reduces the need for centralized data storage. It ensures local compliance with security protocols and regulatory mandates.

Benefits for Healthcare (Data Privacy, Bandwidth Savings, Generalization)

- Data Privacy: Raw patient data is not transferred to preserve confidentiality.
- Bandwidth Savings: Only model parameters are transmitted to reduce communication overhead.
- Generalization: Exposure to heterogeneous datasets enhances robustness and model applicability across populations.

Beyond the standard FL, additional approaches have emerged. Structured FL reduces the communication and storage constraints on model updates. Instead of sending full parameter sets, clients transmit compressed updates, such as sparse vectors, low-rank matrix approximations, or quantized weights. This reduces the size of communication payloads, lowering bandwidth requirements. Clustered FL is another approach that addresses statistical heterogeneity by grouping clients with similar data distributions into clusters and training separate models for each cluster. This mitigates the adverse impact of non-IID data on global model convergence by ensuring that model updates are aggregated among clients with aligned objectives and distributions. Clustering can be performed using metrics such as cosine similarity between model updates or Euclidean distance between feature representations. Other variations include Personalized FL, which modifies models for individual clients to fit patterns within their unique data. Hierarchical FL, which describes an approach where updates are aggregated through intermediate nodes (for example, through hospital networks) before reaching a central server. Each of these variants can also play a key role in ensuring that models are accurate, efficient, and adaptable across different clinical situations.

FL helps meet principles in HIPAA/GDPR, but legal compliance requires additional measures:

- Data minimization: Only essential data (e.g., weights) is transmitted.
- Consent and control: Data remains under the control of its origin institution.
- Accountability: Auditable processes support transparency and legal compliance.

FL is being applied in radiology, pathology, genomics, and wearable-based health monitoring. NVIDIA's Clara FL platform is enabling multi-hospital collaborations for cancer and cardiac imaging (Brisimi et al., 2018). The Federated Tumor Segmentation (FeTS) challenge has further highlighted FL's role in real-world medical AI. FL is now also being extended to EHR tabular data and ICU time-series data, making it central to future healthcare AI architectures. Moreover, integration with Explainable AI (XAI) is increasing to ensure interpretability and clinical adoption (Dayan et al., 2021).

3. SECURITY ARCHITECTURES IN FEDERATED LEARNING

FL is a decentralized systems approach that develops models while keeping raw data at the client or institution (e.g., organization). FL mitigates the risks of direct exposure to sensitive data. However, clients using FL may have exposure in the aspects of inference attacks, model inversion attacks, gradient leakage, and poisoning attacks (McMahan et al., 2017, p. 1274). Privacy is a concern for many areas, but it is a paramount concern in the domain of health care. Because health care data is sensitive in nature and often legislated against, "just" going decentralized is insufficient.

Figure 3. Federated Learning Architecture in a Hospital Network

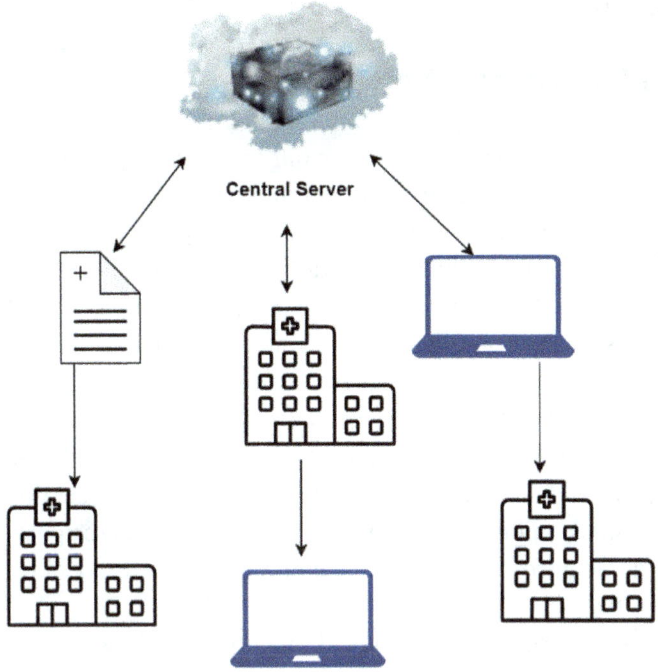

Figure 3 displays an example of Federated Learning architecture within a hospital network. In this model, many host hospitals hold sensitive patient data locally and train local models concurrently with one another. The hospitals can train the models on-site with their sources of patient data, using any computer or laptop (node), and sending only encrypted model updates to a central server. The central server gathers the updates to improve the global model and redistributes the new model to the hospitals. Therefore, there is no direct data sharing, still enabling collaborative intelligence across health care institutions.

The central federated learning system does not depend on a single security model, but rather a layered security model for the entire system. It is a good idea to combine statistical protocols with cryptographic protocols for more secure protection. The four pillars of security in FL include:

1. Secure Aggregation Protocols - ensuring that individual model updates remain confidential during aggregation
2. Differential Privacy - injecting noise to limit the leakage of individual data points
3. Homomorphic Encryption - allowing computation on encrypted data

4. Blockchain - providing an immutable and auditable log of transactions for accountability

3.1 Secure Aggregation Protocols

With secure aggregation, the server can only view the aggregate model updates that the clients have conducted, and not their individual contributions. This is especially important in health care scenarios, as a single update might capture patterns associated with a specific individual's data (Bonawitz et al., 2017). The standard protocol is essentially for each client to encrypt their local model updates using a pairwise shared key. Then the client sends its encrypted model updates to the cloud. The server then only sees the aggregate of all the clients encrypted model updates, so only the aggregate itself is revealed. No individual gradients, staleness, or values are revealed, thus ensuring that all updates are secure, even when the server has become compromised. Examples of applications in the health care domain include secure tumor segmentation tasks using the BraTS dataset, where updates from MRI images were aggregated securely to create one generalized model (Sheller et al., 2018, pp. 100–102).

A standard secure aggregation protocol functions as follows:

- Each client i computes a local model update Δw_i, then encrypts it using a mask or key shared with other participants.
- Specifically, each client generates pairwise random masks $r_{\{ij\}}$ with every other client j, and the final encrypted update is $\widehat{w}_i = \Delta w_i + \sum_j r_{\{ij\}} - \sum_j r_{\{ji\}}$, ensuring the random values cancel out during aggregation.
- These masked updates are sent to the server, which computes $\sum_i \widehat{w}_i$. The masks cancel out due to symmetric sharing, and the server only sees the sum $\sum_i \Delta w_i$, with no access to the individual Δw_i.

This approach supports dropout resilience, allowing the system to proceed even if some clients fail to send their updates. However, it introduces communication overhead and requires coordination to share masking keys securely.

Figure 4. Secure Aggregation & Encrypted Update Flow

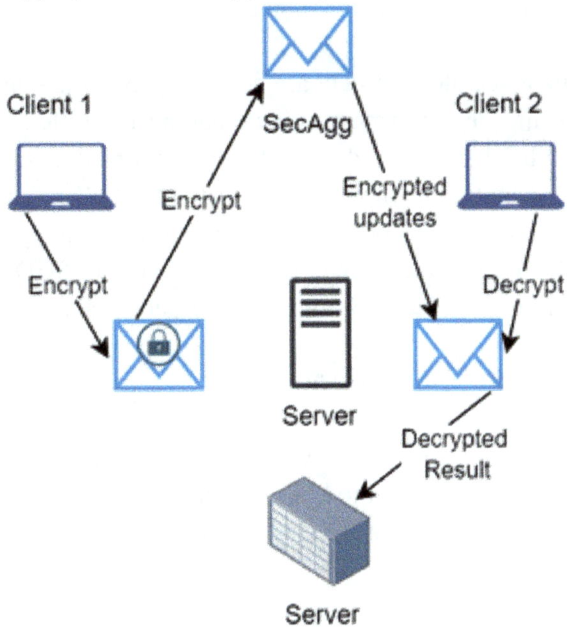

The Secure Aggregation and Encrypted Update Flow is represented in Figure 4. In this workflow, multiple clients (e.g., hospitals) encrypt their local model updates and send them to a secure aggregation module (SecAgg). SecAgg can add the encrypted updates and send the aggregated result to the central server.

3.2 Differential Privacy

Differential privacy (DP) is the mathematical approach of adding noise to data or model gradients prior to sharing the data or model gradients so that the contribution of a single data point to the model output is limited (Dwork et al., 2006). The DP mechanism in FL typically involves:

- Gradient Clipping: Local gradients g is clipped to a predefined norm C:
- $\tilde{g} = \frac{g}{\max\left(1, \frac{\|g\|^{2}}{C}\right)}$
- Noise Addition: Add calibrated Gaussian noise $N(0, \sigma^2 C^2 I)$ to the clipped gradients:

$$\hat{g} = \tilde{g} + N(0, \sigma^2 C^2 I)$$

- Privacy Accounting: Privacy loss is tracked using parameters (ε, δ) over multiple rounds using tools like the moment's accountant or Rényi DP.

The trade-offs associated with DP are between privacy and utility. Adding too much noise can impede performance, while adding too little noise can compromise privacy. DP has been utilized to predict hospital readmission in a healthcare FL context while maintaining the privacy of patient data (Brisimi et al., 2018, pp. 60–61). More advanced forms of DP are becoming increasingly common, including Differentially Private Stochastic Gradient Descent (DP-SGD), which are more readily usable within deep learning workflows (Abadi et al., 2016).

3.3 Homomorphic Encryption

Homomorphic encryption (HE) allows for computation on encrypted data without decrypting it. This allows a server to aggregate encrypted model updates and return the encrypted global model to the clients who decrypt it with their keys (Acar et al., 2018). In practical terms:

- Each client encrypts its model update Δw_i using a public key under a homomorphic encryption scheme (e.g., Paillier or BFV).
- The server performs homomorphic addition on the ciphertexts:
- $Enc\left(\sum_i \Delta w_i\right) = \bigoplus_i Enc\left(\Delta w_i\right)$
- The resulting encrypted aggregate is returned to the clients, who decrypt it using a shared or private decryption key.

There are two main categories in homomorphic encryption. Firstly, partially homomorphic encryption (PHE), supports only one operation (e.g., addition in Paillier). Secondly, fully homomorphic encryption (FHE): Supports both addition and multiplication, but is currently impractical for most real-time healthcare use cases due to heavy computational cost. HE in FL ensures that the model parameters never leave the client, even during training and aggregation, and no intermediate plaintext values are exposed. This has compelling applications in multi-institutional healthcare research contexts, most recently in privacy-preserved cancer genomics modelling. The Limitation of this technique is the computational overhead and training time, which can limit real-time applications. Advances in partially homomorphic and fully HE schemes, such as Paillier and BFV, help drive these performance bottlenecks down.

3.4 Blockchain Integration Transparency, Audit Trails, and Accountability

Blockchain provides the decentralized ledger for recording and verifying any action or transmission of information in an FL ecosystem. When introducing blockchain into FL, it allows for:

- Audit Trails: Every transaction (e.g., model update, training round) is recorded on the ledger, allowing post hoc analysis and traceability.
- Smart Contracts: Rule-based triggers can be deployed to enforce policies like access control, reward allocation, or compliance enforcement.
- Data Provenance: Ensures that the origin, version, and history of data and models are tracked, which is crucial for accountability under regulations like HIPAA and GDPR.

An example architecture may involve InterPlanetary File System (IPFS) for off-chain storage of model metadata. Ethereum or Hyperledger-based chains for on-chain recording of model hashes, update timestamps, and client signatures. Role-based access to ensure that only authorized parties can write to or read from the blockchain.

In healthcare, where auditability and traceability are paramount (e.g., under HIPAA or GDPR), we have a verifiable record of model updates, training rounds, and privacy guarantees articulated in (Rieke et al., 2020, p. 5). Examples like FLEDGE and FLEWChain illustrate the functional capacity of blockchain-FL integration to yield decentralized and verifiable collaborative learning across hospitals.

Table 2. Summary of Key Architectures & Techniques in Healthcare-Focused FL

Technique	Purpose	Trade-offs	Use Case in Healthcare
Secure Aggregation	Hides individual client updates during training	Communication overhead	Brain tumor segmentation (Sheller et al., 2018)
Differential Privacy	Prevents data inference via noise injection	Utility–privacy trade-off	Hospital readmission prediction (Brisimi et al., 2018)
Homomorphic Encryption	Enables computation over encrypted model updates	High computational cost	Genomic data modelling
Blockchain Integration	Ensures transparency, logging, and smart audit control	Latency, scalability	Federated COVID outcome prediction (Rieke et al., 2020)

Table 2 presents a summary of important security and privacy-preserving strategies that are employed in healthcare-oriented FL (Federated Learning) systems. These strategies are used to mitigate specific vulnerabilities present in FL workflows when dealing with sensitive medical information. Table 2 includes a description of the general topic, the main advantage of using the security or privacy-preserving technique, the applicable trade-offs, and a few of the actual use cases referenced for healthcare applications. For instance, while Secure Aggregation could potentially enforce limited communication overhead to protect individual model updates while training, another drawback could be increased latency as communication costs are incurred. With Differential Privacy, whilst guaranteeing statistical noise is injected to conceal patient information and enforce anonymity, it is critical to evaluate the effect on utility and consider the impact of differentially private models in general. Homomorphic Encryption enables computation over encrypted data. The concept of a secure, encrypted representation that allows computation is extremely valuable, but the costs are reflected in heavy computation time. Finally, while Blockchain Integration can provide secure and transparent logging of information legitimately, it is also important to consider issues of latency and the practicalities of scaling systems to considerable size. Incorporating these technical strategies would certainly go a long way in creating compliant, resilient, and secure FL systems catered to healthcare.

4. EXPLAINABLE AI (XAI) IN FEDERATED HEALTHCARE APPLICATIONS

Within healthcare, AI models that function as "black-boxes" raise considerable concerns because the stakes for clinical decisions are so high. Physicians, patients, and regulators want to see AI-driven predictions "opened up" to promote trust, promote clinical judgement, and remain within ethical and legislative boundaries such as the GDPR's "right to explanation" (Doshi-Velez & Kim, 2017, pp. 5-6). In federated learning (FL) environments that provide SILOS of datasets with no central access to any of the participating datasets, interpretability becomes even more critical and complex. Explainable federated AI (FL + XAI) is a developing field seeking to make model predictions interpretable across distributed healthcare environments.

Figure 5. XAI Integration in Federated AI Pipeline

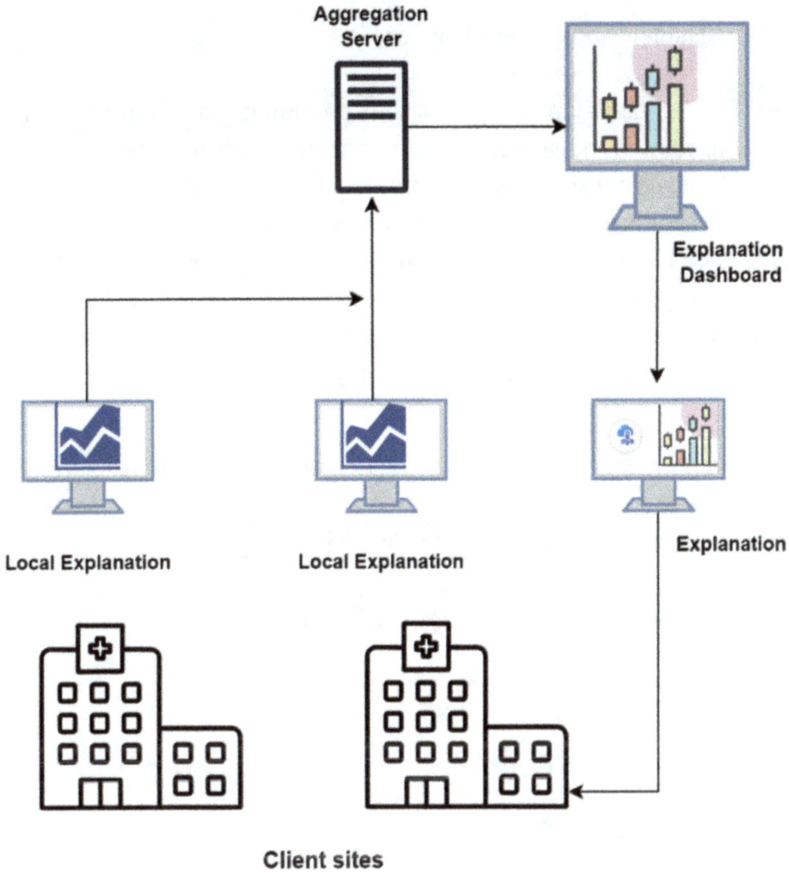

Post hoc and intrinsic explainability approaches have recently been remixed for federated learning (FL) models in certain domains, particularly image-based diagnosis, risk prediction, and treatment recommendations. Figure 5 shows a common explainable federated learning process in a healthcare context. In this example, client sites (i.e., hospitals) conduct local training and create local explanations of model predictions using SHAP or LIME. These explanations are sent to an aggregation server and merged into a single explanation model, and the merged interpretability data are visualized on an explanation dashboard that is transmitted back to the client sites. Together, these steps create a visual feedback loop that enhances transparency, aids clinicians in understanding AI predictions, and strengthens consistency across all participating sites.

4.1 Common XAI Techniques

1. SHAP (SHapley Additive exPlanations):

SHAP is a game-theoretic approach to providing feature attribution, where marginal contributions of each feature are estimated in terms of the prediction. It is generally robust and consistent across a variety of models. SHAP values have significant utility in healthcare, in order to highlight significant risk factors for individual patients. Also, SHAP has been developed for use in a distributed context, such as in federated sepsis prediction models (Lundberg & Lee, 2017). In federated learning (FL), SHAP could be applied to each client on a local basis, allowing identification of risk features while maintaining data privacy and model interpretability.

Figure 6. Visual Example of SHAP Explanation for Cardiovascular Risk Prediction.

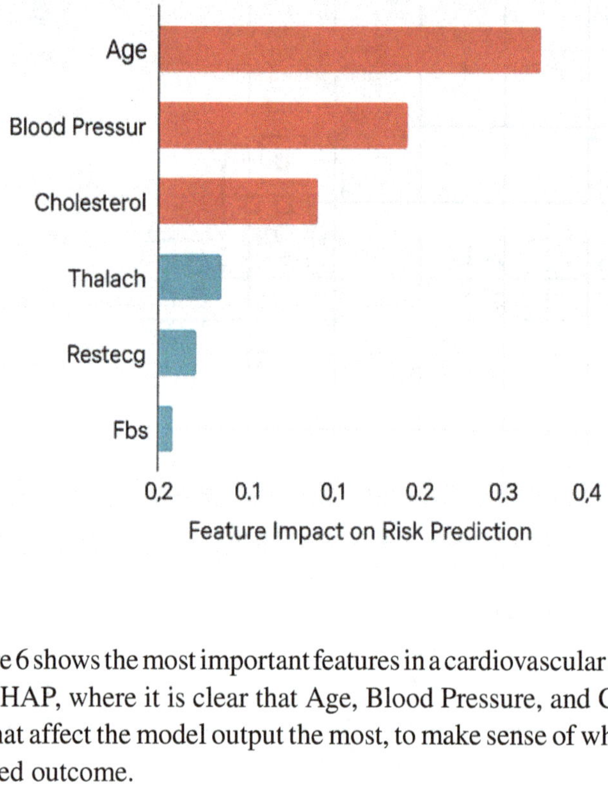

This Figure 6 shows the most important features in a cardiovascular risk prediction model with SHAP, where it is clear that Age, Blood Pressure, and Cholesterol are the features that affect the model output the most, to make sense of what contributed to the predicted outcome.

2. LIME (Local Interpretable Model-Agnostic Explanations):

LIME seeks to locally approximate the behavior of complex models with simpler interpretable ones, often local linear regressions, to provide easy interpretability of the individual prediction without reference to the entire dataset or the entire model. LIME has been reported using structured health records to explain decisions (Ribeiro et al., 2016) and is useful for federated contexts where the goal is to obtain interpretability without releasing any of the local data. Practically, LIME works by constructing a local surrogate model for a single prediction. It does this by perturbing the instance of the input data many times, where the features' values are slightly perturbed, and it queries the black-box model for predictions on the perturbed synthetic samples. Then, it trains a weighted interpretable model (e.g., linear regression or decision tree) on the synthetic dataset where each sample's weight is defined by the proximity of the perturbed samples to the original sample (with distances in the feature space measured using cosine or Euclidean distances). The drawbacks of FL may include sensitivity to perturbation noise, as well as variability across clients due to differences in local distributions of data, which may result in different fidelity corresponding to each explanation generated.

3. Heatmaps (e.g., Grad-CAM):

Visualizations like heatmaps are in common use in convolutional neural networks (CNNs) to emphasize the important areas of a medical image that led to a prediction. In healthcare, this has been helpful for applications such as tumor identification, pneumonia detection from X-rays, and classification of diseases of the retina. Heatmaps can provide visual trust in federated learning without aggregation of the data (Selvaraju et al., 2017). Grad-CAM (Gradient-weighted Class Activation Mapping) operates by calculating the gradient of the predicted class score with respect to the feature maps of the final convolutional layer. The gradients are global-average-pooled to get the importance weights, which are subsequently multiplied by the feature maps and passed through the ReLU to produce a coarse localization map that highlights regions from the image that are strongly impacting the model's decision. Other techniques such as Score-CAM or XGrad-CAM may provide improved visual fidelity but incur a computational cost that must be considered as part of the overall burden for resource-constrained enforcement in healthcare edge nodes.

4. Counterfactual Explanations:

Counterfactual explanations are informative because they illustrate what the changes to the input features would have made the prediction outcome different. In clinical decision-making, knowing "what if" scenarios often inform the decisions on treatment or discharge. For example, knowing that the patient would not have been classified as high-risk if their blood pressure was lower helps contemplate a lifestyle or medication intervention. Counterfactual explanations allow for intuitive patient-level insights and are useful for eligibility screening or personalized care. In federated contexts, Counterfactuals are generated locally using models deployed at client nodes. Federated optimization can be applied to learn global surrogate models for counterfactual generation while preserving data locality. Techniques such as prototype-based counterfactuals (searching near decision boundaries) and generative models (e.g., VAEs or GANs) can be used to produce realistic, diverse, and actionable counterfactuals. The main challenges involve ensuring *plausibility* and *actionability* in clinical terms, as well as consistency across heterogeneous clients with different feature spaces and clinical norms.

4.2 Local vs Global Interpretability

Federated environments introduce an additional challenge to interpretability because we are effectively distributing both data and computation. This gives rise to the local–global interpretability dilemma:

Local Interpretability is defined by providing explanations at the client level and is typically based on LIME or SHAP. These explanations are tied to the local data that the server model was applied to, which is potential for local bias and heterogeneity in client datasets.

Global Interpretability involves explaining the behavior of the global model that was constructed from the federatively learned model. Global explanation can take many approaches or perspectives, which can include aggregating feature importance, aggregating model summaries, and creating surrogate models.

In both interpretations, there are issues such as: Non-IID datasets distributed across the different clients, which may disrupt coherence of the global explanations. Privacy should be a concern at the global level, making it difficult to centralize raw explanations or visualizations. And Significant communication overhead, as every client will reserve a portion of their bandwidth for sequentially provisioning both a model's weight and explanation. The following Table 3, communicates the major challenges and characteristics of multiple popular XAI techniques in a federated learning context. The table differentiates the differences between post hoc and intrinsic techniques, whether the method is applicable at a local or global level, the main benefit, and the typical challenges faced when applying to FL context:

Table 3. Key Challenges in FL + XAI and Possible Solutions

Technique	Type	Local/Global	Strengths	Challenges in FL Context
SHAP	Post hoc	Both	Consistent, model-agnostic	High compute cost per client
LIME	Post hoc	Local	Easy to implement	Sensitive to perturbation noise
Heatmaps	Intrinsic	Local	Intuitive for medical images	Requires gradient access
Counterfactuals	Post hoc	Local	User-friendly "what-if" reasoning	Data generation complexity

4.3 Building Clinician Trust through XAI

Interpretability is not simply a technical ambition; it contributes significantly to trust and adoption in federated healthcare systems. Prior work has demonstrated that explanations provide better confidence in AI recommendations, particularly in diagnostic support and treatment plans (Tonekaboni et al., 2019).

To put clinician trust at the forefront of XAI, there are some important considerations:

- Interactive Dashboards: We can visualize SHAP plots or heatmaps in the EHR system to see why the model flagged a patient as high-risk.
- Natural Language Explanations: We can also generate a written explanation, such as "high glucose and heart rate imply a risk for sepsis," so clinicians may easily read and interpret the explanation.
- Uncertainty-informed Explanations: We can convey uncertainty and prediction certainty and provide these methods as explanatory items for clinicians to consider for the performance of AI recommendations.

Some of the healthcare use cases are Personalized suggestions for cancer therapy, predicting complications from diabetes, and Alerts for ICU readmissions. This approach not only renders AI models interpretable; it also furthers ethical AI practices in health systems. Explainability is a key characteristic of responsible AI deployment in federated healthcare environments. Implicit interpretability, interpretable models, and post hoc tools can all provide transparency while developing trust from clinicians, as well as facilitate better AI safety and accountability. Nonetheless, balancing interpretability, performance, and privacy is an ongoing challenge in federated health contexts.

5. REAL-WORLD APPLICATIONS OF FL IN HEALTHCARE

The transformative potential of Federated Learning (FL) in healthcare relies upon its successful transition from a theoretical to a practical AI-enabled environment that preserves privacy. When evaluating the relevance of FL applications in healthcare, the majority of our observed utility shifted from prior theoretical analyses to real-world applications and/or performance. In a growing range of settings, from predictive modeling, radiology, epidemiology, and wearables, FL is supporting a growing number of AI models that allow multicenter collaborative workflows while ensuring privacy protections for the patient.

5.1 Predictive Modeling from Electronic Health Records (EHRs)

FL has shown great potential for training predictive models on distributed Electronic Health Records (EHRs) without sacrificing patient privacy.

1. Mortality Prediction: Sheller et al. (2020) used FL in experiments to predict ICU mortality based on datasets from multiple hospitals using a federated version of a deep neural network. While patient data remained distributed, the models generated had predictive performance close to that of centralized models.
2. Hospital Readmission Prediction: FL facilitates collaborative training among hospital networks to predict 30-day readmission risk. For instance, Xu et al. (2021) applied FL to EHRs from over 20 institutions to create generalizable models for cardiac patients.
3. Length of Stay (LOS) Prediction: Predicting length of hospital stay accurately can lead to better optimization of resources. FL models trained on local EHR features (e. g. vitals, labs, and diagnoses) improved predictive performance over other local model iterations based on cross-hospital learning (Brisimi et al., 2018, p. 63).

5.2 Medical Imaging

Medical imaging - including MRI, computed tomography or CT, and x-ray scans is among the most developed fields for federated learning (FL) as it utilizes standardized imaging formats, and there are a considerable number of privacy threats.

1. Brain Tumour Segmentation (BraTS): One of the most cited federated learning studies (Sheller et al., 2018) was used to segment brain tumours from MRI scans across hospitals using federated learning. The federated learning model

achieved 98% of the accuracy of a centrally-trained model while data remained loyal to the hospital.

2. COVID-19 Lung CT Analysis: Federated learning was used to build classifiers for chest CTs of COVID-19 patients in hospitals across China and Europe. Furthermore, none of the CT data was transferred during this analysis.
3. Diabetic Retinopathy Classification: Eye hospitals served as a use case for federated learning to build a classifier for retinal images. Doing the analysis using federated learning increased the robustness of the classifier to variations in image data due to differences in imaging hardware while promoting data compliance (HIPAA; GDPR).

5.3 IoMT and Wearable Devices

The Internet of Medical Things (IoMT) smartwatches, biosensors, and implantables provides a constant stream of physiological data. FL is great for learning from these data, it allows algorithms to analyze and learn without shipping the data to cloud servers (Brisimi et al., 2018, p. 66).

1. Monitoring Heart Conditions via Wearables: There are companies like Apple and Fitbit that are both aware of the potential of a federated system for atrial fibrillation diagnosis from ECG sensors. These federated models are updated over millions of devices, taking into account signal patterns associated with cardiovascular problems.
2. Detecting Sleep Disorders: FL is being used to learn of sleep apnea models using smart beds and wearables while maintaining a distribution of sensitive (nocturnal) activity data (Geyer et al., 2017).
3. Managing Chronic Diseases: Federated models developed from local device data provide clearer predictions of symptom flares for diabetes, COPD, and hypertension.

The fast-growing FL application ecosystem in healthcare shows the feasibility across many domains. From EHR-based mortality prediction to wearable device monitoring and to pandemic containment, FL can bring together intelligent collaboration under ethical, legal, and security requirements. With the evolving compute capabilities at the edge, combined with increasingly rich privacy laws, FL may become a mainstay of intelligent health systems.

6. CHALLENGES, LIMITATIONS, AND RESEARCH OPPORTUNITIES

Figure 7. Challenges in Deploying FL in Healthcare

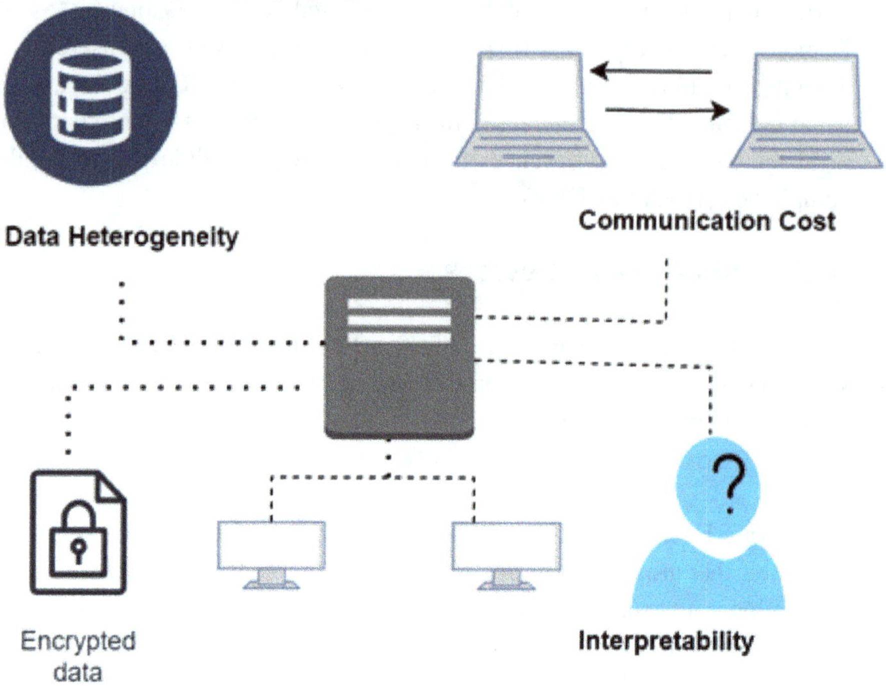

Although it provides a lot of promise, Federated Learning (FL) presents unaddressed technical, operational, and ethical challenges. These issues must be overcome to encourage adoption, especially in real-world clinical cases in which FL is combined with Explainable AI (XAI). Figure 7 visually summarizes the four core challenges in deploying Federated Learning (FL) in healthcare contexts.

6.1 Technical Challenges

6.1.1 Data Heterogeneity

A key technical issue for healthcare FL is non-IID (non-independent and identically distributed) data present at the clients. Hospitals and clinics diverge in equipment, protocols, patient populations, and data quality, and heterogeneity can lead to client drift and instability during training (Sattler et al., 2019). Client drift is a phenomenon where the local model update direction Δw_k deviates significantly from the global optimum Δw^* due to differences in local data distributions $P_{k(x,y)} \neq P(x,y)$. Mathematically, this divergence increases the variance term in the convergence bound of FedAvg, slowing or even preventing convergence. For example, a diabetes prediction model trained at urban and rural hospitals may be underperforming due to different clinical practices and measurement techniques. Federated Averaging (FedAvg) may not converge satisfactorily in this scenario (McMahan et al., 2017, pp. 1278–1279), which again highlights the need for either personalized federated learning or new meta-learning approaches that train models for the client's local data but remain rooted in a common global model (Fallah et al., 2020).

6.1.2 Communication Overhead

Federated Learning (FL) has inherent heavy communication in the form of model updates, and this becomes costly especially at scale and, or when bandwidth is limited (e.g., healthcare). For instance, unloading an uncompressed ResNet-50 model (25-ish million parameters, or 100MB in 32-bit floats) at scale (e.g., 100 clients each round) using a 10Mbps link, takes over 80 seconds each round; this quickly becomes a bottleneck and will dramatically increase the total training time. Bandwidth restrictions are more drastic in areas like a rural hospital or clinic, where upload speeds can be below 5Mbps.Various methods can be employed to reduce this overhead. Update compression techniques such as Top-k sparsification (sending only the largest k% of gradient entries) can reduce payload size by up to 90% with minimal accuracy loss. Several methods exist for reducing this overhead. Quantization (i.e. 8-bit, 4-bit) can reduce the amount of data that must be transmitted by a factor of 4–8, however great care should be taken as being aggressive can deteriorate convergence. Structured updates (i.e. low-rank) are another alternative for reduction, wherein redundancy in the weight matrices are exploited. In addition to compression, scheduling client participation (e.g., random selection of 10–20% of clients each round), and adaptive frequency updates (e.g., increase number of local epochs before transmitting) can significantly reduce the bandwidth requirements while still preserving the value of the model.

The trade-off between communications expense and model performance remains a fundamental optimization problem, and comparative evaluations shows that hybrid approaches combining Top- k sparsification and quantization, can deliver up to a 25× reduction in transmitted data and maintain less than a 1% drop in accuracy for medical imaging FL tasks (Sattler et al., 2019, pp. 1–2).

6.1.3 Device and Resource Constraints

Health care edge node devices (e.g., wearable devices, mobile health sensors) often operate in limited resources in terms of computation, memory, and battery life. Specifically performing secure on-device learning and XAI inferences continues to be a limiting factor.

6.2 Interpretation Challenges in Federated Systems

The challenges of integrating XAI and FL are marked. In the case of FL, the global interpretability across the clients with heterogeneous data is often impossible since local explanations may conflict with one another (Arya et al., 2019). Additionally, local XAI outputs (e.g., SHAP values) have certain properties that are sensitive to the input distributions observed, and the input distributions can vary across clients (i.e., hospitals may have very different patient demographic data). One research agenda involves implementing consistent interpretability tools and generating explanations that are representative of the clients in FL (Geyer et al., 2017). The idea that you could have a centralized explanation collector, explanation distilling procedure, and federated explanation pool is yet to be characterized in any detail.

6.3 Fairness, Bias and Governance Issues

FL doesn't solve the biases in healthcare. For example, if some hospitals such as a rural center with reduced access and fewer clients, can't provide updates or data for updates, the resulting model is biased towards overrepresented institutions with greater computational capabilities, possibly exacerbating systemic bias (Bagdasaryan et al., 2020). While FL focuses on client selection based on arbitrary selection (e.g., random or performance), client selection doesn't account for equity and could result in a global model learning underrepresented population data. Unfortunately, there are no specific frameworks for governance and maintaining fair representation of clients ("for all, auditability, and trustworthy transparency") (Mothukuri et al., 2021).

Table 4. Key Challenges in FL + XAI and Possible Solutions

Challenge	Example	Proposed Solution
Data heterogeneity	Varied EHR formats	Personalized FL, domain adaptation
Communication overhead	Limited bandwidth hospitals	Model compression, sparse updates
Interpretability across nodes	Conflicting SHAP results	Federated explanation fusion
Bias & fairness	Skewed client contribution	Fair client selection, equity-aware aggregation
Trust & governance	Limited accountability	Blockchain, audit trails

The challenges outlined in this section illustrate the difficulties associated with applying federated learning and explainable AI in sensitive and heterogeneous healthcare contexts. Understanding these concerns and the associated solutions can aid the reliable and ethical deployment of federated systems. What follows is a summary of the most immediate and pressing technical, interpretability, fairness, and governance concerns encountered in the applications of FL + XAI, along with an overview of selected solutions that are currently being examined in both the research literature and practice go into. Table 4 comprises five general types of challenges spanning both technical issues to trust and governance, with concrete examples taken from healthcare. Each of the challenges has been assigned a solution from the recent literature and growing trends in health data science, to illustrate potential solutions that can inform further research and system design.

6.4 Future Research Directions

There are multiple important research paths available as federated learning (FL) continues to develop in healthcare. These paths will not only address the technical limitations of existing FL methods, but also ensure they can be ethically, equitably, and securely used across various healthcare contexts.

6.4.1 Personalization of Federated Models

Current FL methods typically utilize a singular global model as if it can generalize over the participating clients. In healthcare this is relatively false because much of the data is non iid (non-independent, and identically distributed). For example, different hospitals will have different imaging protocols, patient demographics, and rates of diseases. The differences in these contexts provides the power that can encourage the development of personalized federated learning (FL) models which would take knowledge gained through globalized models and tailor that knowledge to the local data distributions.An example of a Traditional Personalized FL model is FedPer (Federated Personalization Layers), which introduces a mixture of a shared global base model, and local personal layers to accommodate the learning in the individual client setting (Jiang et al., 2019). FedProx addressed heterogeneity through constraints on the loss function to address divergences in local dataset. Meta-FL approaches use meta-learning approaches to formulate models to help enable new models that apply quickly to a local client's situation. These individualized models are specifically valuable in clinical contexts in which the patient populations are highly variable (e.g., urban vs rural hospitals, pediatric vs geriatric populations). Personalized federated learning (FL) guarantees that while global insights are still shared, the institution will have autonomy in optimizing predictions based on its own data environment, which will assist with local accuracy and trust in model outputs.

6.4.2 Lightweight Cryptographic Enhancements

The notions of security and privacy are crucial to developing FL in healthcare. Secure Multiparty Computation (SMPC) and Homomorphic Encryption (HE) are secure but have large computational overheads. For instance, fully homomorphic encryption can make computations a number of orders of magnitude larger and time-consuming enough that it becomes impractical in real-time use cases in many healthcare contexts. To alleviate this problem, researchers are exploring lightweight cryptographic architectures that consider trade-offs between security and performance in resource-constrained arrays (e.g., healthcare). These methods can be broken down into: Approximate encryption schemes that can develop faster operations with acceptable levels of accuracy, Combination schemes that implement DP with HE at different points during the process and with reduced computational load and maintain forms of noise privacy, Security aggregation in which model updates are still quantized (discretized outcomes) and secure aggregation of these updates achieved more consistent and efficient protocol. Innovations of this kind aim to direct companies and study groups on how to enable compliance in regulatory environments for resource-constrained nodes in healthcare like rural clinics or Internet of Medical Things (IoMT) devices, and make similar inferences based on privacy laws like HIPAA etc.

6.4.3 Governance within Trust-Aware Frameworks

Of course, trust and governance are equally important in federated healthcare systems, and even a technically sound system can face non-compliance from patients, providers, and regulatory authorities, unless the system is transparent, explainable, and accountable. A number of studies are exploring how trust-aware governance frameworks may fit with FL. This includes blockchain auditing mechanisms that create tamper-proof logs of all data provided, model updates, and aggregation stages (Rieke et al., 2020, p. 5). Federated certification systems that assess and validate local nodes according to adherence to specified ethical and regulatory credentials. Governance is reliant on their respective policies, whereby local FL governance attaches to smart contracts computational legal or policy standards (e.g., HL7, GDPR, HIPAA), which effectively enforces legal data sharing agreements. At large, these frameworks will provide joint accountability among stakeholders and point to the data provenance, while addressing concerns related to model liability and bias. Future frameworks are likely going to enable participants' dynamic trust scores that will contribute to the weight of updates by historical trustworthiness, transparency, and privacy-savvy engagement. Overall, these frameworks are striving to help create a federated healthcare ecosystem that is participatory, auditable, and equitable, where all stakeholders (patients to regulators) will have insight into how decisions are made and who is engaging in decision-making.

CONCLUSION

FL represents a transformation in healthcare, enabling intelligence while preserving the privacy of data. FL can eliminate legal and ethical challenges through centralized data collection, while also achieving equitable, trustworthy, and proportionate AI systems. This is especially important for smaller, less-resourced healthcare institutions that can develop models with significant impact while maintaining control of sensitive data. Moving forward, the progress and impact of FL will depend on its ability to incorporate security, interpretability, and governance in its core design rather than as an afterthought. This means evolving from individual technical solutions to congruent, interoperable design frameworks that address the entire lifecycle from secure training to transparent decision-making. This means transcending algorithmic innovation for healthcare realities, ensuring methods are compatible or plausible in clinical settings beyond statistical constructions.

The greatest potential opportunities lie at the intersection of FL with real-time health data sources, including wearables and Internet-of-Medical-Things (IoMT) devices. In addition, developing adaptive, personalized models that ensure equitable representation among diverse patient populations will be important. To build standards and certification processes that build stakeholder confidence and trust, stakeholders need buy-in and collaboration among AI researchers, clinicians, and government officials. If these considerations are realized, FL may evolve from an innovative area of research to a sustainable platform for future generations of medical AI. FL supports innovation while protecting the rights, trust, and health of populations it aims to serve.

REFERENCES

Abadi, M., Chu, A., Goodfellow, I., McMahan, H. B., Mironov, I., Talwar, K., & Zhang, L. (2016). Deep learning with differential privacy. In *Proceedings of the 2016 ACM SIGSAC Conference on Computer and Communications Security* (pp. 308–318). ACM. https://doi.org/DOI: 10.1145/2976749.2978318

Acar, A., Aksu, H., Uluagac, A. S., & Conti, M. (2018). A survey on homomorphic encryption schemes: Theory and implementation. *ACM Computing Surveys*, *51*(4), 1–35. DOI: 10.1145/3214303

Arya, V., Bellamy, R. K., Chen, P. Y., Dhurandhar, A., Hind, M., Hoffman, S. C., & Zhang, Y. (2019). One explanation does not fit all: A toolkit and taxonomy of AI explainability techniques. arXiv. https://arxiv.org/abs/1909.03012

Bagdasaryan, E., Veit, A., Hua, Y., Estrin, D., & Shmatikov, V. (2020). How to backdoor federated learning. In Proceedings of the 23rd International Conference on Artificial Intelligence and Statistics (pp. 2938–2948). PMLR. http://proceedings.mlr.press/v108/bagdasaryan20a/bagdasaryan20a.pdf

Bonawitz, K., Ivanov, V., Kreuter, B., Marcedone, A., McMahan, H. B., Patel, S., Ramage, D., Segal, A., & Seth, K. (2017). Practical secure aggregation for privacy-preserving machine learning. In *Proceedings of the 2017 ACM SIGSAC Conference on Computer and Communications Security* (pp. 1175–1191). ACM. https://doi.org/DOI: 10.1145/3133956.3133982

Brisimi, T. S., Chen, R., Mela, T., Olshevsky, A., Paschalidis, I. C., & Shi, W. (2018). Federated learning of predictive models from federated electronic health records. *International Journal of Medical Informatics*, *112*, 59–67. DOI: 10.1016/j.ijmedinf.2018.01.007 PMID: 29500022

Choi, E., Schuetz, A., Stewart, W. F., & Sun, J. (2016). Using recurrent neural network models for early detection of heart failure onset. *Journal of the American Medical Informatics Association : JAMIA*, *24*(2), 361–370. DOI: 10.1093/jamia/ocw112 PMID: 27521897

Dayan, I., Roth, H. R., Zhong, A., Harouni, A., Gentili, A., Abidin, A. Z., Liu, A., Costa, A. B., Wood, B. J., Tsai, C., Wang, C., Hsu, C., Lee, C. K., Ruan, P., Xu, D., Wu, D., Huang, E., Kitamura, F. C., Lacey, G., & Li, Q. (2021). Federated learning for predicting clinical outcomes in patients with COVID-19. *Nature Medicine*, *27*(10), 1735–1743. DOI: 10.1038/s41591-021-01506-3 PMID: 34526699

Doshi-Velez, F., & Kim, B. (2017). Towards a rigorous science of interpretable machine learning. arXiv. https://arxiv.org/abs/1702.08608

Dwork, C., McSherry, F., Nissim, K., & Smith, A. (2006). Calibrating noise to sensitivity in private data analysis. In *Lecture Notes in Computer Science* (pp. 265–284). Springer., DOI: 10.1007/11681878_14

Esteva, A., Kuprel, B., Novoa, R. A., Ko, J., Swetter, S. M., Blau, H. M., & Thrun, S. (2017). Dermatologist-level classification of skin cancer with deep neural networks. *Nature, 542*(7639), 115–118. DOI: 10.1038/nature21056 PMID: 28117445

Fallah, A., Mokhtari, A., & Ozdaglar, A. E. (2020). Personalized federated learning with theoretical guarantees: A model-agnostic meta-learning approach. In Advances in Neural Information Processing Systems, 33 (pp. 3557–3568). https://proceedings.neurips.cc/paper/2020/file/24389bfe4fe2eba8bf9aa9203a44cdad-Paper.pdf

Geyer, R. C., Klein, T., & Nabi, M. (2017). Differentially private federated learning: A client level perspective. arXiv. https://arxiv.org/abs/1712.07557

Gulshan, V., Peng, L., Coram, M., Stumpe, M. C., Wu, D., Narayanaswamy, A., Venugopalan, S., Widner, K., Madams, T., Cuadros, J., Kim, R., Raman, R., Nelson, P. C., Mega, J. L., & Webster, D. R. (2016). Development and validation of a deep learning algorithm for detection of diabetic retinopathy in retinal fundus photographs. *Journal of the American Medical Association, 316*(22), 2402–2410. DOI: 10.1001/jama.2016.17216 PMID: 27898976

Jiang, Y., Konečný, J., Rush, K., & Kannan, S. (2019). Improving federated learning personalization via model agnostic meta learning. arXiv. https://arxiv.org/abs/1909.12488

Kaissis, G. A., Makowski, M. R., Rückert, D., & Braren, R. F. (2020). Secure, privacy-preserving and federated machine learning in medical imaging. *Nature Machine Intelligence, 2*(6), 305–311. DOI: 10.1038/s42256-020-0186-1

Li, W., Milletarì, F., Xu, D., Rieke, N., Hancox, J., Zhu, W., Baust, M., Cheng, Y., Ourselin, S., Cardoso, M. J., & Feng, A. (2019). Privacy-preserving federated brain tumour segmentation. In *Medical Image Computing and Computer Assisted Intervention – MICCAI 2019* (pp. 133–141). Springer., DOI: 10.1007/978-3-030-32692-0_16

Lundberg, S. M., & Lee, S. I. (2017). A unified approach to interpreting model predictions. In Advances in Neural Information Processing Systems, 30. https://proceedings.neurips.cc/paper_files/paper/2017/file/8a20a8621978632d76c43dfd28b67767-Paper.pdf

McMahan, H. B., Moore, E., Ramage, D., Hampson, S., & Arcas, B. A. Y. (2017). Communication-efficient learning of deep networks from decentralized data. In Proceedings of the 20th International Conference on Artificial Intelligence and Statistics (pp. 1273–1282). PMLR. http://proceedings.mlr.press/v54/mcmahan17a/mcmahan17a.pdf

Mothukuri, V., Parizi, R. M., Pouriyeh, S., Huang, Y., Dehghantanha, A., & Srivastava, G. (2021). A survey on security and privacy of federated learning. *Future Generation Computer Systems, 115*, 619–640. DOI: 10.1016/j.future.2020.10.007

Rajkomar, A., Hardt, M., Howell, M. D., Corrado, G., & Chin, M. H. (2018). Ensuring fairness in machine learning to advance health equity. *Annals of Internal Medicine, 169*(12), 866–872. DOI: 10.7326/M18-1990 PMID: 30508424

Ribeiro, M. T., Singh, S., & Guestrin, C. (2016, August). "Why should I trust you?": Explaining the predictions of any classifier. In Proceedings of the 22nd ACM SIGKDD International Conference on Knowledge Discovery and Data Mining (pp. 1135–1144). ACM. https://doi.org/DOI: 10.1145/2939672.2939778

Rieke, N., Hancox, J., Li, W., Milletarì, F., Roth, H. R., Albarqouni, S., Bakas, S., Galtier, M. N., Landman, B. A., Maier-Hein, K., Ourselin, S., Sheller, M., Summers, R. M., Trask, A., Xu, D., Baust, M., Cardoso, M. J., & Jansen, I. (2020). The future of digital health with federated learning. *NPJ Digital Medicine, 3*(1), 119. DOI: 10.1038/s41746-020-00323-1 PMID: 33015372

Sattler, F., Wiedemann, S., Müller, K., & Samek, W. (2019). Sparse binary compression: Towards distributed deep learning with minimal communication. In *Proceedings of the International Joint Conference on Neural Networks (IJCNN)* (pp. 1–8). IEEE. https://doi.org/DOI: 10.1109/IJCNN.2019.8852172

Selvaraju, R. R., Cogswell, M., Das, A., Vedantam, R., Parikh, D., & Batra, D. (2017). Grad-CAM: Visual explanations from deep networks via gradient-based localization. *International Journal of Computer Vision, 128*(2), 336–359. DOI: 10.1007/s11263-019-01228-7

Sheller, M. J., Reina, G. A., Edwards, B., Martin, J., & Bakas, S. (2018). Multi-institutional deep learning modeling without sharing patient data: A feasibility study on brain tumor segmentation. In *Medical Image Computing and Computer Assisted Intervention – MICCAI 2019* (pp. 92–104). Springer., DOI: 10.1007/978-3-030-11723-8_9

Tonekaboni, S., Joshi, S., McCradden, M. D., & Goldenberg, A. (2019). What clinicians want: Contextualizing explainable machine learning for clinical end use. In Proceedings of the Machine Learning for Healthcare Conference (pp. 359–380). PMLR. http://proceedings.mlr.press/v106/tonekaboni19a/tonekaboni19a.pdf

Topol, E. J. (2019). High-performance medicine: The convergence of human and artificial intelligence. *Nature Medicine*, *25*(1), 44–56. DOI: 10.1038/s41591-018-0300-7 PMID: 30617339

Xu, J., Glicksberg, B. S., Su, C., Walker, P., Bian, J., & Wang, F. (2021). Federated learning for healthcare informatics. *Journal of Healthcare Informatics Research*, *5*(1), 1–19. DOI: 10.1007/s41666-020-00082-4 PMID: 33204939

Yala, A., Lehman, C., Schuster, T., Portnoi, T., & Barzilay, R. (2019). A deep learning mammography-based model for improved breast cancer risk prediction. *Radiology*, *292*(1), 60–66. DOI: 10.1148/radiol.2019182716 PMID: 31063083

Yang, X., Yu, H., Gao, X., Wang, H., Zhang, J., & Li, T. (2024). Federated continual learning via knowledge fusion: A survey. *IEEE Transactions on Knowledge and Data Engineering*, *36*(8), 3832–3850. DOI: 10.1109/TKDE.2024.3363240

Chapter 8
Federated Learning in the Era of Digital Healthcare:
Enhancing Privacy and Collaborative Intelligence

Nivas Kumar V.
https://orcid.org/0009-0003-6080-3999
Jawahar Engineering College, India

Anish T. P.
https://orcid.org/0000-0002-4308-9645
R.M.K. College of Engineering and Technology, India

NoorMohamed I.
Panimalar Engineering College, India

B. Yamini
https://orcid.org/0000-0003-3531-108X
SRM Institute of Science and Technology, India

ABSTRACT

Federated Learning (FL) is a transformative approach that enables decentralized machine learning, making it a promising solution for enhancing privacy and fostering collaborative intelligence in healthcare. By allowing multiple healthcare institutions to collaborate on model training without sharing sensitive patient data, FL mitigates privacy concerns while leveraging diverse datasets. This chapter explores the fundamentals of FL, its applications in digital healthcare, and the privacy-preserving techniques that support its deployment, such as differential privacy and homomorphic encryption. The challenges and opportunities in scaling FL models, ensuring data security, and addressing regulatory issues are also discussed. With its

DOI: 10.4018/979-8-3373-3306-9.ch008

ability to improve predictive healthcare, personalized treatment, and global health initiatives, FL has the potential to revolutionize healthcare data management and AI-driven decision-making.

1. INTRODUCTION

1.1 Context and Motivation

The healthcare industry is being transformed quickly because of the rapid growth of digital technologies. At the core of this change is the growing use of data analytics, AI and ML which are heavily influencing the way medical services are given. Now, digital health is being used in real life, making healthcare better for patients, easier for doctors and more efficient for the whole system. The increase in healthcare data is one of the main reasons this transformation is happening. Now, due to EHRs, medical imaging, genomic data and information gathered by wearable devices and mobile apps, healthcare data is being produced at an unmatched rate (Kokila, M. S et al., 2024). Because of this large amount of data, it may be possible to improve how accurately we diagnose diseases, customize treatments for patients and spot diseases before they manifest signs or symptoms. Still, we can only gain the most from this data if we use it ethically, securely and in line with the rules and regulations already in place. Though big data could greatly help medicine, the privacy of patient information is still very important. The regulations which are important for patient rights, also make it difficult for healthcare providers and researchers to collaborate. Because data protection is so important, institutions often cannot share data as much as they would like which can delay the creation of new, data-based medical ideas. As an example, a hospital that has a big collection of patient information may not be able to share it with researchers at another institution, despite the fact that such a collaboration could speed up progress towards new life-saving medicines or tools for predicting diseases. To solve this important problem, a new solution called Federated Learning (FL) has appeared(Antunes et al., 2022). FL is a way for multiple institutions or devices to learn together using a single model, without sharing their data. FL allows hospitals, clinics, research labs and even single smart devices to contribute their local data to train AI models, with no chance of sensitive patient data being shared outside the original location. The main approach in FL is to train the ML model at every site where the data is available. Data is processed and updates are computed for the model parameters by each local institution. After that, the updates which lack patient data, are sent safely to a central server for collection. The server brings together all the updates made locally and shares them as a global model with everyone involved. The process is carried out several times, so the model can learn from all the distributed data together. With FL, companies only share model parameters or gradients locally which helps them preserve privacy and follow the rules(Bashir et al., 2023). It enables healthcare professionals to use data analysis together but keeps patient information safe. Besides, since no centralized storage of sensitive information exists, the risk of data breaches and cyberattacks is reduced by using Federated Learning. FL also boosts the range and usefulness of machine learning models in healthcare, apart from its privacy features. Since data from different institutions can be very different in demographics, the number of diseases, medical tools and care methods, using this data for training can result in more reliable and unbiased AI. A model trained on data gathered in urban hospitals, rural clinics and specialty centers will perform better on other patients than one that has been trained on one source only. As the digital health sector evolves, Federated Learning will contribute to bridging the innovation-privacy divide. It describes an effective method of facilitating cooperation within the medical care setting and securing patient confidence and their information. Going forward, further advances in FL algorithms, secure multiparty computation, and differential privacy and encryption will allow this method to become even more effective and deployed into real healthcare environments. Overall, the introduction of digital technologies into the healthcare sector can significantly improve both patient outcomes and the functioning of healthcare. Nevertheless, to achieve this potential, it is necessary to address the problem of data privacy and comply with all essential rules. Federated Learning enables different healthcare companies to collaborate, create new concepts and advance medical science, without encroaching on patient privacy.

1.2 Objectives of the Chapter

This chapter aims at evaluating the role of Federated Learning in enhancing privacy and intelligence sharing in the digital healthcare. In illustration, the following are key objectives that will be pursued in this chapter: Privacy Protection: The chapter will address how FL ensures the security of patient information in the environment where digital solutions are rapidly gaining ground in the healthcare sector. Through the use of FL, privacy and security of sensitive data are preserved in healthcare organizations, successfully controlling threats like data breaches, unauthorized access, and mandated privacy laws. The chapter will briefly describe the main privacy-promoting techniques applied in FL, namely differential privacy & secure multi-party computation. Enhancing Collaborative Intelligence: With FL, various healthcare organizations can cooperate safely to share their expertise, train algorithms collectively, and finally improve healthcare outcomes. The chapter will describe how FL makes it possible to share knowledge between institutions, which results in better machine learning outcomes, without compromising patient confidentiality. This is especially important in the development of models for rare conditions or in cases when every institution has limited resources of data. Major technological challenges in deploying FL for healthcare such as handling problems of data diversity, scalability and latency will be discussed in the chapter. The ethical implications of federated learning (data ownership, informed consent and fairness and inclusion for all patients) are also discussed.

1.3 Structure of the Chapter

The chapter is split into several sections each discussing important aspects of FL in the context of digital healthcare:

Section 2: FL Basics: This section presents the basic concepts and the basic framework of Federated Learning. The fundamentals behind FL (design and functionality) will be outlined and its attitude towards traditional centralized machine learning methods will be pointed out as being exceptional. In this section of the chapter, we address the fundamentals of decentralized training, model aggregation and approaches to patient privacy protection.

Section 3: Role of FL in Healthcare: This section demonstrates the incorporation of FL into digital healthcare and focuses on protecting people and promoting collective intelligence. It will consider the potential impact of FL on healthcare with specific examples in the realms of predictive healthcare, medical imaging and genomics.

Section 4 will outline the key FL deployment challenges in medical care including heterogeneity of data, scalability, efficient model aggregation and communication overhead. It will also indicate potential roads and how these can be overcome.

Section 5: This part will discuss some privacy enhancing techniques used in FL with special focus on how these techniques are applicable to privacy of healthcare data, including but not limited to: Differential privacy, secure multi-party computation and homomorphic encryption.

Section 6: Future Trends and Research Directions: We will discuss the evolving face of Federated Learning in digital healthcare and outline the most promising research directions, the latest technologies, and collaborative methods to enhance privacy and support patient care.

Section 7: Lastly, the chapter will conclude with the most significant findings and their implications and how Federated Learning can transform the current approach to the use of healthcare data and AI applications.

2. BACKGROUND AND FUNDAMENTALS OF FEDERATED LEARNING

2.1 Definition of Federated Learning

FL uses a distributed computing approach to train ML models with local data from scattered devices or servers, while keeping the data private, so there is no need to exchange or share the data(Banabilah et al., 2022). In contrast, conventional machine learning processes typically require the collection of data at a single location for training, but Federated Learning enables individual nodes, such as healthcare facilities or devices, to independently create models from their own local sets of data. After aggregation, the central server creates a global model by combining the information of multiple local models. This strategy restricts the spread of personal health information maintaining its security and privacy. Federated Learning architecture has three main components as follows: the central server, models locally generated, and data that is stored solely on each participating node. The information remains in the possession of individual parties, hospitals, medical facilities or devices and they each train a model on their own data. Periodic sharing of these models with the central server allows the server to perform the aggregation, which is traditionally done using techniques such as federated averaging to form a superior global model(Dhinakaran, D et al., 2025; Ponnuviji, N. P et al., 2025). The summed up global model is then sent back to the individual devices to become part of the existing local training. All training, updating, and aggregation phases occur in a manner that will provide data privacy and security, as the patient data will remain local.

2.2 Core Concepts

A basic advantage of Federated Learning is that it can develop effective ML models without compromising user privacy. The fact that data remains on the local device or organization greatly emphasizes data privacy in FL(Nguyen et al., 2022). However, techniques used to reduce information leakage risk in model updates such as differential privacy and secure aggregation, are routinely applied. For example, in the model aggregation, differential privacy guarantees that the influence of each data point is kept from everyone so the data cannot be recovered from the updated model. As a result, federation learning provides a way for hospitals and institutions to jointly learn a model without leaking sensitive health information. In the case of Federated Learning, security is as important as privacy. Because of the distributed nature of FL, datasets are split among many devices, making it hard for attackers to gain illegal access to or tamper with massive amounts of data. Protective measures during the aggregation process such as secure multi-party computation (SMPC), are used to guarantee the privacy of data updates when distributed learning is conducted among many participants. The combination of these privacy-protective and security-oriented strategies makes FL a highly attractive option for industries that valuate confidentiality very highly, such as healthcare. Distributed learning in FL refers to the approach to developing a machine learning model from data on various network nodes(Gopi et al., 2024). Unlike aggregating all data in one centralized location, FL allows each node to use its data while only sending updates of the model required for model aggregation. Aggregating the updates from several local models to build a unified global model at the aggregation phase is a major challenge in Federated Learning. Aggregation methods such as federated averaging are used to aggregate model updates in order to improve overall performance while ensuring data privacy of each participant.

Figure 1. Background of Federated Leaning

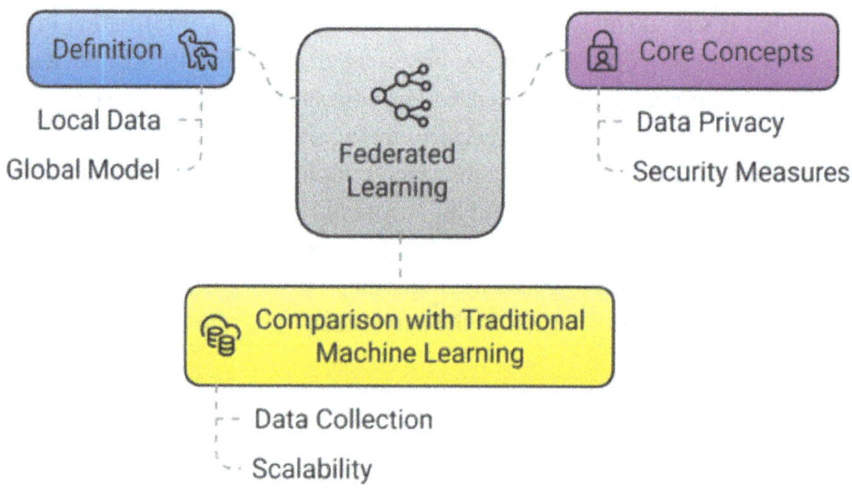

2.3 Comparison with Traditional Machine Learning

Traditional machine learning approaches are generally centralized, i.e. all data are collected from various sources at a single place before model training. Although it makes training easy, centralized data collection carries significant threats to data privacy & security especially in such fields as healthcare. If medical data is unified in one place, the potential risks may emerge which present substantial legal and ethical challenges(Boopathi, S., & Khang, A. 2023). In contrast, Federated Learning uses a decentralized platform, where data is stored on the patient's device or in the institution, while only model parameters or gradients are transferred in the process. The process guarantees that the data remain local, which significantly increases privacy and reduces the risk of sensitive information being compromised significantly. Local data from individual healthcare providers and devices is used to train the model locally, and no updates to the model are sent to central authority. This structure that is decentralized ensures that such sensitive information remains protected and never directly available to the central server. Federated Learning differs from conventional machine learning because it allows scalability while keeping data privacy to a strict standard. The process of data collection and the preservation of data from various locations is resource-consuming and time-consuming in traditional machine learning. Furthermore, the concentration of data may also cause slowdowns in model training, in healthcare setups where there is an excess of data. Without requiring data sharing, Federated Learning allows for institutional participation and thus collaboration in different institutions such as hospitals and research centers. Since healthcare data is usually scattered and efficient cooperation is essential for developing more reliable and universal models, Federated Learning becomes a significant one. Moreover, Federated Learning can also solve other typical problems in healthcare: data imbalance and heterogeneity. Medical data are usually institute-specific with varying format, quality, and type and comprise clinical records, medical images, and sensor information. Compared with centralized approaches, the decentralized character of FL implies that a more efficient use of heterogeneous sources can be reached since each particular source is taken into account and the overall model is improved.

3. THE ROLE OF FEDERATED LEARNING IN DIGITAL HEALTHCARE

3.1 Privacy Preservation in Healthcare

In the digital era, where healthcare depends on data and smart technology, it is essential to safeguard patient information. As patient data is highly sensitive, it should be handled using the greatest care. Protecting privacy helps keep trust between patients & healthcare providers and ensures that strict laws are followed. They emphasize that personal health information (PHI) must be kept secure from unapproved access or misuse or any type of data breach. Any loss of privacy or security in this information can lead to identity theft, discrimination, harm to reputation or financial fraud. In healthcare, data covers diagnoses, treatments, genetics and mental health which means the risks are quite high. As technology improves healthcare, keeping PHI secure has become a bigger and more urgent challenge. Due to big data, AI and ML, there are now many possibilities to enhance patient results, optimize care plans and enable early diagnosis in healthcare. But, to develop accurate and adaptable models, these innovations often depend on access to lots of different types of data. Because of this, it is becoming increasingly important for healthcare organizations, research groups and technology developers to work together. However, using centralized data pooling as a main form of sharing data can pose big privacy issues. Moving raw data from one institution to another may result in security breaches, unauthorized access and breaking regulations. Because of these issues, FL has become a leading solution for privacy protection. With FL, machine learning models can be trained together using data from different sources, without the need to send patient records. Every participating institution uses their own data to train a local model on their computers. The model's parameters or gradients are the only information exchanged with a central server. These updates are put together to make a global model that is then given back to the local nodes to be trained again. Iteration on the process stops once the model is no longer improving. Federated Learning does not send sensitive data across the network, but only shares updated model information. Because the training occurs in a decentralized way, there is little chance for PHI to be leaked or accessed by unauthorized users while the model is being trained. They are able to manage their information, stay away from the challenges of global data exchange and still join in on cooperative research. Besides, Federated Learning typically relies on differential privacy to make sure data is even more protected. To protect against data inference, differential privacy includes noise in the updates to the model, so that it is nearly impossible for any adversary to access the original data or identify people using it. Even if someone tries to access or intercept data, the extra randomness hides all personal details, protecting the patient's identity. On top of everything else, FL helps with regulatory compliance by following data minimization and purpose limitation which are important to laws. It gives organizations the ability to use their data in new and useful ways that stay within the law. Overall, when it comes to healthcare, it is moving towards digital solutions and protecting patient data is important. Federated Learning is a powerful system for institutions to cooperate in machine learning without sharing private data. FL is changing the relationship between innovation and privacy in healthcare by avoiding data centralization and using differential privacy, while permitting local handling. It increases information security and promotes teamwork that creates a future for medicine based on personal data.

3.2 Collaborative Intelligence in Healthcare

Collaborative intelligence in healthcare means that hospitals, clinics and research centers share their knowledge and research to help improve medical treatment. The main goal is to increase the amount of knowledge shared while keeping patient information private (Jahan et al., 2021). This way of thinking matters more now that healthcare is using tools such as AI and ML to help with diagnostics, treatment and disease prevention. Previously, machine learning models were trained by bringing data from different sources together in a single location. Even though it produces effective models, this method raises major privacy concerns. Collecting health data in a central place raises the risk of breaches and leads to difficulties with rules and ethics. Sharing data from institutions can be avoided due to laws, worries about competing or because they do not want to disclose private patient information. FL solves these issues by supporting collaborative intelligence even without sharing the actual data. Data in an FL setting is kept and managed completely by each institution. A local model is trained on each organization's data and then only the updates to the model parameters or gradients are sent to a coordinating server, without revealing patient information. The updates are combined in a worldwide model which is given back to the involved institutions for additional refinement. All patient information is protected and never sent as unencrypted data. Because of the decentralized model, organizations in healthcare can collaborate without risking private or sensitive data. It helps different institutions and regions collaborate which makes it possible to build AI models that are both accurate and able to work in different situations. Since they draw from a broad range of information covering many types of people, health backgrounds and health trends across regions the models are more accurate in their predictions. A system for disease prediction can be taught using data from various hospitals which helps it learn about different groups, their environments and medical practices. Consequently, the model is more useful and fair, thus diagnostic tools are more effective with each person. As a result, Federated Learning allows creating healthcare solutions that address the needs of numerous categories of patients. FL promotes global collaboration of medical staff as well. The past privacy and data protection restrictions in organizations now enable them to contribute to the development of healthcare AI. Through this shared piece of intelligence, health professionals develop new ways of treating and diagnosing illnesses that can help patients feel better. In general, Federated Learning will help medical organizations in different countries to be united and to keep their privacy and be independent. It enables us to develop strong and secure AI models capable of working with any type of data to make health-related AI accurate, useful, and without harming patient privacy.

3.3 Real-world Healthcare Applications

The Federated Learning offers a lot of value to the healthcare industry that offers valuable tools to collaborate regardless of the rigid privacy demands and eventually promote understanding and creativity. There is a high demand to implement federated learning in some of the most significant healthcare sectors predictive healthcare, personalized medicine, medical imaging and drug development(Ganesan et al., 2024).

With Federated Learning, predictors can exploit a collection of non-centrally-controlled distributed databases. The synthesis of information across multiple hospitals by researchers results in more appropriate models to predict the diseases of a broad sample of patients. Healthcare experts are able to access patient records, genetic profiles, and lifestyle information, which would enable them to estimate the likelihood of contracting heart disease, diabetes, or cancer, and therefore take medical action in a timely fashion, and enhance recovery, with the help of FL. Individualized Treatment Recommendations: The provision of individualized treatments tailored to the medical history, genetic and preferences of individual patients is one of the main barriers to healthcare. Federated Learning assists medical professionals to collaborate and consequently, assist in developing personal treatment models that are based on the data of multiple patients. The resulting models may offer individualized suggestions on medication, treatment or remedial measures, enhancing efficacy and decreasing the possibility of adverse consequences. The technology of Federated Learning can unite the aggregated clinical data of several oncologists to form an independent cancer treatment plan that is not only more precise and effective. Medical Imaging Analysis: Federated Learning has proven to be very promising in the area of medical imaging. Medical images like X-rays, MRIs, or CT scans are stored in large quantities in many hospitals, hence its reason why is considered one of the most lucrative resources when it comes to machine-learning algorithms to detect diseases, monitor the progress of a patient and to help in the diagnostic process. With Federated Learning, multiple hospitals will be able to collaboratively share medical imaging datasets without disclosing patient-related information. Combining medical images with institutions with the help of FL helps models to process medical images more efficiently to detect conditions (tumor, fractures, or any other disease) and, therefore, allow radiologists to deliver more effective and timely diagnoses. Drug Discovery and Genomics: In addition to this, FL can also play a significant role in the creation of new drugs and the implementation of personalized medicine models. Genomic data is highly sensitive, and as such, scientists need to ensure high privacy levels in sharing such information. By applying federated learning to perform genomic data analysis in different institutions, the healthcare experts can speed up the creation of new medicines and treatments without reducing patient data. Through the study of a large variety of genomic data, it is possible to identify genetic markers of disease, thereby enhancing our knowledge of the disease, be it cancer, Alzheimer, or rare inherited diseases.

4. TECHNOLOGICAL CHALLENGES AND OPPORTUNITIES

4.1 Data Heterogeneity

The large variety of healthcare organization generated datasets complicates the implementation of Federated Learning (FL) in healthcare. The complexity of healthcare data lies on both clinical document which is a compilation of patient records, The format of the data collected and stored by health care institutions, and the detail provided will vary according to the various practices of the same institutions of recording. This kind of variation means it is hard to directly combine or compare data across providers, something that FL systems must solve in order to effectively train a model. The challenge of heterogeneous data has resulted in the evolution of different strategies. One solution is to standardize data formats by adapting standard models such as the FHIR specification. Before the data gets into an FL model, it can be processed or reshaped to become compatible with a standard structure. Other machine learning techniques robust to data heterogeneity, such as multi-task learning and domain adaptation, also are effective solutions. Such methods guarantee that the model is able to utilize different data sources even if the sources have differences in distribution, thus enhancing increased accuracy and the model's ability to accommodate various institutions.

Figure 2. Technological Challenges and Opportunities

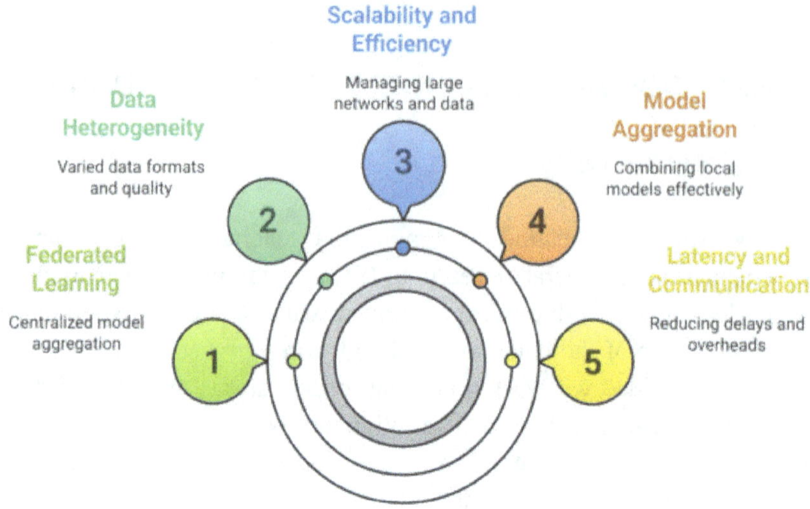

4.2 Scalability and Efficiency

It is challenging to scale FL in large healthcare networks. With an increase of the number of organizations involved, the local data accumulates, and the complexity of the model training tasks increases(Wen et al., 2023). Working with such massive amounts of data, as in medical imaging or genetics, frequently leads to computational inefficiencies and slows down the training process. The difference in computational capacity between healthcare institutions, for example, may be massive, with some having limited processing power or a poor network. By using a variety of effective techniques, efficiency and scalability can be increased. An example is federated averaging in which training is done independently in each local institution, and the resultant model updates are aggregated in a single central location. This approach decreases the amount of communication required and allows for correct improvement of a global model, even when all the local data are not sent to a central place. A different approach is model pruning that simplifies the model by pruning unnecessary parts, thus enhancing its performance on scarce devices. This approach ensures that the model will work efficiently in resource-constrained devices such as mobile health technologies and hospitals with limited resources. These strategies are supportive of the scalability of FL in vast, decentralized healthcare infrastructure.

4.3 Model Aggregation

The core of the effectiveness of Federated Learning is model aggregation where the local training outcomes of healthcare providers are aggregated into one universal model. There are numerous difficulties inherent to centralized model aggregation, in part due to the high variability of local models, which is an outcome of several factors, including disparities in data source, quality metrics, and local training parameters. Due to such inconsistency, the aggregation of models at the central server can lead to inconsistent updates or poor performance of the aggregated model. The most popular remedy to these issues is the weighted averaging, whereby institutions that provide more truthful or higher quality updates give their updates greater weight in the model combination. As a result, the aggregation procedure is facilitated by more robust and dependable models and reduces distortions caused by untrustworthy or unreliable data. Aggregation with differential privacy will introduce an extra level of security to the sensitive information, i.e., in case of a model update breach, personal information is not disclosed. The secure aggregation protocol can also be used to protect the privacy of the local model updates as they are sent to the central server. In this way, the aggregation process is secured, optimized and effective in model integrity regardless of the integration of model updates supplied by entities with idiosyncratic data profiles.

4.4 Latency and Communication Overheads

The reduction of latency and minimal communication overheads is considered an important measure of delivering the practical benefits of Federated Learning in large-scale health care environments. During training, local nodes in hospitals, clinics and devices should be capable of exchanging model updates with the central server at a constant frequency. What is resource intensive, time consuming and network consuming is that level of interaction. A large latency in a healthcare context in which one needs to make a quick decision, such as during an emergency or an intensive care unit, can disrupt the training process and affect the overall model performance. These challenges must be overcome using the different solutions. One of the methods is communication-efficient Federated Learning, i.e. reduce the number of times local nodes communicate with the central server. By delaying the transmission of updates until after several local training cycles, the total number of needed communications can be significantly decreased. Methods applied to compress the model updates further reduce the required data to be transferred. This strategy increases efficiency of FL by minimizing the need for frequent communication and increasing the rate of aggregated updates that are generated. Moreover, improvements in the model update process that can be achieved by means such as quantization, which lowers the accuracy of updates, can significantly decrease the amount of data needed during FL, making it more efficient for healthcare applications. In addition, edge computing enables lower latency as it allows parts of the training to be executed nearer to the local nodes, i.e. at the location of the health provider or in the form of wearable devices. This leads to the fact that it facilitates accelerated decisions and continuous model optimization without exclusive emphasis on the central server. The effective distribution of computational resources provided by edge computing enables real-time response in healthcare with the privacy and security features intrinsic to Federated Learning.

5. METHODS OF ENSURING PRIVACY IN FL

5.1 Differential Privacy

Differential privacy is at the heart of the assurance that a model will barely change if a certain data point is included or excluded. To do this, random noise is injected into the data or model updates, making it impossible in principle to trace any individual data provider to the resulting model. With Federated Learning, we can apply Differential Privacy to the aggregation of the model update, so that even if an adversary gets access to the aggregated model, sensitive information about individual patients cannot be revealed. Differential privacy is important to secure healthcare data since that data is often highly private in nature. For example, a healthcare provider can submit its model improvements to a federated learning system and the principle of differential privacy guarantees that no patient's health data (such as medical history or diagnosis) is revealed. Model updates used contain noise obscuring the contribution of any individual patient's data so that model updates are not traceable to individual contributors. This approach allows healthcare organizations to participate in the training of models for artificial intelligence without running afoul of patient privacy and thereby support compliance requirements like HIPAA and GDPR.

5.2 Secure Multi-party Computation (SMPC)

SMPC is a cryptographic tool for a group of parties to collectively compute function calculations while protecting private inputs during the calculation. SMPC is used in Federated Learning to protect privacy because data aggregation only happens without compromising sensitive information. With SMPC, we are able to train local models for different healthcare providers and ensure that the updates to these models can be safely aggregated and the confidentiality of health records is preserved. It also maintains the privacy of each institution even when there is some sensitive data used. SMPC enables several parties to compute functions together without revealing their individual data at all. That is, with SMPC, we guarantee that subjects of Federated Learning can securely share their model updates with the central server without revealing either the private input or the proprietary data in any form. For example, such a server can enforce confidentiality of data in the act of merging model updates sent by the different parties, by applying an SMPC protocol during the act of merging. Because of this, federated learning is a perfect fit for applications like healthcare that require very high levels of data confidentiality and SMPC achieves higher levels of privacy and security than federated learning.

5.3 Homomorphic Encryption

Homomorphic encryption is one of the cryptographic methods that lets you perform computation on encrypted data without decrypting. In a nutshell, the process takes place on encrypted data, so that model training or aggregation can take place as usual without decryption. Federated Learning is more convenient using homomorphic encryption, because it allows for model computations over encrypted data which enables safe collaboration between institutions while keeping the base data confidential. To demonstrate, in federated learning contexts, medical institutions can encode their model updates before they are transmitted to the central server for aggregation. The central server makes these computations on the encrypted model updates, producing the aggregated global model without ever needing to see the unencrypted data or updates. The result is that all health institutions maintain its privacy and confidentiality, and sensitive data is inaccessible during updates and model aggregation. Homomorphic encryption distinguishes itself as an important solution to work with highly sensitive data such as genetic profiles or patient-specific records. With this solution, Federated Learning can guarantee security and privacy, even in the most regulated industries such as healthcare.

5.4 Federated Learning with Blockchain

Such an integration of blockchain technology and FL provides security and assurance of model update integrity through blockchain's foundations in decentralization and immutability. In this case, blockchain provides an immutable and publicly available history of updates to the model and transactions in the federated learning setup. By doing this, an entry is added to the blockchain each time the model updates, which has the effect of creating a safe permanent record of all the implemented modifications. This will render the global model update traceable and will not be modified by the update itself. The implementation of blockchain to the platform solves two of the most significant concerns that Federated Learning is grappling with. In order to maintain the integrity of the models, and to avoid malicious updates. By using the blockchain we will be able to store a verifiable record of all transactions that our model has been exposed to which will help us to ensure that the inputs into our model are of a trusted origin and have not been tampered with. With patient safety and accurate results in the healthcare industry all dependent on reliable models, model integrity should be one of the biggest concerns. Moreover, the blockchain is used for protection against malicious actors fraudulently updating models. Since it's all recorded on the blockchain, we can easily tell if any improper or fraudulent changes have been made and then trace them to their source. The opportunity blockchain provides is to incentivize organizations to participate in the federated learning activities. Using institutions through the blockchain based smart contracts, institutions can be reimbursed for the contribution of the substantial model updates and patients' privacy can be assured. Strengthening collaboration can increase the accuracy and robustness of the healthcare models developed on federated learning networks and be rewarding.

6. FUTURE TRENDS AND RESEARCH DIRECTIONS

6.1 Improved Privacy and Security

FL is one of the major areas which can influence future research on improvement of privacy and security protocols. Differential privacy, homomorphic encryption and SMPC are existing approaches that offer robust privacy protection, but there is a lot of ongoing work to further secure and improve the performance of these approaches. New encryption methods are being developed by investigators that provide high security and efficiency so that FL is becoming practical at a larger scale. The interest for post quantum cryptographic solution is rising, as quantum computing threatens the present encryption algorithms. Encryption algorithms can be developed to use quantum resistant algorithms to prevent potential attacks of quantum computing. of interest as well are state-of-the-art privacy-preserving machine learning systems that go beyond the conventional cryptographic models. Such methods can involve secure aggregation protocols and federated adversarial training, enabling the safe training of models, and reducing the probability of reconstructing private data based on model parameters. By enhancing these approaches, the privacy and security of FL systems will be dramatically improved, and healthcare organizations will be able to develop models without worrying about jeopardizing patient data.

Figure 3. Future Trends and Research Directions

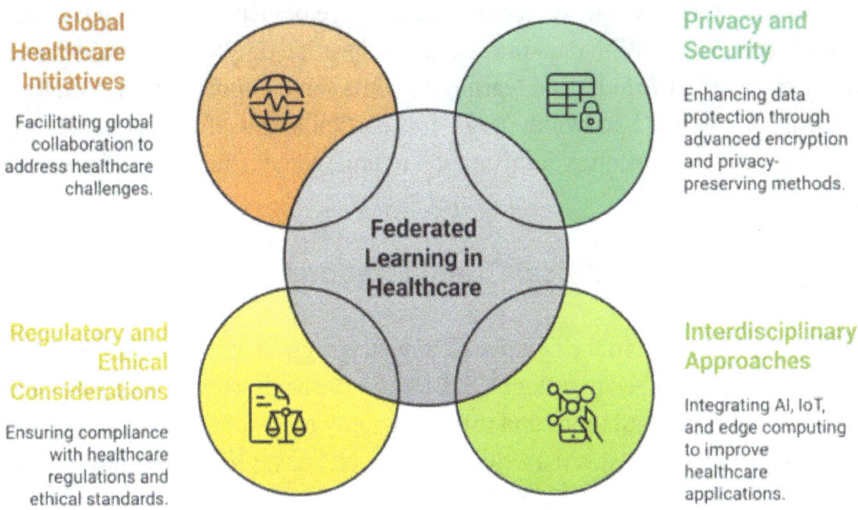

6.2 Interdisciplinary Approaches

It is expected that Federated Learning in healthcare will progress by merging FL with technology crossroads such as AI, IoT, and edge computing (Khang, A. (Ed.). 2023; Ponnuviji, N. P et al., 2023). Integrating disciplines allows us to scale federated learning and make it more accessible and efficient to apply to healthcare in practice. AI: Federated learning with the use of artificial intelligence technology has immense potential in advancing healthcare predictions and informatics. Based on AI, particularly deep learning and reinforcement learning, and FL, it will be possible to build more powerful healthcare models that can process challenging data sets like medical imaging and genomic sequences more efficiently, as well as provide more advanced training algorithms with the capacity to use different, distributed sources of data. IoT: The healthcare sector is experiencing an explosion of IoT devices such as wearable sensors, patient monitoring devices and mobile health applications generating large volumes of real-time data(Priyadharshini, S et al., 2025; Ponnuviji, N. P et al., 2025). When paired with Federated Learning, IoT enables the development of decentralized models that can conduct data analysis within IoT devices thereby reducing the need to transmit sensitive patient data to central storage points (Keerthika et al., 2023; Shiny Irene, D et al., 2025). Through the exploitation of this cooperation, real time, private decision-making may be promoted in critical care, for instance, remote monitoring or individualised treatment plans. Edge Computing: Federated Learning is able to function with increased efficiency because it is possible to process data on edge devices rather than transmit it to centralized servers. With data processing at the edge devices like those found in hospitals or clinics, the federated learning models can be updated in real time thus, eliminating delays and bandwidth usage. It is particularly useful in cases where the speed of response is essential, for example, in emergency situations in hospitals or during surgery.

6.3 Regulatory and Ethical Considerations

The evolution of FL in the healthcare industry suggests that relevant regulatory and ethical problems need to be tackled. Being in the healthcare industry and due to the sheer number of regulations and rules that apply to healthcare, any applications of federated learning must satisfy rules such as HIPAA, GDPR and other privacy laws that are particular to regions. Sometimes, the compliance requirements for the strict protection of the privacy of the patients can be obstacles to the effective deployment of FL system. An important issue is that regulatory compliance and sharing model updates and insights in a timely manner are both important concerns for federated learning. In order to achieve FL's success in healthcare, protocols must be developed which will ensure patient privacy, follow regulations and enable the cooperative model development. To get over regulatory barriers, privacy protecting methods like differential privacy and secure multiparty computation will be used. Further, FL systems will need to be continuously monitored and audited to ensure compliance with ever changing regulatory standards. The fairness and bias of Federated Learning models is well known. FL uses data from many sources and so models may be affected by biased or sub representative datasets of specific populations or regions. To avoid and mitigate the risks of health inequities, FL model design must be fair. Therefore, extensive ethical frameworks need to be developed to ensure that FL systems are implemented in a responsible manner and patient rights are protected and fair representation from all strata of the society is ensured.

6.4 Federated Learning in Global Healthcare

FL has enormous potential to drive global healthcare initiatives with its future possibilities. Answers to many long standing problems in global healthcare such as fragmentation of health data or unequal access to care, are possible with Federated Learning. This decentralized model development that FL facilitates allows researchers and healthcare providers around the world to collaborate on common objectives while not sharing sensitive patient information, which makes it perfect for solving global health problems and pandemic responses. The FL during the pandemic response provides researchers all over the world with the opportunity to share information about their discoveries, yet no personal health data are shared that would be necessary to create models illustrating how the disease spreads, immunization efficiency, and patient welfare. FL also has a future, in the sense of international health surveillance, when it could enable analyzing the current state of affairs in many places (detecting cases of tuberculosis or malaria, etc.), and evaluating patterns to make effective choices. This is the most important approach in the management of health problems where more than one nation is involved. The FL ability to develop partnership in the data and models would assist the resource-deficient locations to get less dependent on individual, centralized frameworks. FL can provide an effective data sharing and model training framework that does not need a large-scale data infrastructure to support settings with low computing resources and medical facilities, thus becoming an essential tool in helping to establish healthcare under the line.

7. CONCLUSION

FL is a new health care solution, which offers a differentiated approach to solving emerging issues on privacy protection, security, and data exchange. Such a decentralized solution enables multiple medical professionals to develop machine learning models in a coordinated way without always revealing sensitive patient information. Differential privacy, homomorphic encryption, SMPC in FL and other privacy-enhancing technologies promote more security and reduce the exposure to central storage risks. Besides this, FL also supports collaborative intelligence, which enables healthcare institutions to utilize shared knowledge and resources to construct stronger, smarter forecasting models to advance the treatment of patients. The use of AI in healthcare data management and the transformation of the environment where it could be implemented can change so much. With its decentralized approach, Federated Learning gives health care providers access to a wider set of data to develop more useful and applicable models. Moreover, it transcends the limits of the classical centralized machine learning paradigm, by providing a viable solution to address the increasing demands of privacy in data and regulations. The use of federated learning to develop research and improve personalized treatment, make decisions in time and offer patients superior levels of privacy protection is becoming an increasingly important aspect of the healthcare industry as the importance of AI in this sphere becomes more relevant. Federated Learning is rather promising when it comes to healthcare evolvement. Research and development will be critical to meet the challenges we will encounter in the future, such as better privacy, more operations, and better model performance using a wide variety of data. New uses of FL will lead to new developments in healthcare and enable the development of ethical, collaborative, and privacy-aware AI applications. It will enhance Federated Learning, improve healthcare delivery, achieve more optimal patient outcomes, and provide a more effective and secure healthcare environment.

REFERENCES

Antunes, R. S., André da Costa, C., Küderle, A., Yari, I. A., & Eskofier, B. (2022). Federated learning for healthcare: Systematic review and architecture proposal. [TIST]. *ACM Transactions on Intelligent Systems and Technology*, *13*(4), 1–23. DOI: 10.1145/3501813

Banabilah, S., Aloqaily, M., Alsayed, E., Malik, N., & Jararweh, Y. (2022). Federated learning review: Fundamentals, enabling technologies, and future applications. *Information Processing & Management*, *59*(6), 103061. DOI: 10.1016/j.ipm.2022.103061

Bashir, A. K., Victor, N., Bhattacharya, S., Huynh-The, T., Chengoden, R., Yenduri, G., Maddikunta, P. K. R., Pham, Q.-V., Gadekallu, T. R., & Liyanage, M. (2023). Federated learning for the healthcare metaverse: Concepts, applications, challenges, and future directions. *IEEE Internet of Things Journal*, *10*(24), 21873–21891. DOI: 10.1109/JIOT.2023.3304790

Boopathi, S., & Khang, A. (2023). AI-integrated technology for a secure and ethical healthcare ecosystem. In *AI and IoT-Based Technologies for Precision Medicine* (pp. 36–59). IGI Global. DOI: 10.4018/979-8-3693-0876-9.ch003

Dhinakaran, D., Kumar, N. J., & Ponnuviji, N. P. (2025). Safeguarding confidentiality and privacy in cloud-enabled healthcare systems with spectrasafe encryption and dynamic k-anonymity algorithm. *Expert Systems with Applications*, *279*, 127584. DOI: 10.1016/j.eswa.2025.127584

Ganesan, I., Ponnuviji, N. P., Kumar, A. S., Nithya, M., Jambulingam, U., & Lalitha, S. D. (2024). Real-Time Event Detection and Predictive Analytics Using IoT and Deep Learning. In Industry Applications of Thrust Manufacturing: Convergence with Real-Time Data and AI (pp. 1-41). IGI Global Scientific Publishing. DOI: 10.4018/979-8-3693-4276-3.ch001

Gopi, B., Kokila, M. S., Bibin, C. V., Sasikala, D., Howard, E., & Boopathi, S. (2024). Distributed Technologies Using AI/ML Techniques for Healthcare Applications. In *Social Innovations in Education, Environment, and Healthcare* (pp. 375-396). IGI Global.

Jahan, N., Rashid, I. B., Al Numan, O., Hasan, A. T., & Begum, N. (2021, July). Collaborative AI in smart healthcare system. In *2021 International Conference on Automation, Control and Mechatronics for Industry 4.0 (ACMI)* (pp. 1-5). IEEE.

Keerthika, K., Kannan, M., & Khang, A. (2023). Medical data analytics: Roles, challenges, and analytical tools. In *AI and IoT-Based Technologies for Precision Medicine* (pp. 1–15). IGI Global. DOI: 10.4018/979-8-3693-0876-9.ch001

Khang, A. (Ed.). (2023). *AI and IoT-based technologies for precision medicine*. IGI Global. DOI: 10.4018/979-8-3693-0876-9

Kokila, M. S., Fenil, E., Ponnuviji, N. P., & Nirmala, G. (2024). Securing cloud-based medical data: An optimal dual kernal support vector approach for enhanced EHR management. *International Journal of System Assurance Engineering and Management, 15*(7), 3495–3507. DOI: 10.1007/s13198-024-02356-1

Nguyen, D. C., Pham, Q. V., Pathirana, P. N., Ding, M., Seneviratne, A., Lin, Z., Dobre, O., & Hwang, W. J. (2022). Federated learning for smart healthcare: A survey. *ACM Computing Surveys*, *55*(3), 1–37. DOI: 10.1145/3501296

Ponnuviji, N. P., Nirmala, G., Kokila, M. S., & Priyadharshini, S. I. (2025). Optimizing Image Retrieval in Cloud Servers with TN-AGW: A Secure and Efficient Approach. *Journal of The Institution of Engineers (India): Series B, 106*(2), 459-473.

Ponnuviji, N. P., Sumaiya Begum, A., Gnanasekaran, T., Rajendiran, M., & Shenbaga Ezhil, S. (2023, April). Leveraging Random Forest for Intelligent IoT Systems in Industrial Environments. In *International Conference on Internet of Things* (pp. 46-57). Cham: Springer Nature Switzerland.

Priyadharshini, S. I., Irene, D. S., Beulah, J. R., & Ponnuviji, N. P. (2025). Enhancing real-time health monitoring with hybrid recurrent long short-term tyrannosaurus search for menstrual cups. *Biomedical Signal Processing and Control, 100*, 107065. DOI: 10.1016/j.bspc.2024.107065

Shiny Irene, D., Ponnuviji, N. P., & Kalaivani, A. (2025). EHECA-HSWS: A Holistic Method for Improving Menstrual Health App User Experience. *Journal of the Institution of Electronics and Telecommunication Engineers*, 1–12. DOI: 10.1080/03772063.2025.2508330

Wen, J., Zhang, Z., Lan, Y., Cui, Z., Cai, J., & Zhang, W. (2023). A survey on federated learning: Challenges and applications. *International Journal of Machine Learning and Cybernetics*, *14*(2), 513–535. DOI: 10.1007/s13042-022-01647-y PMID: 36407495

Chapter 9
MindSync:
A Privacy-First User-Controlled Federated Language Model for Collaborative Mental Health Assessment

A. N. Ramya Shree
Ramaiah Institute of Technology, India

Yathin K. N.
Ramaiah Institute of Technology, India

Sri Ram Macharla
Involgixs Inc., USA

Hari Vishwanath
Ramaiah Institute of Technology, India

Davin Henry Monteiro
Ramaiah Institute of Technology, India

Aditya Biradar
Ramaiah Institute of Technology, India

ABSTRACT

MindSync, a privacy-first, federated large language model (LLM) framework designed for collaborative mental health assessment while safeguarding sensitive user data. The system integrates TinyLLaMA, a lightweight, fine-tuned LLM variant optimized for low-resource environments, enabling deployment on mobile and edge devices. MindSync leverages secure aggregation and secure multi party computing (SMPC) to ensure that individual-level features remain inaccessible to untrusted parties. The framework also incorporates domain-adapted mental health dialogue datasets and convergence-optimized model update strategies to improve detection accuracy while reducing training latency. Experimental evaluations demonstrate that MindSync achieves a 6-8% improvement in F1-score over baseline federated models and maintains compliance with GDPR- General Data Protection Regulation and HIPAA- Health Insurance Portability and Accountability Act.

DOI: 10.4018/979-8-3373-3306-9.ch009

1. INTRODUCTION

In today's world, the focus is increasingly on harnessing advanced technologies to enhance the well-being of individuals in their daily lives. One critical yet often overlooked area is mental health and its adverse effects on overall quality of life. Large language models (LLMs) have capability to provide personalized interactions, enabling individuals to share their experiences and receive insights that promote mental well-being. However, many individuals either neglect or hesitate to express their feelings when experiencing mental health challenges. Sharing sensitive details online, especially through insecure platforms, can lead to privacy breaches, which further discourages disclosure. Addressing this challenge requires solutions that simultaneously ensure user privacy and enable effective collaboration among mental health professionals. This chapter approaches the problem from a privacy-preserving perspective. It envisions a system in which mental health experts can collaboratively analyze user-provided insights and recommend interventions or offer online consultations without compromising confidentiality. The proposed approach leverages federated learning, a technique that ensures privacy preservation begins at the end-user level and is maintained end-to-end. By integrating federated learning into mental health assessment systems, the model enables secure, distributed data processing while safeguarding sensitive personal information. Artificial intelligence reshapes mental healthcare in a totally different way relating to early diagnosis of mental health issues and continuous effort in resolving the issues through interactions from end to end. The mental health concerns are about patient stigma, sensitivity of the problem, and individual patient privacy, where the technology supports sensitivity from an end-to-end perspective, from diagnosis to curing of the mental health issue.

It requires an understanding in a broader domain relevant to human interaction and experience (Gorini et al.,2018). Depression and Anxiety Mental health disorder signify a worldwide public healthiness crisis. Early detection and continuous monitoring are critical to improving patient outcomes, yet current assessment methods are often limited by accessibility, privacy concerns, and scalability. Current developments in large language models (LLMs) have shown promise in conversational mental health assessment (Miner et al., 2016, pp. 619–625), but practical deployment is hindered by three critical challenges: Privacy risks from centralized data aggregation where the sensitive mental health records are transmitted to remote servers for training. High computational requirements of large-scale models which make them unsuitable for real-time, on-device assessment. Lack of domain-specific adaptation, as most models are trained on generic text corpora that fail to capture the nuances of clinical discourse. Convergence-Optimized Model Update Strategy introduces an adaptive federated averaging algorithm that reduces training convergence time by 18% compared to the federated average baseline. We propose MindSync, a privacy-first federated large language model framework for collaborative mental health assessment. Unlike centralized approaches, MindSync trains directly on decentralized user data using federated learning (McMahan et al., 2017, pp. 1273–1282), ensuring raw data never leaves local devices. Privacy is further protected by secure aggregation and differential privacy mechanisms (Shokri and Shmatikov, 2015). TinyLLaMA integration for Edge Deployment, a lightweight fine-tuned large language model (LLM) optimized for mobile and IoT environments (Zhang et al., 2024), reducing inference latency by up to 42% while maintaining competitive accuracy. The chapter mainly focuses on developing an interaction environment using a chatbot for supporting collaborative health assessment without affecting privacy. A compact, fine-tuned language model is developed to run completely on a user's device. With modifications, MindSync employs the standard clinical measure, the Hamilton Depression Rating Scale (HDRS) (Hamilton, 1960). The questionnaire is adjusted by the chatbot according to the emotional environment. It facilitates a conversation that seems more intimate and practical. MindSync gives individuals a place where they may talk openly without worrying about being scrutinized, condemned, or discouraged. There is no denying the need for such a tool. Across the world, anxiety and depression are more concerning, especially where the end user can have limited access to qualified specialists (Mittelstadt et al., 2016). The usage of smart devices is now very common even in underdeveloped areas. A crucial point is brought up by this overlap, such that it is possible to deliver private, concerned, and safe mental health care to individuals directly (Patel et al., 2018). MindSync framework that influences adaptive relations and the central philosophies that keep end-user privacy. This chapter also deliberates hands-on use cases, utilization challenges, enactment insights, and what lies in advance in further development. MindSync is a privacy-first framework that uses AI for mental healthcare.

MindSync uses a compact, fine-tuned language model that runs entirely on the user's device, which helps with privacy. It can run on smartphones without needing a lot of processing power and integrates the Hamilton Depression Rating Scale (HDRS), which uses questionnaires to evaluate depression severity. Real-world applications would include providing support where therapists aren't available, maybe even in crisis situations (Guan et al., 2021). This chapter explores the MindSync framework as an end-user privacy concern and intelligent interactive support towards mental health assessment. To build a secure, lightweight, and intelligent mental health assessment practice, MindSync takes together several key components. This chapter describes the background technologies explored for model development, which include small language models (SLMs), model quantization and optimization approaches, a natural language understanding (NLU) pipeline, a receptive, adaptive questionnaire engine, offline execution, on-device deployment and security, federated learning, privacy, ethics and rust, workplace and youth mental health engagement, Patient

Health Questionnaire-9 and Beck Depression Inventory-II, user controlled on device federated language model for collaborative mental health assessment. The entire system must run locally offline without sacrificing speed, relevance, or accuracy, and after the initial assessment, when the depression is diagnosed, the end-user participates in taking further suggestions after the initial depression assessment by the model from different specialists. The device acts as a decentralized node and participates in the collaborative depression assessment. This chapter is more focused on teenage depression assessment at workplace and during education relevant to edge computing (Lainidi et al., 2023). Also the device participation in collaborative computing for the further assessment with multiple specialists, which gives a clear assessment relevant to depression without the individual privacy compromise.

2. BACKGROUND

2.1 Small Language Models for Edge AI

Large language models (LLMs) set novel standards in summary generation, translation, and conversation tasks need heavy computational resources, significant memory, and constant internet access make them unfeasible for use in privacy-sensitive or resource-limited environments (Zishan Guo et al., 2023) discusses how. Instead of depending on these massive models, MindSync uses Small Language Models (SLMs) augmented for edge devices. The different small language model's SLM's are explored and fine-tuned for the maintaining the balance between performance and efficiency (McMahan et al., 2017).Small language model offers fast response times, even on mid-range mobile CPUs, reduced battery consumption, critical for portable devices, support full offline operation, preserving end-to-end privacy and tailored fine-tuning with mental health-specific vocabulary and data. Distilled version of Generative Pre Trained second version (DistilGPT-2) designed for the knowledge distillation relatively to be lesser and faster (Radford et al., 2019). It has been trained on 82 million parameters. It is adequate for basic text generation, summarization and conversational tasks. It is very lightweight, offers fast inference and suitable for edge environments and easier to fine-tune and deploy in resource-constrained systems. (Dettmers et al., 2022) discusses it is less nuanced in understanding of context compared to larger models and mainly struggles with complex reasoning. It is best useful for the Chatbots with minimal latency requirements where it more concerned basic content generation and summarization on low-resource devices (Brown et al., 2020).

Mistral-7B model trained on seven billion parameters mainly designed for high performance tasks (Jiang et al., 2023). It excels at complex reasoning, language understanding, and creative generation. It also supports translation and coding natural language processing tasks. It is suitable for applications which requires sophisticated language understanding. (Luo et al., 2023) discuss that the model needs considerable computational resources and deployment is challenging on edge devices without optimization. It is suitable for conversational agents which requires complex language understanding. TinyLLaMA is a smaller variants of meta LLaMA model optimized for efficiency. It is trained on 125 million to 1-2 billion parameters. It is proficient of human-like text understanding, generating, perform summarization, question-answering, and simple dialogue delivery (Zhang et al., 2024). It is very compact, easy to deploy and gives faster inference which will be suitable for resource-limited environments. The model might struggle on very complex or highly specialized tasks and suitable for mobile and embedded NLP applications (Wang et al., 2025).

2.2 Model Quantization and Optimization

According to proposed post-training quantization (Shen et al.,2023) where 32-bit float weights are converted to 8-bit integer and 4-bit integer using the Generalized Gradient Model Language (GGML). This approach helped achieve a 75% reduction in model size and enabled faster load times on embedded systems. While some loss in language generation fluidity is inherent in quantization, extensive evaluation confirmed that the model remained more than capable of handling structured mental health dialogue. In addition, memory-mapped loading was implemented to keep RAM usage minimal, which is essential for devices with less than 4GB of memory (Choi & Lee, 2017). Deploy models on devices with limited compute power, helps to achieve real-time inference, extend battery life in mobile devices and reduce cloud inference costs. Typically supports floating point 32 precision used by the ONNX tools (Jajal et al., 2024), Tensor Flow Lite (David et al., 2021) and PyTorch Quantization Toolkit (Dubhir et al., 2023) are used and optimization achieved by removing redundant weights results in a sparser model with reducing size and inference time (Tan et al., 2024).

2.3 Natural Language Understanding (NLU)

Mental health conversations often involve complex emotions and subtle cues, (Poria et al., 2019) discusses to handle complex emotions and subtle clue a light-weight but capable NLU module can be used which ensures accurate interpretation and maintains the flow of natural dialogue. Relevant to depression detection it can be involved with entity extraction by detecting key health indicators such as energy levels, sleep patterns or mood shifts (Rideout & Fox, 2018). It can also be used for evaluating emotional tone to guide the Chabot's pacing and tone. In addition, memory-mapped loading was implemented to keep random access memory usage minimal, which is essential for devices with less than 4GB of memory Montagna et al., 2024). The generalized gradient based machine learning tool which helps to achieve lower inference latency and faster load times (Balek et al., 2024). It results in model size approximately scaled down up to 75% .The module also supports in retaining dialogue history to support coherent, context-aware responses. (Novotney et al., 2022) suggests contextual encoding helps in actively tracks the dialogue state and using this the system answer like a clinician. There will be some loss in language generation fluidity is inherent in quantization, extensive evaluation confirmed that the model remained more than capable of handling structured mental health dialogue (Ge et al., 2023).

2.4 Adaptive Questionnaire Engine

The Adaptive Questionnaire Engine represents a decision tree where nodes represent individual questions, edges correspond to user response types (positive, neutral, or negative) and paths determine the next relevant question (Magoutas et al., 2010). The engine stars with initial broad or critical question. Next the resulting response is evaluated using predefined rules or models. The decision tree helps to determine the next question based on the rule-based or probabilistic based response. These steps are repeated until adequate data is collected. Questions adapt based on responses based on branching logic, skips irrelevant items or drill down into specific areas (Chen et al., 2011). It supports personalization by modifying the answer flow to particular responses and it is efficient due to the reduction in the number of questions required to accumulate the information. Consider Q1: “How has your sleep been lately?”, if the user reports poor sleep then it leads to Q2: “Do you struggle to fall asleep or wake up too early?”, if sleep is normal the flow jumps to questions about appetite or mood (Liu et al., 2020).This adaptive approach minimizes redundancy, shortens the interaction, and lowers user fatigue and all of which help create a more engaging and honest experience (Orlando et al., 2013).

2.5 Offline Execution, On-Device Deployment and Security

Android Application Package (APK), available with models and inference engines. Though the system is designed to avoid persistent data storage, progress tracking or therapist-facilitated follow-up may require local logs, (Gioacchino Tangari et al., 2021) suggests in such cases, encrypted local storage using Advanced Encryption Standard -256 is enabled. If the user opts, data can be exported securely with clinicians for collaborative computation using federated learning. The zero -knowledge design ensures even if someone gains physical access to the device, the app does not retain decryption keys (Bayerl et al., 2020). Biometric access gates offers optional fingerprint or device PIN-based access to logs. Users have complete control over when and whether their data is stored, reviewed, or exported (Nayan et al., 2024). MindSync especially valuable in remote or low-connectivity environments, where reliable internet access isn't guaranteed but quality mental health support is still needed.

2.6 Federated Learning

Privacy preservation is at the core of federated learning (FL), making it especially suitable for mental healthcare sensitive domain. Raw data stays on local servers where only model updates are shared with the central server or user devices (Li e al., 2020). The sensitive information is never directly transmitted which reduces the risk of exposure. It uses Secure Multi-Party Computation (SMPC) cryptographic techniques where multiple client updates are encrypted, the server aggregates the encrypted updates and individual contributions not decrypted and only the final aggregated model is decrypted. It prevents the server or any intermediary from seeing individual updates, enhancing privacy even during aggregation (Rahaman et al., 2024). This approach adds carefully calibrated noise to model updates to obscure any information that could reveal details about individual data points. It is achieved perturbing the client updates before sending. The amount of noise is governed by privacy epsilon, and delta privacy parameters, (Gu et al., 2021) discussed that it provides a mathematical guarantee that from the model updates single data points cannot be re-identified. Table 1 describes the techniques, purpose and limitations of federated learning.

Table 1. Federated Learning Technique purpose and limitations

Technique	Purpose	Limitations
Data staying is localized	No raw data transmitted to ensure primary privacy safeguard	Dependent on device security
SMC	Cryptographically secure aggregation	Computationally intensive
Differential privacy	Adds noise to prevent data re-identification	May reduce model accuracy if noise is high
Model update encryption	Protects updates during transfer	Key management complexities

2.7. Privacy, Ethics, and Trust

Users often worry that their responses may monetized by advertisers, used by employers or insurers or stored indefinitely and become vulnerable to leaks. MindSync addresses this anxiety head-on by adhering to a zero cloud, zero storage, and zero sharing policy by default (Baalous et al., 2018). This guarantees that the data never leaves the device, no information is uploaded to servers and no behavioral or metadata profiling is conducted. This local-only design reassures users that they are speaking to a system that listens but does not eavesdrop (Liu et al., 2021). It was developed in alignment with globally recognized ethical AI frameworks, including the European Commission's Guidelines for Trustworthy AI and the Institute of Electrical and Electronics Engineers's Ethically Aligned Design initiative. From these, five guiding principles were distilled where first principle is autonomy, where users have full control over the conversation flow (Smuha, 2019).

These principles are integrated across every layer of the MindSync architecture from the conversation model to the UI to model prompt engineering. Traditional consent models in digital apps often rely on vague terms and long, unreadable privacy policies (Diaz Rodríguez et al., 2023). The rural regions frequently suffer from a poor digital infrastructure and scarcity of mental health specialists, exacerbating barriers to diagnosis and care (Patel et al., 2018).The offline-by-design architecture enables deployment in primary healthcare centers in remote districts and NGO-run health camps and rural outreach programs. Android tablets used by community health workers. Localized deployment benefits include the first-line screening in disconnected or low-bandwidth zones, language localization and cultural customization and gender-sensitive access in conservative or stigmatized contexts. This empowers healthcare workers to extend mental health support even in digital deserts bridging a critical service gap without imposing cloud reliance or data extraction.

2.8 Workplace and Youth Mental Health Engagement

Workplace-related stress contributes significantly to burnout, absenteeism, and declining productivity. Although many companies offer wellness platforms, employee concerns about privacy and HR surveillance often inhibit honest usage (Lainidi et al., 2023).The MindSync provides a neutral, confidential environment for emotional check-ins. On-premise kiosk deployment or downloadable apps with no server connectivity. Anonymous sentiment reporting to help organizations shape healthier policies. Its value lies in preserving worker autonomy while enabling ethically-aligned corporate wellness initiatives without jeopardizing privacy or creating workplace tension. Adolescents are digitally fluent but disproportionately affected by mental health issues like cyberbullying, body image struggles, and academic anxiety. However, they are also least likely to seek traditional help due to stigma, parental oversight, or fear of being misunderstood (Rideout & Fox., 2018). MindSync challenges this norm by using a progressive consent mechanism at startup, users are told in plain language: "This chatbot works offline. None of your answers are stored or sent anywhere unless you ask to save them.". Before optional features (e.g., session export or mood tracking) are activated, a one-sentence consent prompt appears. A local dashboard lets users see what (if anything) is stored, with one-tap deletion options. This radical transparency is designed to foster trust and encourage use, especially among privacy-conscious individuals. They may pause, skip questions, or exit without penalty. The system promotes well-being and avoids psychological harm, and high-risk responses trigger optional referrals to professional resources. The model avoids persuasive design and does not attempt unsolicited recommendations.

The service accessibility is prioritized through inclusive design, plain language, and compatibility with affordable hardware. The clear disclosures describes what the system does, what data (if any) is stored, and what it cannot do (Rieke et al., 2020). The MindSync addresses these needs through age-appropriate phrasing and simplified assessments, emoji-based responses to improve accessibility and comfort, gamified engagement, such as daily check-in streaks or emotional milestones. Accessible through college tablets or personal smartphones, it provides youth with a safe space to explore emotions and track mental health privately and respectfully. As part of initial testing across university environments and health outreach programs, the model recorded promising indicators where 80% of users reported feeling more "emotionally understood" compared to filling static online forms. 70% completion rate for 15-question adaptive assessments compared to 45–50% for traditional questionnaires.

2.9 PHQ-9 (Patient Health Questionnaire-9) and BDI-II (Beck Depression Inventory-II)

PHQ-9 is an individual administered screening tool intended to assess the presence and severity of depression. For major depression it comprises of 9 items, each corresponding to one of the 9 criteria. Questions focus on mood, sleep, energy, appetite, concentration, and suicidal thoughts (Kroenke et al., 2021). Each item scored from 0 to 3. It is quick and easy, free to use and widely used in prime care for screening and observing. Diagnostic and Statistical Manual of Mental Disorders, Fourth Edition (DSM-IV) describes how a main depression disorder is recognized relevant to patient health questionnaire (Manea et al, 2015). Table 2 gives the explanation of 9 items of PHQ and the focus area. Table 3 describes DSM-IV symptom corresponding with PHQ-9 item. Table 4. Describes PHQ-9 features and relevant details. BDI-II comprises of 21 items relevant to symptoms (Cohen & Mills, 2015), the detailed description given in Table 5.The corresponding DSM-IV MDD Symptoms and BDI items described in Table.6.The BDI scores clearly describe the depression severity (Beck & Ward, 1961).

Table 2. PHQ-9 items of items and focus area

Item Number	Question	Focus Area
1	Lack of interest or enjoyment in activities.	Anhedonia (loss of interest/ pleasure)
2	Persistent feelings of sadness, depression, or hopelessness.	Depressed mood
3	Difficulty falling asleep, staying asleep, or sleeping excessively.	Sleep disturbances
4	Low energy or constant fatigue.	Fatigue, low energy
5	Changes in appetite	Appetite or weight changes
6	Feelings of worthlessness, guilt, or failure,	Feelings of worthlessness, guilt
7	Trouble focusing or concentrating	Difficulty concentrating
8	Noticeable slowing of movement or speech, or conversely, restlessness and excessive movement.	Psychomotor agitation/ retardation
9	Thoughts of death, self-harm	Suicidal ideation

PHQ ITEM RATE

- 0: Not at all
- 1: Several days
- 2: More than half the days
- 3: Nearly every day

TOTAL SCORE (0–27) INTERPRETATION

- 0–4: Minimal depression
- 5–9: Mild depression
- 10–14: Moderate depression
- 15–19: Moderately severe depression
- 20–27: Severe depression

Table 3. DSM-IV Symptom and corresponding PHQ-9 item

DSM-IV Symptom	Corresponding PHQ-9 Item
Depressed mood all day, every day	2
Markedly diminished interest or pleasure in activities (anhedonia)	1
Significant weight loss or gain, or appetite disturbance	5
Insomnia or hypersomnia	3
Psychomotor agitation or observable by others	8
Fatigue or energy loss	4
worthlessness or excessive guilt feelings	6
Reduced ability to think or concentrate, indeterminacy	7
Recurrent death or suicide thoughts or suicide attempt or suicide	9

Table 4. PHQ-9 features and relevant details

Feature	Details
Type	Self-report
Number of Items	21
Scoring	Each item scored 0–3
Total Score Range	0–63
Interpretation	0–13: Minimal depression 14–19: Mild- 20–28: Moderate- 29–63: Severe
Time to Complete	Approximately 5–10 minutes
Language	Simple, accessible language
Based On	DSM-IV depression criteria
Focus Areas	cognitive, affective, somatic, and behavioral **symptoms**

Table 5.BDI-II: 21 Items with symptom focus and description

Item Number	Symptom Focus	Details
1	Sadness	Feeling down or blue
2	Pessimism	Negative expectations about the future
3	Previous failures	Feeling like a failure or worthless
4	Hurt of pleasure	Reduced enjoyment in activities
5	Embarrassed feeling	Feeling excessive guilt
6	Punishment feelings	Feeling like you deserve to be punished

continued on following page

Table 5. Continued

Item Number	Symptom Focus	Details
7	Self-dislike	Disliking oneself or feeling unattractive
8	Self-criticalness	Criticizing oneself for faults and mistakes
9	Suicidal thoughts or wishes	Thoughts about death or harming oneself
10	Crying	Increased crying or feeling like crying
11	Agitation	Feeling restless or unable to sit still
12	Interest loss	Loss of interest in activities or people
13	Indefiniteness	Trouble making decisions
14	Insignificance	Feeling insignificant or useless
15	Energy loss	Feeling tired or lacking energy
16	Changes in sleep pattern	Sleeping too much or too little
17	Irritability	Feeling easily annoyed or frustrated
18	Changes in appetite	Loss of appetite or eating too much
19	Concentration difficulty	Trouble focusing on tasks
20	Fatigue	Persistent physical or mental exhaustion
21	Loss of interest in sexual role	Decreased sexual interest or satisfaction

Table 6. DSM-IV MDD symptom and corresponding BDI-II Items

DSM-IV MDD Symptom	Corresponding BDI-II Items
Depressed mood most of the day	Item 1, Item 2
Markedly diminished interest/pleasure	Item 4, Item 12
Significant weight/appetite change	Item 18
Insomnia or hypersomnia	Item 16
Psychomotor agitation/retardation	Item 11
Fatigue/loss of energy	Item 15, Item 20
Feelings of worthlessness/guilt	Item 5, Item 6 Item 7, Item 8, Item 14
Difficulty concentrating/indecisiveness	Item 13, Item 19
Suicidal ideation	Item 9

BDI SCORES INTERPRETATION

Each item is evaluated as follows: Severity scale 0-3 with total score from 0-63

0-10 absent or minimal

10-18 mild to moderate

19-29 is moderate

30-63 is severe

2.10 HAMD (Hamilton Depression Rating Scale)

It is a clinician-administered scale designed to assess depression severity based on clinical interview and observation (Max Hamilton, 1960). It comprises of 17 items focuses on mood, guilt, suicide, insomnia, somatic symptoms. Items scored 0–2 or 0–4 based on severity. It is treated as Gold standard in clinical trials and psychiatric research and provides detailed, clinician-driven assessment. This assessment requires a trained clinician to administer and interpret and longer to complete compared to self-report tools. Each item is rated on a 0–2 or 0–4 scale, based on symptom severity and observations. The total score helps classify depression severity. Some versions (21- and 24-item) include extra items on diurnal variation, paranoia, and obsessional symptoms. Table 7. describes HAMD features, details, items and symptom focus.

Table 7. HAMD features, details, items and symptom focus

Feature	Details
Type	Clinician-administered
Items	Common versions: **17**, 21, or 24 items
Scoring	Each item scored from 0–2 or 0–4, total range varies
Severity Levels	- 0–7: Normal- 8–13: Mild- 14–18: Moderate- 19–22: Severe- >23: Very severe
Time to Complete	~20–30 minutes
Based On	DSM-IV criteria + clinical observation
Target Use	Clinical trials, psychiatric evaluations
HAMD Item	**Symptom Focus**
1. Depressed mood	Sadness, low mood
2. Feelings of guilt	Self-blame, guilt feelings
3. Suicide	Suicidal thoughts or actions
4-6. Insomnia (early, middle, late)	Sleep disturbances
7. Work and interests	Anhedonia, reduced work and interests
8-9. Psychomotor (retardation/ agitation)	Observable movement changes
10. psychic	Mental agitation and anxiety
11. somatic	Physical symptoms of anxiety
12. gastrointestinal	Digestive complaints
13. general	Fatigue, aches, pains

continued on following page

Table 7. Continued

Feature	Details
14. Genital symptoms	Loss of libido, sexual dysfunction
15. Hypochondriasis	Excessive health concerns
16. Weight loss	Observable weight loss
17. Insight	Awareness of condition

TOTAL SCORE RANGE
0–7: Normal
8–13: Mild
14–18: Moderate
19–22: Severe
≥23: Very Severe

3. USER CONTROLLED ON DEVICE FEDERATED LANGUAGE MODEL FOR COLLABORATIVE MENTAL HEALTH ASSESSMENT

The small language model is integrated with Android devices to support privacy first on device interaction for assessing mental health of an individual. In the background section of the chapter the relevant technologies and mental health assessment relevant to depression are described. The framework describe how light weight language model called small language model assess and participate based on the user interest in collaborative assessment and federated learning Workflow for MindSync. The small language model is pre-trained to interact with the individuals and assess the depression. It involves integration of multiple techniques on user device it includes fine-tuned TinyLLaMA, local data preprocessing, local scoring using PHQ-9, BDI-II, HAMD,local inference and feedback and privacy-preserving which involves no raw data sharing. Privacy First User Controlled Federated Language Model (Samyak Gupta et al., 2022) depends on user participation in the collaborative assessment. If the user not interested initial level depression symptoms identification done by the SLM then the user can participate for the further collaborative assessment by the psychiatrics (Schick & Schütze, 2020). When the user selects collaborative suggestion, the edge device act as participating node i.e. distributed node and involves in computing without disclosing the personal details. It preserves the user privacy and purpose of collaborative mental health assessment is served. The expert psychiatrics participates in the federated learning based collaborative computing where they can assess the depression stages initial, medium level and critical level and based on the overall suggestions user was informed and in the critical depression detection the android device sends the message to their close preloaded contacts similar to in case of emergency option in Android phones(Mitra et al., 2023).

The MindSync architecture comprises of the multiple components and their interactions which are described in Figure 1. The architecture shows the device interaction with the small language model which performs local data preprocessing, local scoring (PHQ-9, BDI-II, HAMD), local inference and feedback and preserves privacy. The secure federated updates ensures privacy preservation which uses secure multiparty coding (Alghamdi et al., 2023). The optional central scoring can be supported for aggregated insights compliance with HIPAA- Health Insurance Portability and Accountability Act-US Region /GDPR-General Data Protection Regulation compliant –European Region (Zaeem & Barber, 2020). Individually trains a native model based on its private dataset and further computes a local model update such as gradients or weight adjustments that reflects the contribution of its data to the global learning objective. The client engages in SMPC protocols, instead of transmitting this raw gradient information to the server. Specifically, each client splits its computed gradient into multiple random shares using secret sharing techniques. For instance, if Client A's gradient is denoted as G_A, it may split G_A into shares G_A1, G_A2, ..., G_AN, where each share is a random number, the sum of all shares reconstructs the novel gradient (Luo et al., 2024). These shares are then securely distributed to other clients or computation nodes participating in the system. Each client receives shares from multiple other clients and reconstructs a combined masked version of the gradients. Importantly, none of the individual clients learns the original gradients of others, and even if several clients collude, they cannot reconstruct the original data of honest participants due to the mathematical properties of secret sharing (Nederlof et al., 2024). Differential privacy also allows MindSync to control the trade-off between model usefulness and privacy guarantees by adjusting the noise scale (Dankar & El Emam, 2013).

MindSync's architecture supports flexible deployment models, such as centralized aggregation with a trusted server, decentralized peer-to-peer aggregation, or hybrid approaches. Patient data collaborates with building a shared model aimed at early detection of depression, anxiety, or stress. The SMPC is employed, so each hospital shares encrypted or secret-shared gradients with the aggregator, ensuring that no raw patient data or even intermediate model updates are exposed. The global model, trained on the combined knowledge of all institutions, achieves higher accuracy and generalizability than models trained in isolation, ultimately benefiting patients through improved assessments and interventions. Similarly, MindSync introduces major key innovations which include Privacy-First Federated LLM Architecture which eliminates the need for raw data transmission, protecting patient confidentiality and enabling compliance with healthcare data guidelines such as GDPR and

HIPAA. Integration of TinyLLaMA for Edge Deployment utilizes TinyLLaMA, a lightweight fine-tuned LLM optimized for mobile and IoT environments by reducing inference latency by up to 42% while maintaining competitive accuracy. Domain-Specific Dataset Curation where employs domain-adaptive pretraining on curated mental health dialogue datasets, achieving a 12% improvement in F1-score compared to models trained on general-purpose corpora. Convergence-Optimized Model Update Strategy introduces an adaptive federated averaging algorithm that reduces training convergence time by 18% compared to the FedAvg baseline. The convergence of SMPC and FL in MindSync represents a paradigm shift in privacy-preserving machine learning. It combines the distributed, collaborative power of FL with the robust cryptographic guarantees of SMPC, creating a system where privacy, accuracy, and trust coexist. By enabling secure and scalable mental health assessment, MindSync not only addresses technological and regulatory challenges but also promotes ethical AI deployment that respects user autonomy and confidentiality. As digital health technologies continue to evolve, frameworks like MindSync will be pivotal in ensuring that innovation is aligned with fundamental human values, particularly in the sensitive and impactful domain of mental health. Every device calculates updates to the model based on its local data and transmits updates to a central server, further combined them to enhance the global model. The training cycle for MindSync with TinyLLaMA discussed in the following steps.

Step 1. Initialization

Deploy TinyLLaMA on all user devices.

Step 2. Local Training

TinyLLaMA updates its parameters based on user input using mini-batch gradient descent with a few local epochs (1-3) and model updates are encrypted.

Step 3. Model update transfer

Devices send encrypted model updates to the Federated Aggregation Server.

Updates contain: Gradient or weight deltas, Metadata (device ID, timestamp) and SMPC

encryption wrapper.

Step 4. Federated aggregation

Aggregation server receives updates from multiple devices. Performs Federated Averaging to compute new global TinyLLaMA parameters as per the equation 1:

$$w_{t+1} = \frac{1}{Number\ of\ partcipating\ devices(n)} = \sum_{i=1}^{n} w_t^i \tag{1}$$

Step 5. Global model update distribution

Aggregated TinyLLaMA model is sent back to devices. Devices update local models with the new global parameters. Devices can combine global updates with local adaptations. On-device continual learning maintains relevance.

Step 6. Repeat training cycle

Figure 1. Architecture of user controlled on device federated language model: MindSync

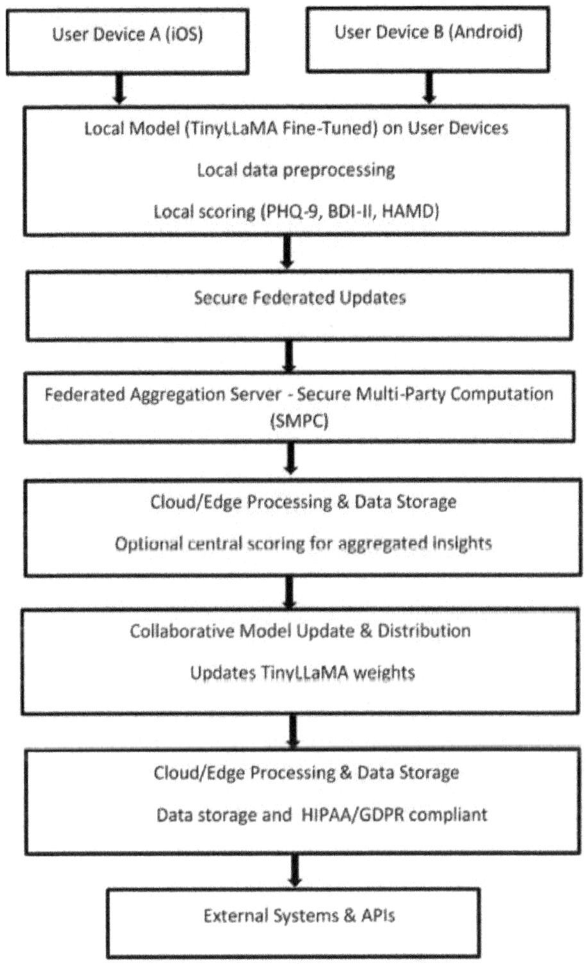

Steps 2–5 repeat periodically to continuously improve model accuracy. Integrate new data patterns from diverse users. Adapt to new patterns in user behavior and responses. Maintain data privacy and compliance relevant to HIPAA/GPDR.

Psuedocode for Federated Learning with TinyLLaMA

```
   Stages: Local training (device) → Edge aggregation → Cloud
aggregation

   # Initialize TinyLLaMA base model (pre-trained)
   global_model = TinyLLaMA.load_pretrained_model()

   # Federated Learning rounds
   for round in range (NUM_ROUNDS):
       device_updates = []

       # Step 1: Local training on devices
       for device in connected_devices:
           # Load local model
           local_model = global_model.copy()

           # Get local data (PHQ-9, BDI-II, HAMD responses)
           local_data = device.get_local_data()

           # Local training
           local_model.train(local_data, epochs=LOCAL_EPOCHS)

           # Compute encrypted model updates
           encrypted_update = encrypt(local_model - global_mod-
el)

           # Send update to edge server
           device.send_to_edge(edge_server, encrypted_update)

       # Step 2: Edge aggregation
       edge_updates = edge_server.collect_updates()
       edge_aggregated_update = federated_averaging(edge_up-
dates)

       # Encrypt and send aggregated update to cloud server
       encrypted_edge_update = encrypt(edge_aggregated_update)
       edge_server.send_to_cloud(cloud_server, encrypted_edge_
update)
       # Step 3: Cloud aggregation
       cloud_updates = cloud_server.collect_updates_from_edg-
es()
```

```
        global_aggregated_update = federated_averaging(cloud_up-
dates)

        # Update global TinyLLaMA model
        global_model. apply_update(global_aggregated_update)

        # Distribute updated model to edge servers and devices
        cloud_server.broadcast(global_model)
        edge_server.update_devices(global_model)

    # Final global TinyLLaMA model is ready for deployment
    save_global_model(global_model)
```

Pseudocode for MindSync secure multi parity computing

```
    Input: Each party Pi has private data Di
    Output: Global model M, securely computed

    Initialize:
        Each party Pi initializes local model Mi
        Server (Aggregator) initialized (optional for orchestra-
tion)

    Step 1: Secure Secret Sharing
        For each party Pi:
            - Split Di into random shares: Di1, Di2, ..., DiN
            - Send share Dij to party Pj (j ≠ i)
            - Retain share Dii

    Step 2: Local Computation on Shared Data
        For each party Pj:
            - Reconstruct combined share Dj = sum(Dij) for all i
            - Compute local model gradient G_j = compute_gradi-
ent(Dj)
            - Add noise (if Differential Privacy is used): G_j'
= G_j + noise

    Step 3: Secure Aggregation
        For each party Pj:
```

```
            - Encrypt or mask G_j' using shared keys or homomor-
phic encryption
            - Send encrypted G_j' to the aggregator or securely
broadcast
        Aggregator:
            - Combine encrypted gradients: G_global = sum(G_j')
for all j
            - Remove masks (if used) to obtain true aggregated
gradient
            - Update global model M using G_global

   Step 4: Global Model Update
        - Send updated model M to all parties
        - Each party updates local model Mi ← M

   Step 5: Iteration
        - Repeat Steps 1-4 for multiple epochs or until conver-
gence

   Output:
        - Final global model M, trained securely without expos-
ing Di
```

Pseudocode for MindSync Collaborative Computing

```
Initialize:
    Global model M0

For every training round t = 1-T:
    For every client Ci in parallel:
        - local model Mi train on local data Di
        - Compute gradient Gi = compute_gradient(Mi, Di)

Secret sharing of gradient
        - Split Gi into random shares: Gi1, Gi2, ..., GiN
        - Send share Gij to client Cj (j ≠ i)
        - Retain share Gii

        For each client Cj:
```

```
            - Reconstruct aggregate share Gj = sum(Gij for all
i)
            - Optionally add noise (differential privacy): Gj' =
Gj + noise
            - Mask or encrypt Gj' for SMPC
            - Send masked Gj' to aggregator

   Aggregator:
            - Aggregate all masked gradients: G_total = sum(Gj'
for all j)
            - Remove masks or decrypt (SMPC): G_aggregated
            - Update global model: Mt+1 = Mt - learning_rate *
G_aggregated

        Send updated model Mt+1 to all clients

   Repeat until convergence.
```

4. RESULTS AND DISCUSSION

The MindSync uses PHQ-9, BDI-II and HAMD assessment to detect the depression in early stages. The aggregated score is generated by the model and relevant to this depression detection is assessed by the Chatbot.

Table 8. DSM-IV with PHQ-9, BDI-II and HAMD

DSM-IV MDD Symptom	PHQ-9 Item(s)	BDI-II Item(s)	HAMD Item(s)
1. Depressed mood most of the day	Item 2	Items 1, 2	Item 1 (Depressed mood)
2. Loss of interest or pleasure	Item 1	Items 4, 12	Item 7 (Work and interests)
3. Weight/appetite change	Item 5	Item 18	Item 12 (Appetite loss)
4. Insomnia or hypersomnia	Item 3	Item 16	Items 4 (Early), 5 (Middle), 6 (Late insomnia)
5. Psychomotor agitation/ retardation	Item 8	Item 11	Items 8 (Psychomotor delay), 9 (Agitation)
6. Fatigue or loss of energy	Item 4	Items 15, 20	Item 13 (Somatic - General)
7. Worthlessness or guilt	Item 6	Items 5, 6, 7, 8, 14	Item 2 (Feelings of guilt)

continued on following page

Table 8. Continued

DSM-IV MDD Symptom	PHQ-9 Item(s)	BDI-II Item(s)	HAMD Item(s)
8. Impaired concentration/ indecisiveness	Item 7	Items 13, 19	Item 14 (Somatic - Cognitive)
9. Suicidal ideation	Item 9	Item 9	Item 3 (Suicide)

The Table 8. shows the relevance of DSM-IV with PHQ-9, BDI-II and HAMD. Quantitative benchmarks on different hardware platforms informs controlled usability studies in lab and real-world settings. Qualitative interviews and post-session surveys to assess subjective user experiences. MindSync tested across three representative device classes which includes mid-range Android, Raspberry Pi 4 (8GB) Cortex-A72 2GB and Entry-level Android (Pardeshi et al., 2017),.The representative device classes outcome described in Table 9.

Table 9. Device representative class outcomes

Device Type	RAM	CPU	Model Size	Average Latency
Mid-range Android	4GB	Snapdragon 678	0.8GB	~1.6s
Raspberry Pi 4 (8GB)	8GB	Quad-core Cortex-A72	1.2GB	~2.2s
Entry-level Android	2GB	MediaTek Helio A22	0.6GB	~3.1s

To assess the quality of the Chabot's output, a scoring framework used based on the following:

- Context relevance: *Does the reply address the user's previous statement?*
- Empathy rating: *Does the reply reflect a supportive, non-judgmental tone?*
- Language fluency: *Are the responses grammatically sound and natural?*

The TinyLLaMA model (quantized 4-bit) model tested the over 2000 simulated conversation pairs, evaluated by ten human annotators with background in psychology and linguistics. Context Relevance score obtained 4.6 out of 5, Empathy / Tone 4.4 out of 5 and Language Fluency 4.3 out of 5. MindSync can ask for evidence by the conversational prompts. The conversation prompts are described as follows.

Conversational prompt: *"You mentioned feeling low this week. Can you tell me more about when it started?"*

Clarification request: *"You said you've been sleeping poorly. Is this happening every night or just occasionally?"*

Conversation Prompt: *"I haven't been sleeping well. I wake up a lot."*

Clarification request: "*That sounds exhausting. Has it been affecting your energy during the day?*"

MindSync deployed with a test group of 60 users which includes (college students, health volunteers, and young professionals) over a two-week period. They were asked to complete a session with the chatbot without any prior guidance. Table 10. describes evaluation metrics and relevant outcome. After their sessions, users completed a feedback form rating aspects of usability, trust, and comfort. The feedback form outcomes described in Table 11. The MindSync performance on different operating systems described in Figure 2, iphone13 and Pixel 5 device has been tested with the processing components as user input response, NLP preprocessing,context and sentiment analysis finally SLM inference in terms of response time in milliseconds for both devices across these components. Table 12. describes MindSync performance assessment across PHQ-9, BDI-II, and HAMD. Figure 3. describes about text generation speed i.e how many tokens the model generates per second.The model which exhibits higher token generation rate is preferable for the development.The tested models varied from from compact (1.1B) to larger (8B) models (Fatima et al., 2025). A light green representation is a lightweight edge AI device, delivering moderate performance (Jetson Orin Nano Scalcon et al., 2024). A dark green representation is a high-performance edge AI device, offering significantly faster generation rates (Karumbunathan, 2022).

Table 10. Evaluation metrics outcome relevant with user interaction

Metric	Result
Completion Rate (15 Q sessions)	72%
Average Session Duration	6 minutes
Abandonment before Q5	12%
Voluntary Repeat Sessions	41%

Table 11. Feedback Assessment with agreement rate

Feedback Item	Agreement Rate (%)
"I felt comfortable being honest with the chatbot."	83%
"The questions felt thoughtful and relevant."	88%
"I trust that my data stayed private."	100%
"I would recommend this to a friend."	74%

Figure 2. MindSync performance comparison on iPhone 13 vs Pixel 5

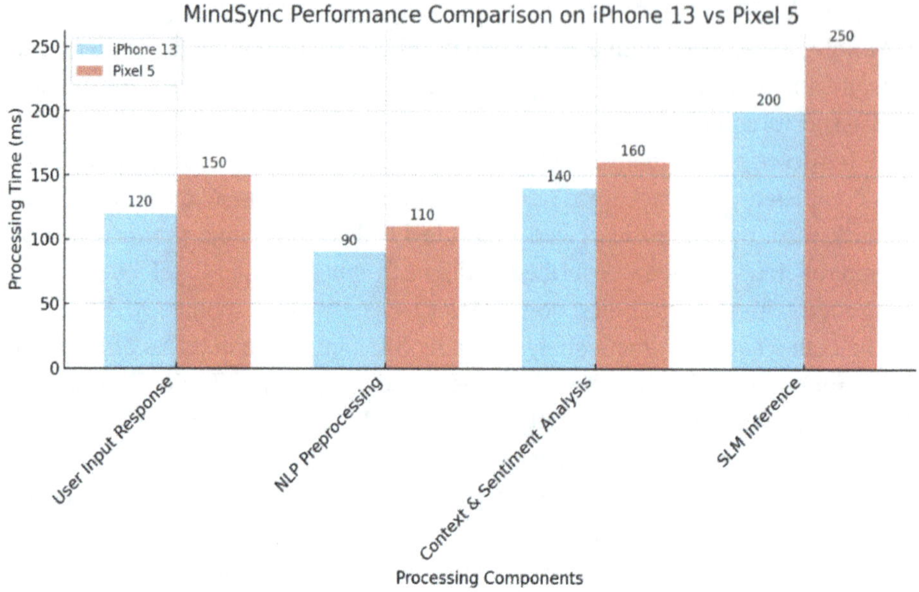

The MindSync ensures that sensitive mental health data is kept private and secure, especially in offline models, can be complex. Handling edge cases where user consent or data deletion is required might pose a challenge in an offline setting. While lightweight models like the ones used in chatbot i.e. SLM-based models are efficient, their accuracy and adaptability to diverse user inputs can be a challenge. The balance between resource efficiency and performance needs constant evaluation. MindSync uniquely combines federated learning, secure mutiparity coding, edge compatibility, and domain adaptation within a single LLM-based framework for mental health assessment. This integration addresses limitations in scalability, privacy, and domain specificity observed in prior work. The proposed MindSync framework compared against Woebot (Fitzpatrick et al., 2017) and MentalBERT (Shaoxiong Ji et al., 2022), systems. The comparison w.r.t to privacy methods, model type, edge deployability, domain adaption capabilities, F1-score, and training convergence factors. Table 13 summarizes that the Woebot system lacks edge deployment capabilities and is based on centralized proprietary. Convergence took up to 32 epochs, and its performance yielded an F1-score of 72.48%. The MentalBERT, a BERT-based architecture with a special domain adaptation which operates under a centralized paradigm with limiting scalability and privacy. MentalBERT achieved a relatively higher F1-score of 80.62% with faster convergence in under 25 epochs. The proposed MindSync framework based on federated learning architecture augmented with secure aggregation and secure multiparty computation .It also supports privacy preservation and ensures collaborative learning across decentralized nodes with domain adaptation and edge deployment .The proposed framework attained the highest F1-score of 84.67%, converging in fewer than 20 epochs.

Table 12. MindSync Performance analysis across PHQ-9, BDI-II, and HAMD

Feature	PHQ-9	BDI-II	HAMD
Integration	High	High	Moderate
Data Type	Self-reported text	Self-reported text	Clinician notes
NLP Preprocessing	short responses	longer responses	extraction of context from transcripts
Context Analysis	Direct analysis	Richer analysis	conversion from interview format to text
Sentiment Analysis	identifying mood states	complexity with nuanced terms	careful context extraction
SLM Inference (Model)	efficient	efficient	complex input
Processing Time (Hypothetical)	~200ms	~300–350ms	~400–500ms
Accuracy Potential	High	High	High

FUTURE RESEARCH DIRECTIONS

Federated learning is about to change MindSync and other privacy-sensitive AI applications. In response to escalating data privacy concerns HIPAA and GDPR, federated learning offers a scalable, decentralized paradigm where personal data stays local and only model updates are safely exchanged. MindSync is a privacy first user controlled federated language model for collaborative mental health assessment where collaborative computing participation computation is depend on the individual interest. If the individual not interested to participate and obtain a collective opinion then individual can block the operation. Handling edge cases where user consent or data deletion is required might pose a challenge in an offline setting. In case of severe depression where the individual don't behave in normal manner and how the application will handle the interaction, depression assessment engaging the individual, hardware limitations of smart devices and limited computing ability of the end devices are the limitations. These limitations opens up the new research directions in the domain of privacy first on device user controlled federated learning.

Figure 3. Text generation speed of model relelvant to Jetson Orin Nano and Jetson AGX

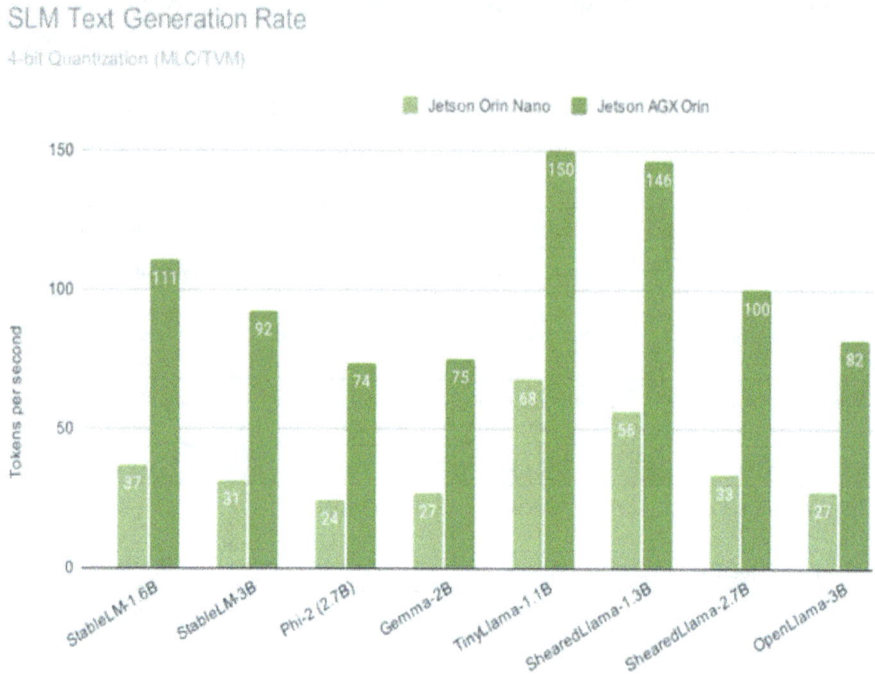

Table 13. The comparative analysis between MindSync and existing systems

System	Privacy Mechanism	Model Type	Domain Adaptation	Edge Deployable	F1 Score (%)	Training Convergence
Woebot (2019)	Centralized Processing	Proprietary	Partial	No	72.48	<32 epochs
MentalBERT (2021)	Centralized Processing	BERT-based	Yes	No	80.62	<25 epochs
MindSync	Federated Learning + Secure Aggregation + SMPC	TinyLLaMA LLM	Yes	Yes	84.67	<20 epochs

5. CONCLUSION

The MindSync as a federated learning-based, privacy-preserving LLM system for mental health assessment. By integrating TinyLLaMA, the framework maintains high predictive accuracy on resource-constrained devices while enabling on-device inference, minimizing data exposure risks. The combination of secure aggregation and SMPC ensures that model updates preserve user confidentiality without sacrificing the performance. Unlike prior approaches that rely on centralized processing or generic LLMs, MindSync is specifically tailored for domain-specific conversation analysis in mental health, supporting both early detection and longitudinal assessment. It helps to detect depression from the conversations and behavior cues from end user without transmitting the raw user data. It aggregates encrypted model updates from diverse local datasets and compliance with GDPR and HIPAA standards. MindSync offers transparent, context-aware insights to support clinicians in diagnosis and treatment planning by considering evidences choice of words and conversation flow, sleep patterns, activity logs and interaction frequency. Future work will explore adaptive personalization layers and multi-modal input integration to further enhance diagnostic precision. There is a need of balancing accuracy and privacy for real-world deployment.

REFERENCES

Alghamdi, W., Salama, R., Sirija, M., Abbas, A. R., & Dilnoza, K. (2023). Secure multi-party computation for collaborative data analysis. E3S Web of Conferences, 399, 04034. https://doi.org/DOI: 10.1051/e3sconf/202339904034

Baalous, R., Poet, R., & Storer, T. (2018, April). Analyzing privacy policies of zero knowledge cloud storage applications on mobile devices. In 2018 Institute of Electrical and Electronics Engineers International Conference on Cloud Engineering (IC2E) 218-224. Institute of Electrical and Electronics Engineers. https://doi.org/DOI: 10.1109/IC2E.2018.00047

Balek, V., Sýkora, L., Sklenák, V., & Kliegr, T. (2024). LLM-based feature generation from text for interpretable machine learning. arXiv preprint arXiv:2409.07132. https://arxiv.org/pdf/2409.07132

Bayerl, S. P., Frassetto, T., Jauernig, P., Riedhammer, K., Sadeghi, A. R., Schneider, T. & Weinert, C. (2020, March). Offline model guard: Secure and private ML on mobile devices. In 2020 Design, Automation & Test in Europe Conference & Exhibition, 460-465. Institute of Electrical and Electronics Engineers https://doi.org/.DOI: 10.23919/DATE48585.2020.9116560

Beck, T., & Ward, H. (1961). An inventory for measuring depression. *Archives of General Psychiatry*, *4*(6), 561–571. DOI: 10.1001/archpsyc.1961.01710120031004 PMID: 13688369

Brown, T. B., Mann, B., Ryder, N., Subbiah, M., Kaplan, J., Dhariwal, P., & Amodei, D. (2020). *Language models are few-shot learners* (Vol. 33). Advances in Neural Information Processing Systems, https://arxiv.org/abs/2005.14165

Chen, K., Chen, H., Conway, N., Hellerstein, J. M., & Parikh, T. S. (2011). Usher: Improving data quality with dynamic forms. *IEEE Transactions on Knowledge and Data Engineering*, *23*(8), 1138–1153. DOI: 10.1109/TKDE.2011.31

Choi, J., & Lee, S. (2017). *Efficient memory-mapped file I/O for in-memory file systems*. In *Proceedings of the 9th USENIX Workshop on Hot Topics in Storage and File Systems (HotStorage '17)*. USENIX Association.

https://www.usenix.org/system/files/conference/hotstorage17/hotstorage17-paper-hoi.pdfUsenix

Cohen, B. M., & Mills, A. (2015). The Diagnostic Drawing Series (DDS) at thirty: Art therapy assessment and research. The Wiley handbook of art therapy, 558-568. https://doi.org/DOI: 10.1002/9781118306543.ch53

Dankar, F. K., & El Emam, K. (2013). Practicing differential privacy in health care: A review. *Transactions on Data Privacy*, 35–67. https://www.tdp.cat/issues11/tdp.a129a13.pdf

David, R., Duke, J., Jain, A., Janapa Reddi, V., & Jeffries, N., Li, Rhodes, R. (2021). Tensorflow lite micro: Embedded machine learning for tinyml systems. *Proceedings of Machine Learning and Systems*, *3*, 800–811. https://proceedings.mlsys.org/paper_files/paper/2021/file/6c44dc73014d66ba49b28d483a8f8b0d-Paper.pdf

Dettmers, T., Pagnoni, A., Holtzman, A., & Smith, N. A. (2022). QLoRA: Efficient fine-tuning of quantized LLMs. *Proceedings of the 2023 International Conference on Machine Learning (ICML)*. https://arxiv.org/abs/2305.14314

Diaz-Rodríguez, N., Del Ser, J., Coeckelbergh, M., de Prado, M. L., Herrera-Viedma, E., & Herrera, F. (2023). Connecting the dots in trustworthy Artificial Intelligence: From AI principles, ethics, and key requirements to responsible AI systems and regulation. *Information Fusion*, *99*, 101896. DOI: 10.1016/j.inffus.2023.101896

Dubhir, T., Mishra, M., & Singhal, R. (2023, December). Benchmarking of quantization libraries in popular frameworks. In 2021 Institute of Electrical and Electronics Engineers International Conference on Big Data (Big Data) (pp. 3050-3055). https:// Institute of Electrical and Electronics Engineersxplore.Institute of Electrical and Electronics Engineers.org/document/9671500

Fatima, E., Dhanda, N., & Zaidi, T. (2025, March). AI-Driven Detection of Stress, Anxiety, and Depression: Techniques, Challenges, and Future Perspectives. In 2025 3rd International Conference on Disruptive Technologies (ICDT) 118-123. Institute of Electrical and Electronics Engineers.

Fitzpatrick, K. K., Darcy, A., & Vierhile, M. (2017). Delivering Cognitive Behavior Therapy to Young Adults With Symptoms of Depression and Anxiety Using a Fully Automated Conversational Agent (Woebot): A Randomized Controlled Trial. *JMIR Mental Health*, *4*(2), e19. DOI: 10.2196/mental.7785 PMID: 28588005

Ge, T., Hu, J., Wang, L., Wang, X., Chen, S. Q., & Wei, F. (2023). In-context autoencoder for context compression in a large language model. arXiv preprint arXiv:2307.06945. https://arxiv.org/pdf/2307.06945

Gorini, A., Mazzocco, K., Triberti, S., Sebri, V., Savioni, L., & Riva, G. (2018). A P5 mHealth approach: Design rationale and technology components. *JMIR Mental Health*, *5*(3), e10232. DOI: 10.3389/fpsyg.2018.02066 PMID: 30429810

Gu, X., Li, M., & Xiong, L. (2021). PRECAD: Privacy-preserving and robust federated learning via crypto-aided differential privacy. *arXiv preprint arXiv:2110.11578*. https://arxiv.org/abs/2110.11578

Guan, Y., Li, Y., Zhang, T., & Liu, L. (2021). A federated learning framework for privacy-preserving prediction of mental health disorders. *Institute of Electrical and Electronics Engineers Journal of Biomedical and Health Informatics*, *25*(8), 3088–3097. DOI: 10.3390/s25082374

Guo, Z., Jin, R., Liu, C., Huang, Y., Shi, D., & Supryadi, Yu. L., Liu, Y., Li, J., Xiong, B., & Xiong, D. (2023). Evaluating large language models: A comprehensive survey. arXiv. https://arxiv.org/abs/2310.19736

Gupta, S., Huang, Y., Zhong, Z., Gao, T., Li, K., & Chen, D. (2022). Recovering private text in federated learning of language models. Advances in neural information processing systems, 35, 8130-8143. https://proceedings.neurips.cc/paper_files/paper/2022/file/35b5c175e139bff5f22a5361270fce87-Paper-Conference.pdf

Hamilton, M. (1960). A rating scale for depression. *Journal of Neurology, Neurosurgery, and Psychiatry*, *23*(1), 56–62. DOI: 10.1136/jnnp.23.1.56 PMID: 14399272

Jajal, P., Jiang, W., Tewari, A., Kocinare, E., Woo, J., Sarraf, A., & Davis, J. C. (2024). Interoperability in deep learning: A user survey and failure analysis of onnx model converters. In Proceedings of the 33rd Association for Computing Machinery SIGSOFT International Symposium on Software Testing and Analysis 1466-1478) https://dl.acm.org/doi/pdf/10.1145/3650212.3680374

Ji, S., Zhang, T., Ansari, L., Fu, J., Tiwari, P., & Cambria, E. (2022). MentalBERT. In *Proceedings of the Thirteenth Language Resources and Evaluation Conference*, pages 7184–7190, Marseille, France. European Language Resources Association.

Jiang, A. Q., Sablayrolles, A., Mensch, A., Bamford, C., Chaplot, D. S., de las Casas, D., Bressand, F., Lengyel, G., Lample, G., Saulnier, L., Lavaud, L. R., Lachaux, M.-A., Stock, P., Le Scao, T., Lavril, T., Wang, T., Lacroix, T., & El Sayed, W. (2023). *Mistral 7B*. arXiv. https://arxiv.org/abs/2310.06825

Karumbunathan, L.S. (2022). Nvidia jetson agx orin series. https://www.nvidia.com/content/dam/en-zz/Solutions/gtcf21/jetson-orin/nvidia-jetson-agx-orin-technical-brief.pdf

Kroenke, K., Spitzer, R. L., & Williams, J. B. (2021). The PHQ-9: Validity of a brief depression severity measure. *Journal of General Internal Medicine*, *16*(9), 606–613. https://onlinelibrary.wiley.com/doi/pdf/10.1046/j.1525-1497.2001.016009606.x. DOI: 10.1046/j.1525-1497.2001.016009606.x PMID: 11556941

Lainidi, O., Jendeby, M. K., Montgomery, A., Mouratidis, C., Paitaridou, K., Cook, C., Johnson, J., & Karakasidou, E. (2023). An integrative systematic review of employee silence and voice in healthcare: What are we really measuring? *Frontiers in Psychiatry*, *14*, 1111579. DOI: 10.3389/fpsyt.2023.1111579 PMID: 37304444

Liu, X., Li, H., Xu, G., Chen, Z., Huang, X., & Lu, R. (2021). Privacy-enhanced federated learning against poisoning adversaries. *IEEE Transactions on Information Forensics and Security*, *16*, 4574–4588. DOI: 10.1109/TIFS.2021.3108434

Liu, Y., Ott, M., Goyal, N., Du, J., Joshi, M., Chen, D., & Stoyanov, V. (2020). RoBERTa: A robustly optimized BERT pretraining approach. arXiv preprint arXiv:1907.11692. https://arxiv.org/abs/1907.11692

Luo, H., Sun, Q., Xu, C., Zhao, P., Lou, J., Tao, C., Geng, X., Lin, Q., Chen, S., Tang, Y., & Zhang, D. (2023). WizardMath: Empowering mathematical reasoning for large language models via reinforced Evol-Instruct. arXiv. https://arxiv.org/abs/2308.09583

Luo, J., Zhang, Y., Zhang, Z., Zhang, J., Mu, X., Wang, H., & Xu, Z. (2024, August). SecFormer: Fast and Accurate Privacy-Preserving Inference for Transformer Models via SMPC. In Findings of the Association for Computational Linguistics ACL 2024 13333-13348. https://aclanthology.org/2024.findings-acl.790.pdf

Magoutas, B., Schmidt, K. U., Mentzas, G., & Stojanovic, L. (2010). An adaptive e-questionnaire for measuring user perceived portal quality. *International Journal of Human-Computer Studies*, *68*(10), 729–745. DOI: 10.1016/j.ijhcs.2010.06.003

Manea, L., Gilbody, S., & McMillan, D. (2015). A diagnostic meta-analysis of the Patient Health Questionnaire-9 (PHQ-9) algorithm scoring method as a screen for depression. *General Hospital Psychiatry*, *37*(1), 67–75. DOI: 10.1016/j.genhosppsych.2014.09.009 PMID: 25439733

McMahan, H. B., Moore, E., Ramage, D., Hampson, S., & Arcas, B. A. (2017). Communication-efficient learning of deep networks from decentralized data. Proceedings of the 20th International Conference on Artificial Intelligence and Statistics (AISTATS), 54, 1273–1282. http://proceedings.mlr.press/v54/mcmahan17a.html

McMahan, H. B., Moore, E., Ramage, D., Hampson, S., & Arcas, B. A. (2017). Communication-efficient learning of deep networks from decentralized data. *Proceedings of the 20th International Conference on Artificial Intelligence and Statistics (AISTATS)*, 54, 1273–1282. https://arxiv.org/abs/1602.05629

Miner, A. S., Milstein, A., Schueller, S., Hegde, R., Mangurian, C., & Linos, E. (2016). Smartphone-Based Conversational Agents and Responses to Questions About Mental Health, Interpersonal Violence, and Physical Health. *JAMA Internal Medicine*, *176*(5), 619–625. DOI: 10.1001/jamainternmed.2016.0400 PMID: 26974260

Mitra, A., ... "Orca 2: Teaching small language models how to reason." arXiv preprint arXiv:2311.11045 (2023). https://arxiv.org/abs/2311.11045

Mittelstadt, B. D., Allo, P., Taddeo, M., Wachter, S., & Floridi, L. (2016). The ethics of algorithms: Mapping the debate. *Big Data & Society*, *3*(2), 1–21. DOI: 10.1177/2053951716679679

Montagna, S., Aguzzi, G., Ferretti, S., Pengo, M. F., Klopfenstein, L. C., Ungolo, M., & Magnini, M. (2024, March). LLM-based solutions for healthcare Chatbots: a comparative analysis. In 2024 Institute of Electrical and Electronics Engineers International Conference on Pervasive Computing and Communications Workshops and other Affiliated Events, 346-351, Institute of Electrical and Electronics Engineers. DOI: 10.1109/PerComWorkshops59983.2024.10503257

Nayan, T., Guo, Q., Al Duniawi, M., Botacin, M., Uluagac, S., & Sun, R. (2024). {SoK}: All You Need to Know About {On-Device} {ML} Model Extraction-The Gap Between Research and Practice. In 33rd USENIX Security Symposium (USENIX Security 24) pp. 5233-5250. https://www.usenix.org/system/files/usenixsecurity24-nayan.pdf

Nederlof, M., Stoker, L. J., Egberts, T. C., & Heerdink, E. R. (2024). Instructions for clinical and biomarker monitoring in the Summary of Product Characteristics (SmPC) for psychotropic drugs: Overview and applicability in clinical practice. *Journal of Psychopharmacology (Oxford, England)*, *29*(12), 1248–1254. DOI: 10.1177/0269881115609016 PMID: 26464457

Novotney, S., Mukherjee, S., Ahmed, Z., & Stolcke, A. (2022). CUE vectors: Modular training of language models conditioned on diverse contextual signals. https://arxiv.org/pdf/2106.01978

Orlando, L. A., Buchanan, A. H., Hahn, S. E., Christianson, C. A., Powell, K. P., Skinner, C. S., & Henrich, V. C. (2013). Development and validation of a primary care-based family health history and decision support program (MeTree). *North Carolina Medical Journal*, *74*(4), 287–296. https://pmc.ncbi.nlm.nih.gov/articles/PMC5215064/pdf/nihms838194.pdf. DOI: 10.18043/ncm.74.4.287 PMID: 24044145

Patel, V., Saxena, S., Lund, C., Thornicroft, G., Baingana, F., Bolton, P., & Unützer, J. (2018). The Lancet Commission on global mental health and sustainable development. *Lancet*, *392*(10157), 1553–1598. DOI: 10.1016/S0140-6736(18)31612-X PMID: 30314863

Poria, S., Cambria, E., Hazarika, D., & Vij, P. (2019). A deeper look into conversational AI: A survey of open-domain dialogue systems. *Information Fusion*, *54*, 124–144. DOI: 10.1016/j.inffus.2019.07.001

Radford, A., Wu, J., Child, R., Luan, D., Amodei, D., & Sutskever, I. (2019). Language models are unsupervised multitask learners. OpenAI. https://cdn.openai.com/better-language-models/language_models_are_unsupervised_multitask_learners.pdf

Rahaman, M., Arya, V., Orozco, S. M., & Pappachan, P. (2024). Secure multi-party computation (SMPC) protocols and privacy. In Innovations in Modern Cryptography, pp. 190-214. IGI Global. https://doi.org/DOI: 10.4018/979-8-3693-5330-1.ch008

Rideout, V., & Fox, S. (2018), Digital Health Practices, Social Media Use, and Mental Well-Being Among Teens and Young Adults in the U.S.1-96, https://digitalcommons.providence.org/publications/1093/

Rieke, N., Hancox, J., Li, W., Milletarì, F., Roth, H. R., Albarqouni, S., & Cardoso, M. J. (2020). The future of digital health with federated learning. *NPJ Digital Medicine*, *3*(1), 119. DOI: 10.1038/s41746-020-00323-1 PMID: 33015372

Scalcon, F. P., Tahal, R., Ahrabi, M., Huangfu, Y., Ahmed, R., Nahid-Mobarakeh, B., & Emadi, A. (2024, June). AI-Powered Video Monitoring: Assessing the NVIDIA Jetson Orin Devices for Edge Computing Applications. In 2024 Institute of Electrical and Electronics Engineers Transportation Electrification Conference and Expo (ITEC) pp. 1-6. Institute of Electrical and Electronics Engineers.

Schick, T., & Schütze, H. "It's not just size that matters: Small language models are also few-shot learners." arXiv preprint arXiv:2009.07118 (2020). https://arxiv.org/pdf/2009.07118

Shen, H., Chang, H., Dong, B., Luo, Y., & Meng, H. (2023). Efficient llm inference on cpus. arXiv preprint, https://arxiv.org/pdf/2311.00502

Shokri, R., & Shmatikov, V. (2015). Privacy-preserving deep learning. In *Proceedings of the 22nd ACM SIGSAC Conference on Computer and Communications Security (CCS '15)*. Association for Computing Machinery, New York, NY, USA, 1310–1321. https://doi.org/DOI: 10.1145/2810103.2813687

Smuha, N. A. (2019). The EU approach to ethics guidelines for trustworthy artificial intelligence. Computer Law Review International, 20(4), 97-106. https://www.europarl.europa.eu/cmsdata/196377/AI%20HLEG_Ethics%20Guidelines%20for%20Trustworthy%20AI.pdf

Tan, X., Jiang, Y., Yang, Y., & Xu, H. (2024). Teola: Towards end-to-end optimization of llm-based applications. arXiv preprint arXiv:2407.00326. https://arxiv.org/pdf/2407.00326

Tangari, G., Ikram, M., Sentana, I. W. B., Ijaz, K., Kaafar, M. A., & Berkovsky, S. (2021). Analyzing security issues of android mobile health and medical applications. *Journal of the American Medical Informatics Association : JAMIA*, *28*(Issue 10), 2074–2084. https://doi.org/. DOI: 10.1093/jamia/ocab131 PMID: 34338763

Wang, R., Gao, Z., Zhang, L., Yue, S., & Gao, Z. (2025). Empowering large language models to edge intelligence: A survey of edge efficient LLMs and techniques. *Computer Science Review*, *57*, 100755. https://chinaxiv.org/abs/202411.00258V1. DOI: 10.1016/j.cosrev.2025.100755

Zaeem, R. N., & Barber, K. S. (2020). The effect of the GDPR on privacy policies: Recent progress and future promise. [TMIS]. *ACM Transactions on Management Information Systems*, *12*(1), 1–20. DOI: 10.1145/3389685

Zhang, P., Li, Y., Zhou, Z., & Wang, J. (2024). TinyLLaMA: Compact and efficient language models for edge NLP applications. Proceedings of the 2024 International Conference on Computational Linguistics (COLING). https://arxiv.org/html/2401.02385v1

ADDITIONAL READING

Ataccama. (2024). Small language models: A beginner's guide. https://www.ataccama.com/blog/small-language-modelsataccama.com

Chen, J., Yan, H., Liu, Z., Zhang, M., Xiong, H., & Yu, S. (2024). When federated learning meets privacy-preserving computation. *ACM Computing Surveys*, *56*(12), 1–36. DOI: 10.1145/3679013

Cramer, R., Damgård, I., & Nielsen, J. B. (2015). *Secure multiparty computation.* Cambridge University Press. DOI: 10.1017/CBO9781107337756

DataCamp. (2024). Small language models: A guide with examples. https://www.datacamp.com/blog/small-language-modelsDataCamp

Ghosh, A., & Chaudhuri, S. S. (2021, August). Iot based portable image de-hazing machine. In 2021 8th international conference on signal processing and integrated networks (SPIN) pp. 31-35. IEEE, https://doi.org/DOI: 10.1109/SPIN52536.2021.9565998

https://proceedings.mlr.press/v54/mcmahan17a/mcmahan17a.pdf.

IBM. (2024). What are small language models, https://www.ibm.com/think/topics/small-language-modelsMicrosoft Azure

Li, T., Sahu, A. K., Talwalkar, A., & Smith, V. (2020). Federated learning: Challenges, methods, and future directions. Institute of Electrical and Electronics Engineers signal processing magazine, 37(3), 50-60. https://doi.org/DOI: 10.1109/MSP.2020.2975749

McMahan, B., Moore, E., Ramage, D., Hampson, S., & Arcas, B. A. (2017, April). Communication-efficient learning of deep networks from decentralized data. In *Artificial intelligence and statistics 1273-1282*. PMLR.

Pardeshi, V., Sagar, S., Murmurwar, S., & Hage, P. (2017, February). Health monitoring systems using IoT and Raspberry Pi—a review. In 2017 international conference on innovative mechanisms for industry applications (ICIMIA) 134-137. IEEE. https://ieeexplore.ieee.org/iel7/7966475/7975508/07975587.pdf

Radford, A., Wu, J., Child, R., Luan, D., Amodei, D., & Sutskever, I. (2019). Language models are unsupervised multitask learners. OpenAI Blog. https://cdn.openai.com/better-language-models/language_models_are_unsupervised_multitask_learners.pdf

Splunk. (2024). LLMs vs. SLMs: The differences in large & small language models. https://www.splunk.com/en_us/blog/learn/language-models-slm-vs-llm.html

Wang, R., Lai, J., Zhang, Z., Li, X., Vijayakumar, P., & Karuppiah, M. (2022). Privacy-preserving federated learning for internet of medical things under edge computing. Institute of Electrical and Electronics Engineers journal of biomedical and health informatics, 27(2), 854-865. https://doi.org/DOI: 10.1109/JBHI.2022.3157725

Zhang, C., Xie, Y., Bai, H., Yu, B., Li, W., & Gao, Y. (2021). A survey on federated learning. *Knowledge-Based Systems*, *216*, 106775. DOI: 10.1016/j.knosys.2021.106775 PMID: 34909232

KEY TERMS AND DEFINITIONS

Personal Privacy: It involves the protection of personal data, communications, behaviors, and identity from being exposed or misused without consent. Its related to an individual right towards protection of personal information and only consent relevant data sharing. Personal Privacy refers to an individual's right to control access to their personal information and the ability to keep their private life and data free from unauthorized intrusion or disclosure.

Personal Health Information and HIIPA: PHI refers to an individual right to manage who has access to their personal data. It concerns about protection of individual private life and information from illegal access or exposure. PHI is confidential and is protected by HIPAA regulations to ensure privacy and security. PHI includes Names, Addresses, Dates, Contact details, Medical records and health conditions, Payment information. It refers to any health-related data that can be used to identify an individual and that is protected under the Health Insurance Portability and Accountability Act (HIPAA) in the United States.

PHI and GDPR: PHI refers to an individual right to manage who has access to their personal data. It concerns about protection of individual private life and information from illegal access or exposure. PHI is confidential and is protected by GDPR regulations to ensure privacy and security. General Data Protection Regulation is a comprehensive data protection law enacted by the European Union (EU). GDPR regulates how organizations collect, store, and process personal data of individuals inside the EU, ensuring privacy rights and data protection.

DSM-IV: Diagnostic and Statistical Manual of Mental Disorders (4th Edition).

DISTILGPT-2: The language model is simply the model that predict the next token from given tokens like the prediction that appear to us when using google search or even youtube search. A distilled version of Generative PreTrained Version -2 (~82 million parameters, 6x smaller then GPT2). It is created by Hugging Face to maintain performance with faster inference and less compute/memory usage. Ideal for generating text, summarizing content and chatbots.

MISTRAL-7B: It is a 7-billion parameter dense language model released by Mistral AI. It is an independent AI company. Trained with a focus on efficiency, open access, and performance, it was designed to be compact, fast, and powerful. The Mistral 7B and its tokenizer is loaded in the environment, interact through prompt and generate response.

GGML: General-purpose GPU-friendly Machine Learning: GGML is a low-level tensor library built for efficient inference of large models like LLaMA. Optimized for running models with low memory footprint and high computational efficiency, especially on CPU and small GPUs. It is a cross-platform, low-level, and memory-efficient tensor library for machine learning. It supports integer quantization, automatic differentiation

APK: Android Package Kit: It essentially acts as a container that bundles all the necessary files for an app to run on an Android device and it is the package file format used by the Android operating system for the distribution and installation of mobile apps and middleware.

ONNX: Open Neural Network Exchange: It is an open-source format and framework designed to facilitate the interoperability of machine learning models across different platforms.

Chapter 10

Next-Generation Medical Intelligence:
Harnessing Federated Learning and Collaborative AI for Healthcare Innovation

S. Anusha
Easwari Engineering College, India

J. Balachandar
Chennai Institute of Technology, India

J. Bibija
S.A. Engineering College, India

B. Yamini
https://orcid.org/0000-0003-3531-108X
SRM Institute of Science and Technology, India

T. Thilagam
https://orcid.org/0000-0002-7657-0726
Vel Tech Rangarajan Dr. Sagunthala R&D Institute of Science and Technology, India

Anto Gracious L. A.
https://orcid.org/0000-0003-2386-9182
R.M.K. College of Engineering and Technology, India

ABSTRACT

The combination of Federated Learning (FL) and Collaborative AI has brought significant changes to the healthcare industry due to challenges with data centralization, privacy, and compliance issues. FL allows for decentralized model training in different institutions and does not require raw data to be shared among them, thus protecting patient information while improving the model. Collaborative AI also enhances healthcare innovation through human-AI cooperation, collaboration across institutions, and integration of multiple data modalities. This chapter explores the basics of these paradigms, the technical models, and revolutionary uses of such

DOI: 10.4018/979-8-3373-3306-9.ch010

concepts in diagnosing diseases, imaging, individualized medicine, and remote patient monitoring. Due to the relevance of FL and Collaborative AI, it is possible to develop the next generation of medical intelligence that is smarter, ethical, scalable, and without violating user privacy, ensuring equal access to healthcare for everyone.

1. INTRODUCTION

1.1 Background and Motivation

AI has brought new opportunities for the development of healthcare and has become one of the most rapidly growing fields in recent years. From helping in diagnosis and prognosis of diseases, to robotic surgery, or even in digitalized enabling of proper treatment protocols, AI integration has become the new norm in healthcare applications (Khang 2024). Of them, two of the most popular subsets, ML and DL have shown high efficacy in various pattern recognition tasks that include image classification, NLP of clinical reports, and EHR-based patient prognosis. This has led both researchers and businesses to search for efficient large-scale AI solutions that would be able to process extensive amounts of medical information (Khang et al., 2024). However, there is still a major issue that slows down the more extensive use of AI in the healthcare field: data integration problem. Most of the previous AI models presuppose the accumulation of data from various sources into a single database for training. This is especially important in the field of healthcare as it poses great risks to patients' privacy and data security. However, the data in healthcare is diverse in terms of formatting, quality, the demography of patients, and protocols used at different facilities, and therefore, training a centralized model is not only technically difficult, but also it poses some ethical questions. Therefore, there is a need to look for new approaches that will address the issue of data ownership and at the same time foster concept of collective intelligence and creativity (Kumar, P., & Sharma, M. K. 2024).

1.2 The Need for Federated Learning and Collaborative AI

To address these issues, there is a new decentralized learning approach in the form of Federated Learning (FL) which allows the training of models on distributed machines or institutions without the exchange of data. FL is a method that enables local training of models by local parties (such as hospitals) and only updates (gradients or weights) are shared with a central server for aggregation (Su et al., 2021). This mechanism also protects the privacy of the patient, increases the level of data protection, and meets legal and ethical requirements while using the intelligence of multiple sources. It can be beneficial in such a setting as Federated Learning is designed specifically for situations where data privacy is an issue and where institutions are located in different geographical locations (Mammen, P. M. 2021). With FL, hospitals, research centers and pharmaceutical companies can construct superior and more generalizable patient models without the transfer of raw data. This is not merely an application, but rather is a new form of thinking that can respect privacy of medical technology. The idea of Collaborative AI also broadens the idea of distributed intelligence, which is closely connected with FL. Multi-agent coordination can be defined as the communication between two or more autonomous agents with the aim of achieving some goal by using collaborative AI. In health care, it extends beyond AI-human cooperation into the diagnostic decision process, to institutional cooperation which integrates the wisdom of diverse forms of data, such as genomics, imaging and clinical notes. Collaborative AI can open up a more inclusive, equitable health care AI ecosystem, in which trust, transparency, and interoperability are valued, in addition to accuracy and efficiency, when utilized with FL. Together, Federated Learning and Collaborative AI define the future of what we can refer to as next-generation medical intelligence a decentralized, holistic and privacy-respectful method to build and deploy AI systems in medicine. The new paradigm ensures the safety of the personal patient data in addition to supporting innovation due to the engagement of multiple stakeholders and international cooperation. With the healthcare systems seeking to use the power of AI and overcome ethical and legal limits, FL and Collaborative AI can be incorporated as strategic providers of scalable and responsible remedies.

1.3 Scope and Objectives

The purpose of the survey is to give a thorough and systematic study of the idea of Federated Learning and Collaborative AI integration and its ways of transforming the healthcare sphere. It integrates the most recent developments, latest applications, theoretical foundations, and open research problems to assist readers in navigating this rapidly evolving field. This chapter is aimed at determining the potential and risks of employing decentralized intelligence in medicine based on the existing literature and practice. Specifically, the survey explores about the overall conceptual frameworks and models of Federated Learning, including horizontal and vertical FL, and introduces the technical building blocks of model aggregation and secure computation schemes. It is also an exploration into the broader Collaborative AI space, exploring how multi-agent systems, human-AI collaboration, and cross-institutional collaboration may enhance the capabilities and reliability of healthcare applications. Some areas of its application are expounded further, these include disease diagnosis, medical imaging, the patient individualized treatment and remote patient surveillance systems. Lastly the survey explores possible future developments and directions which include usage of edge AI, blockchain and self-supervised learning in federated systems. In this way, the chapter aims at providing an overview of this landscape to the researchers, and practitioners to help them explore the possibilities of using Federated Learning and Collaborative AI to create the next generation of medical intelligence that is safe, scalable, and socially responsible.

2. FOUNDATIONS OF FEDERATED LEARNING (FL) IN HEALTHCARE

2.1 What is Federated Learning?

FL is an ML approach that allows the training of models on distributed devices or organizations without sharing the original data (Hassan et al., 2024). The traditional machine learning procedures require accumulation and storage of data from different sources before the training is initiated. This concentration is not only costly but it poses several risks to people's privacy and compliance issues especially when it comes to matters affecting peoples' health. FL addresses this challenge by taking the model to the data rather than the data to the model (Krishnan et al., 2024). In the context of FL, a global model is first deployed, and then it is locally trained on the clients' data which could be hospitals/clinics/ edge devices. These local updates (which could be gradients or weights of the model) are then sent back to a central coordinator for the purpose of updating the global model. This is done in a number of rounds until the model is optimized and the results no longer change (Lilhore et al., 2024). The principle of FL is that only the model parameters or updates are exchanged with the other clients but not the patient data, hence the privacy of the patient data and data ownership are preserved. This makes FL particularly useful in environments that have strict laws that govern the use of data as it reduces the chances of data leakage while at the same time allowing for the training of machine learning models on decentralized datasets (Chattopadhyay & Das, 2024; Gracious et al., 2024).

2.2 Types of FL Approaches

FL is not a single method, it has many variations depending on the distribution of the data in the network. The major categories of FL are horizontal FL, vertical FL and federated transfer learning. Sample FL is known as Horizontal FL as well and is best suited for cases where the participating entities have different datasets, yet these datasets have the same features, such as patient records with age, weight, and diagnosis, but are from different hospitals. This is the most common FL setup since different institutions generally gather the same type of data but from different patients. Feature-based FL or Vertical FL is useful when different organizations have the same patients' information but different features. For example, an acute care hospital has EHR data on a patient, whereas a clinical genomic laboratory has DNA sequencing data on the same patient. Vertical FL is used to train a model under a cooperative environment without disclosing the raw data that is usually considered sensitive or proprietary. Federated Transfer Learning is applied in situations where the data sharing is not only limited in the number of samples and features but also does not intersect. In such cases, knowledge transfer methodologies like pretrained models or shared representations are used to build models that are trained from limited but related data resources. This variant is particularly applicable in the cases of international cooperation because datasets may vary from country to country due to population, or approaches to healthcare.

2.3 Technical Components

To effectively apply Federated Learning in the healthcare sector, there is a need to have a strong technological platform. One of the most important parts is the model aggregation, the procedure of updating the global model with the local updates received from the client nodes. The simplest one is Federated Averaging (FedAvg) where the local models are averaged according to their size of the data sample in order to update the central model. The simplest of them all is FedAvg which has been used in many FL systems because of its efficiency, however, it can be slow converging and sensitive to non-IID data distributions. In order to alleviate these problems, there are variations of FedAvg such as FedProx that introduce proximal terms to minimize heterogeneity among the clients. Besides the aggregation techniques, secure computation is crucial in order to protect the privacy of the data in the FL process. The methods such as differential privacy add noise to the model updates that are shared to avoid any possibility of reconstructing the patient's data. On the other hand, homomorphic encryption enables computations on encrypted data so that none of the parties can get hold of the raw model parameters during training. Another approach is secure multiparty computation where the computation is done jointly without exposing the inputs of each party. All these cryptographic and privacy-preserving methods combined guarantee that federated learning other health data regulation and ethical benchmark legal. Another factor is the communication effectiveness especially in transmitting large data in FL as it involves several clients and a central server. Some of the strategies include gradient compression, update sparsification and periodic communication which help to reduce the amount of bandwidth needed, thus making it useful for resource limited settings such as rural clinics or edge devices.

2.4 Advantages Over Centralized Learning

There are several reasons that have made the transition from the centralized learning in healthcare to federated learning possible. Among them, the most important is data locality, which enables the protected medical data to be stored and processed in the local premises of healthcare organizations. This significantly minimizes the threats of data leakage and unauthorized access, and it is compatible with the rules and regulation of laws, which severely restrict the handling and sharing of personal health information. The second notable benefit is the compliance with the legal and regulatory frameworks. The standard models are also repeatedly trained on a homogenous set of data not necessarily representative of global populations of patients. Federated Learning in its turn works with data on various institutions with various demographics and medical practices, which brings its models which are more probable to be implemented to other settings. This diversity does not only improve the predictive power but also renders AI tools more equitable and fairness in medicine. In addition to it, FL will also bring about team innovation whereby the institutions can share with each other the benefits of accessing state of the AI models without compromising proprietary data. It democratizes technology and develops a knowledge-sharing ecosystem, where sharing is not compromised with privacy or autonomy. Overall, Federated Learning is a promising framework to advancing privacy-sensitive, ethical, and technically viable intelligent healthcare. In a modern era where healthcare is struggling to manage the twin engines of innovation and regulation, FL is a key facilitator of medical intelligence of the next generation.

3. COLLABORATIVE AI IN THE MEDICAL DOMAIN

3.1 Concept of Collaborative AI

Collaborative AI is an artificial intelligence system that is not intended to be independent but instead work cooperatively with other actors, be it a human, machine, or institution. In contrast to other, more conventional AI models, which are trained and executed in isolated settings, Collaborative AI is designed to exist in linked spaces, where the prowess of various actors is leveraged to attain collective aims. The application of this method is especially relevant in the sphere of healthcare because the systems are complex, diverse, and interrelated. Among the notable applications of Collaborative AI is in multi-agent systems (MAS) where multiple

AI agents function collectively among themselves in order to accomplish tasks that are too complicated to be delegated exclusively to a particular system. These agents are able to exchange information, knowledge or partial models to arrive at joint decisions. As an example, radiology image, laboratory data, and patient history could be analyzed independently by separate AI systems in a hospital network, and the results could be combined to come up with a single diagnosis or treatment recommendation. This collective intelligence makes it possible to think of patient health in a holistic way and can come up with more informed and rich decisions. The other aspect of collaborative AI is the fact that such systems are capable of learning off other systems. Multi-agent reinforcement and ensemble learning is also being developed so that coordinated behaviors can be achieved among AI agents(Manjunathan et al., 2024). These architectures are human-like collaboration where knowledge is disseminated, communication plays a key role and dynamically shared tasks. The latter systems are most suitable to healthcare, where information is disseminated and non-homogeneous, and in which clinical judgments often require the ability to synthesize different information and knowledge.

Figure 1. **Collaborative AI in the Healthcare**

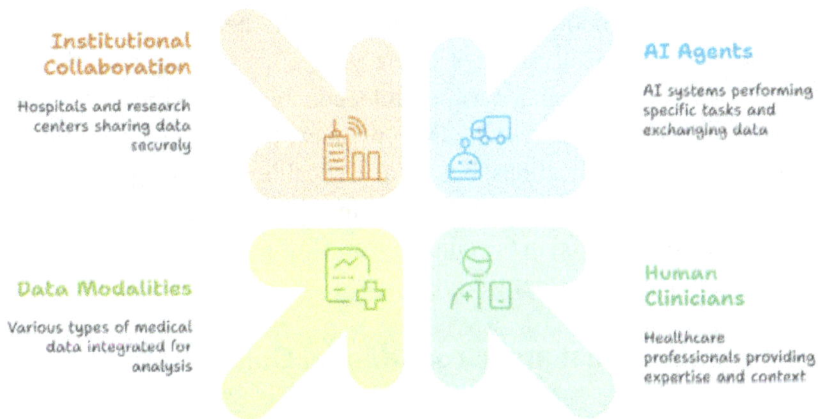

Institutional Collaboration
Hospitals and research centers sharing data securely
AI Agents
AI systems performing specific tasks and exchanging data
Data Modalities
Various types of medical data integrated for analysis
Human Clinicians
Healthcare professionals providing expertise and context

3.2 Human-AI Collaboration

Of all the issues related to Collaborative AI in medicine, the most important is the communication between the human element, particularly clinicians, and AI systems. Currently, the idea of human-AI collaboration focuses on enhancing the decision-making process in clinical practice rather than replacing it. In this model,

AI merely gives the analytical support, risk analysis or treatment recommendations and the final decisions are made by human beings who look at these AI recommendations within the context of the particular case. For instance, in radiological images, algorithms can mark areas that may be cancerous or in EHRs, point out abnormalities that a radiologist or a physician can review based on his or her experience and the patient's record. This form of collaboration decreases diagnostic errors, increases productivity, and allows the clinicians to work on higher level, value-added activities. Distinguishing AI as a supplement to the human experience means that it can add to the cognitive filter rather than replace it, and feels a part of the care optimization process. However, effective human-AI collaboration hinges on three essential factors: trust, transparency, and explainability. It relies on trust- the clinician must have confidence that the AI systems available to him/her are valid, precise and true. This would require building this confidence with a high level of validation on scaled amounts of data, detection of any model anomalies, and ongoing optimization in the performances. The feature of the system to publicly disclose its decision-making is its transparency and the aspect that the system aims at and the rationality that it applies. Explainability has even higher ambitions, and is building tools and techniques, such as attention maps and counterfactual explanations and feature importance scores, to enable AI decisions to be explainable and understandable by non-technical consumers. The health care case example cannot afford transparent black-boxes where people are playing with their lives, and every choice counts. As much as possible, collaborative AI must always tend to be understandable to the extent it can be practical to the degree that clinicians, not only can access AI applications, but are also capable of challenging, perfecting, and refining them over time. Such a dynamic interplay would be the last promise that ensures that AI is utilized in the clinical workflow process and delivers a better user confidence and patient safety.

3.3 Cross-Institutional and Cross-Modal Collaboration

Collaborative AI in medicine is also useful at the institutional level and the data modality level besides the interaction between the individual agent and the clinician. The significance of the cooperation between the institutions is that no single hospital or research center possesses enough data diversity to build universally applicable models. Using privacy-enabling and safe methods, such as federated learning and secure multiparty computation, different institutions can collaborate to develop collaborative AI models without exposing patients to sensitive information. Such an approach will enable a more representative and equitable model development as it is advantageous to everyone involved and does not breach the laws and moral principles. Real-world uses of this concept include multinational cancer registries, pandemic response systems, and collaborative drug discovery. In both cases, AI systems are trained using decentralized datasets donated by many sources, which supports more effective models in different populations and disease manifestation. It is particularly topical to reduce the bias in algorithms, which is typically introduced by having the training models trained on non-representative or non-homogenous datasets. This is as critical as the cross-modality, or the combination of different kinds of data, including medical images, genomic information, pathology reports, monitoring and wearable devices data, EHR data. Most diseases or treatments often involve multiple systems in the human body, and thus, it is common to find information that integrates data from the multiple domains. Collaborative AI helps this integration by synchronizing these various modes of data and making it more accurate and holistic. For example, in the field of oncology, showed that integrating histopathological images with patients' molecular and clinical information can produce substantially superior prognostic coefficient and therapeutic approach. In cardiology, the use of ECG and blood tests and history gives better risk assessment of the heart disease. Such multimodal and Collaborative AI approaches open up new avenues to precision medicine and create possibilities of developing digital twins, state-of-the-art accurate representations of how patients will progress and thus how the therapies should be designed and adapted beforehand in silico.

Thus, the effectiveness of such systems is not only contingent upon the integration of the technical aspects that enable information sharing but also on organizational readiness to cooperate. The institutions will embrace the common data annotation standards, interconnection standards, systems of governance, specifying roles, responsibilities, and ethical guardrails. Collaborative AI is successful in situations where openness, accountability, and mutual benefit are values.

4. APPLICATION AREAS

4.1 Disease Diagnosis and Risk Prediction

The applications of FL and CA are especially apparent in the diagnosis of diseases and prediction of risks in the medical field.

Detecting diseases in their initial stages, for instance, cardiovascular conditions, diabetes, and cancer, enhances patients' treatment chances, decreases the costs of attending to the ailments, and lessens the pressure on the health care systems. However, accuracy of the predictive models is often highly dependent on the availability of large and diverse data set, which is not easy to come by in centralized learning setup due to privacy and data management issues. This is because federated learning models provide a solution to the problem that allows hospitals and clinics to train AI systems on local data while keeping patient data secure. For instance, in cardiovascular disease prediction, several cardiology centers can use FL to train accurate models for risk assessment based on ECG signals, blood pressure, and other personal data. These models do not compromise the disclosing of sensitive health information of the collaborating institutions while leveraging the diversity of data. In diabetes too they have used the federated strategies for the prediction of disease onset, disease progression, and risks of comorbidity based on the data from numerous geographically and demographically dispersed patient groups. This is through the integration of multiple AI systems in cancer clinics that will always facilitate the detection of malignancies via biomarkers, lab data, and imaging of patients' organs and tissues and all this while strictly adhering to the regulations of patient's privacy. Due to the fact that these models are trained on real-world, non-uniform data sets that originate from different environments and populations their generalization and fairness is much enhanced.

4.2 Medical Imaging

Medical imaging is one of the spheres that have benefited from the implementation of Collaborative AI and Federated Learning. Deep learning based AI models particularly have performed very well in interpreting the complex visual data from modalities such as MRI, CT, PET, and X-rays(Sundari V et al., 2024). However, these models entail a need for large annotated datasets for training, which are often stored in different organizations due to legal and other considerations. The practice of collaborative learning has thus allowed joint model development across different departments of radiology and different imaging centers without necessarily sharing large amounts of sensitive data. For instance, in the case of segmentation of brain tumor using MRI, a number of hospitals can have a federated learning framework where each hospital trains a deep neural network locally and the results are contributed to the global model. The obtained model is less sensitive to the variety of tumor presentations, scanning protocols, and patients' characteristics, which in turn enhances its reliability and accuracy. Federated learning methods have also been utilized to detect thoracic diseases based on chest X-ray images and to classify lung nodules on CT scans with the performance that is at par with or even better than that of models trained on centralized data. It also retains the privacy aspect and enables institutions with less data to take advantage of models that they cannot train themselves. Moreover, by combining federated techniques with explainability tools these imaging models can provide visual explanation of the predictions made to the radiologists for their improved trust in the AI-assisted diagnostics.

Figure 2. **Application Areas**

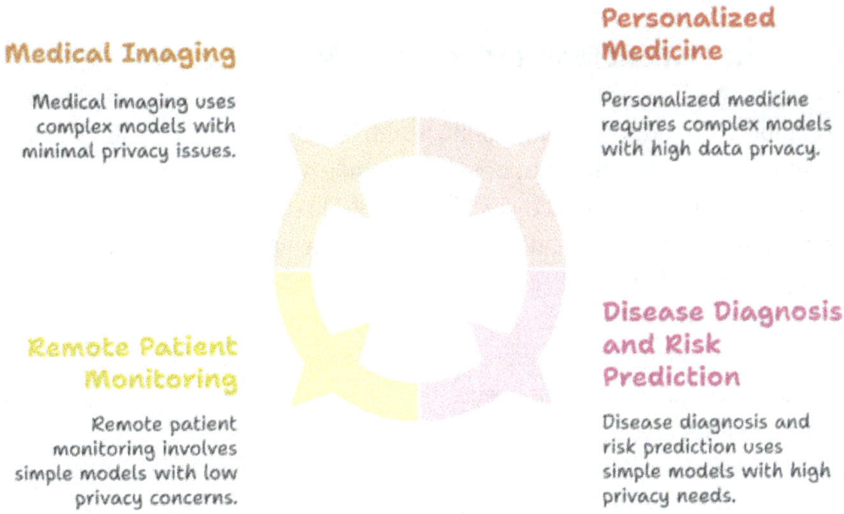

4.3 Personalized Medicine

Personalized medicine is a concept of rendering treatment to patients depending on their genetic make-up, lifestyle, and clinical history. This field is likely to benefit from the implementation of Federated Learning and Collaborative AI especially in the analysis of genomics and pharmacogenomics fields. However, genomic data is considered being one of the most private and personal kinds of health data, and its storage and processing at a central place raise numerous privacy and ethical concerns. Federated Learning solves the problem of data privacy by allowing several medical centres across the country and hospitals to work together to develop artificial intelligence algorithms to analyze the clients' genetic sequences and to look for disease-causing mutations or drug response indicators. For example, institutions from different geographical areas may develop models that estimate the readiness for hereditary diseases, including breast cancer or other hereditary diseases, without using raw genome data. In pharmacogenomics, the federated models are also under consideration to establish the relationship between genetic differences and the effectiveness of medications or their side effects in different populations. These knowledge areas can enable clinicians to choose appropriate drugs and dosages of the drugs to administer to the patients and prevent mistakes in prescriptions. Such models are trained on a larger number of genotypes and phenotypes than individual models, making the whole promise of personalized medicine more achievable.

4.4 Remote Patient Monitoring and IoMT

Wearable health devices and mobile health or mHealth has provided an avenue to monitor patient's health continuously particularly in chronic disorders and after operations. The Internet of Medical Things (IoMT) devices can be used to capture gigantic volumes of real-time health data, heart rate and sleep patterns against the level of glucose and physical activity that can be analyzed by AI to identify abnormalities, predict health decline, and provide relevant solutions. Nevertheless, this streaming of information is of sheer importance in terms of bandwidth, ownership and privacy. Federated Learning meets these obstacles by enabling AI models to be trained either on device or on an edge device like a smartphone, smartwatch or home-based health monitor. This allows creating health insights in the region and safely in aggregate form and remote monitoring is thus scalable and safe. Individual care is one more side that it is possible to provide with the cooperation of collaborative AI in this situation. Indicatively, AI-based systems can identify the initial stages of heart arrhythmias, diabetes-related complications, or respiratory conditions and notify medical professionals or caregivers immediately by examining patterns in the wearable data. Such models get better with time as they are trained on distributed data and do not violate the user's privacy settings. Furthermore, the use of federated wearable data together with the clinical record and the environmental context can form a complete picture of the patient's health status, which will be beneficial for the clinicians. These integrative systems are useful in preventative medicine and chronic disease, which would decrease the rate of readmissions and enhance the quality of life.

5. CHALLENGES AND LIMITATIONS

5.1 Data and System Heterogeneity

The following are some of the challenges that are ever present in the implementation of FL in the context of healthcare: The first challenge is that the data and systems are heterogeneous across institutions. The general assumption that the medical data is independent and independently distributed (non-IID) does not hold as the data can be extremely heterogeneous in terms of structure, quality, labeling, and distribution of features. For instance, patient characteristics, disease incidence, treatment patterns and diagnostic facilities vary from hospital to hospital and from region to region. The model trained with such non-uniform data might have the issue of convergence instability or suboptimal generalization, especially when some clients dominate the training process. The second and major challenge is system heterogeneity which is a technical issue. There is a wide variation in the IT environment and computational resources of health care facilities. Some may possess modern GPUs and strong networks, while some may still use older GPUs or suffer from instable connection. This can cause asynchronous update of the model and worker, stragglers, and workers to have different contribution to the global model. This is so because the communication overhead required to propagate the model updates across multiple clients increases with the size of the models or when the environment is resource limited such as in the rural clinic or mHealth platforms. These need to be addressed by algorithms that can handle data distributions that are not necessarily uniform and participation that may be constantly changing without affecting the quality of the model.

5.2 Privacy and Security Concerns

As mentioned earlier, FL is built with privacy as one of its core principles, nonetheless, it is not invulnerable to complex security threats that can endanger patients' privacy and the model itself. Another classic example is the model inversion, in which the attackers leverage the access to either model gradients or outputs in order to reconstruct certain aspects of the used training data. In a healthcare context, this may refer to the exposure of identifiable data such as x-rays or DNA sequences, even if the actual data is never transmitted from the local machine or organization. Another threat is poisoning attacks, where the participants provide the model with erroneous information that would be detrimental to the global model. In targeted attacks, adversaries may attempt to skew the model's behavior for specific inputs, which could have dire consequences in clinical applications for example, misclassifying a malignant tumor as benign. In the untargeted attacks, it may be to reduce the model's accuracy in general, which affects trust and usefulness of collaborative AI systems.

Figure 3. **Challenges and Limitations**

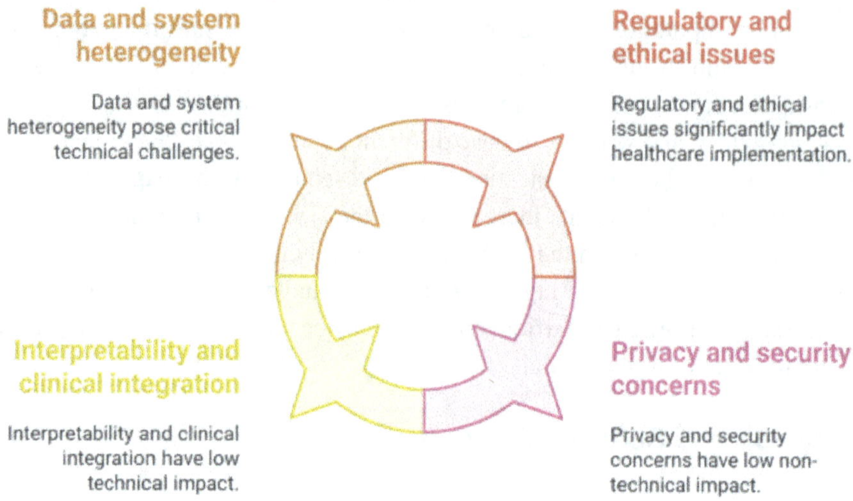

Even though, methodologies like differential privacy, secure multiparty computation, and homomorphic encryption provide some level of protection, they bring the cost of computation and model performance. Moreover, these methods are not completely immune from drawbacks and the choice of parameters in these methods needs fine-tuning in order to bring the level of privacy protection to the necessary amount while not losing the possibility to extract clinical benefits. Security in FL systems should also protect against side-channel attacks and insider threats since the FL systems may be part of a large network involving multiple institutions. Therefore, there is a need to develop more innovative approaches to threat modeling and designing secure protocols to protect the federated healthcare ecosystems.

5.3 Regulatory and Ethical Issues

Another area that is closely connected to FL and requires careful approach is the connection between FL and healthcare regulations and ethical issues. Despite the fact that the federated models strive to meet the data protection laws, legal issues remain ambiguous. For instance, it is still unclear if model updates despite not being raw data could be regarded as personal data under some of the interpretations. This makes cross-border relations challenging and increases the need for laws that recognize FL paradigms by default. Apart from compliance, new concerns of data governance and consent are becoming more important. Even when the patient data is not transferred outside the hospital, patients do not know that their data is being used for AI model training. Obtaining informed consent, providing opt-out mechanisms, and ensuring transparency in data usage policies are critical to maintaining public trust. However, it can be argued that federated learning may perpetuate existing prejudices in the system if the institutions involved are not diverse. If the FL models are trained without any intentional inclusion and bias removal measures, then the performance of the models would be worse particularly for the minority groups. Issues of intellectual property can also come up in a collaborative context. This may not work well if institutions are not willing to contribute their data or computational resources to the shared model because they do not benefit from it in the same proportion. These issues include ownership and attribution, as well as revenue generation in federated research and commerce applications. It is crucial to ensure the fair and clear rules for all the participants in order to create proper motivation.

5.4 Interpretability and Clinical Integration

The last frontier in development of federated learning and collaborative AI in healthcare is the interpretability and implementation into practice. Most of the AI models, particularly those that are based on deep learning, are often referred to as 'black boxes' whereby it is hard for the clinicians to determine how the predictions are made. Such a lack of transparency is a significant issue and could be one of the possible reasons why other consumers do not use this technology. The clinicians who deal with such a situation as cancer diagnosis, sepsis prediction or treatment are supposed to be able to explain and review the algorithmic decision making not only because of ethical consideration but also because of the legal responsibility. It is also intensified in federated settings, where the heterogeneity of data and disseminated training complicates models. Explainable algorithms, including saliency maps, SHAP values, or attention mechanisms, are more difficult to apply and justify in FL examples. In addition, clinicians might lack technical advancement as federated systems might achieve, so they can be cynical or resistant unless the models are supported with well-informed sources and easy interfaces. Other practical considerations like models' versioning, ongoing validation, and real-time responsiveness among other details should be addressed as well to support successful implementation in clinical workflows. The medical places must not only have precision, but reliability, safety and accountability. To make FL work move from pilot projects to clinical tools, there must be integration of various stakeholders such as data scientists, clinicians, ethicists, and policy makers to come up with FL systems that are effective and efficient in their application.

6. EMERGING TRENDS AND FUTURE DIRECTIONS

6.1 Edge AI and On-Device Learning

When looking for the most prospective development in federated learning, it is pertinent to consider the connection of Edge AI and device-embedded learning features significantly in healthcare services since decision-making process in these environments has to be fast. Specifically, traditional FL follows client-server models where the edge devices send updates of the model to an aggregator. However, current advancements in edge computing infrastructures imply that it is now possible to train as well as perform inference on such models directly on the devices like smartphones, wearable sensors or even on the medical devices that are embedded into the system. This shift of paradigm to edge intelligence can greatly decrease reliance on the network connection and minimize the need for communication. For example, fitness bands and health trackers, that can monitor the physiological patterns of a person, can independently develop models specific to the user to identify a new form of abnormality, or predict future health state without any outside input. Such local learning not only improves user experience by providing instant feedback but also strengthens privacy by avoiding exposure of even a little information during the communication. Further, the edge-enabled FL can be used to support continuous learning while not requiring a new central training when there are changes in patients' behavior or treatment schedules. Thus, such areas as remote patient monitoring or Intensive Care Units reveal the potential of Edge AI even more. In this case, systems are capable of responding to changes in patient status, identifying early signs of deterioration and notifying clinicians independently of the cloud. Because of advancements and growing capabilities of edge computing devices, edge devices also are expected to become much more involved in federated architectures across healthcare systems, which in turn will foster the shift toward hyper personalized medicine with high levels of privacy protection.

6.2 Blockchain and Decentralized Trust Mechanisms

Another innovative concept related to federated learning is the blockchain and other has decentralized trust models(Yamini, B et al., 2025). Although FL enables the decentralization of data utilization, the training and aggregation processes are often centralized. It can act as a single point of failure or a trust bottleneck for cross-instutional collaborations whenever more than one stakeholder participates in the process, each having his or her own recognition(Maheshwaran et al., 2024). FL can benefit from Blockchain as a secure and immutable record keeping system that would provide a transparent record of the updates performed on the models.

Smart-contracts applications which are embedded in a blockchain may be applied to automate the trust policies, to define the access rights to data, as well as to manage the compensation or credit split between the involved participants. For instance, a smart contract could guarantee that the institutions providing better quality data to a federated model get the corresponding recognition or incentives(Babu, A et al., 2024) .When applied to healthcare, the main benefit of the proposed FL is the ability to provide secure and transparent data sharing between hospitals, research centers, and pharma companies. It also paves way for patient-level data management where the patient can see how his/her data is used in creating models and control its use. While the application of blockchain also has issues in scalability and computational complexity, sidechains and proof-of-stake protocols are the solutions which are gradually making the blockchain more suitable for the healthcare scale application.

6.3 Self-Supervised and Foundation Models in Federated Settings

The experiences obtained by large foundation models and self-supervised learning in domains like the natural language processing and vision have led to new study on federated settings. These pre-trained models are trained on extremely large and varied datasets using objectives that are self-supervised, hence, they learn general purpose features that can be adapted quickly for other particular tasks given very little labeled data. When integrated with FL, foundation models will be able to transform the medical AI by bringing the pretrained intelligence to the masses. In federated settings, foundation models may be trained cooperatively across institutions on unlabeled data, alleviating the need for limited expert annotations. The hospitals may jointly train a multimodal foundation model on medical images, clinical notes, and genomic data- each with a subset of the training corpus- without actually exchanging raw data. After training, such models can be adapted locally to achieve task-specific performance benefits, with generalization across a wide range of environments. Self-supervised learning (SSL) used in FL also solves the problem of data sparsity and label imbalance typical of medical tasks. Such methods as contrastive learning or masked modeling can be used to utilize unlabeled EHRs, radiology scans, or bio signal streams to create powerful feature extractors in a federated fashion. Also, federated pretraining can be used as a transition to global interoperability by aligning feature spaces across data silos, improving model robustness and transferability. Although their integration into FL frameworks continues to be a technically challenging endeavor, as they are large and highly resource intensive, progress in model compression, distillation, and federated sub model selection is rapidly making them more feasible. This convergence will re-establish collaborative AI, allowing powerful tools generalizable across privacy-respectful and institutionally diverse scales to be developed.

6.4 Towards Federated Clinical Trials and Digital Twins

In the future, there is perhaps one of the most ambitious federated learning uses in the organization of federated clinical trials and the creation of digital twins, artificial replicas of patients, to be used in simulation and precision medicine. The classical clinical trials are time consuming, costly and limited by geography which restricts access and diversity. FL provides the possibility to run distributed trials involving more than one institution in real-time model development, without disclosing patient-level information. By combining the experience of larger and more diverse populations, these federated clinical trials could enhance statistical power, yet also maintain patient privacy. In addition, real-time monitoring of outcomes, adverse events, and the efficacy of treatments can be performed almost instantly with the help of federated analytics. Federated methods can speed up drug development pipelines and enhance the generalizability of medical discoveries by facilitating adaptive trial designs. Meanwhile, the concept of digital twins, dynamic and computation models of individual patients, gained relevance in the field of precision medicine. These twins may mimic disease progression, treatment efficacy or outcome, or assist in the decision of optimally individualized therapy. The proposed federated learning method for training digital twin models across different institutions using the distributed EHR, imaging, genomics, wearables data while keeping the data decentralized. The combination of FL with digital twins can enable fast and individualized interventions at scale – thus, the application of AI in healthcare becomes less futuristic. However, there are some limitations and issues that are associated with the field which are; infrastructure, standardization and ethical use of the field. However, when federated learning is combined with other technologies such as edge computing, blockchain, SSL, and digital twins, it has brought a significant change to how learning and developmental processes can be intelligent, inclusive, and equitable for healthcare systems.

7. CONCLUSION

This study has discussed the possibility of using federated learning and collaborative AI in changing the healthcare industry through solving issues related to the centralization of data processing. Because of the issues of data privacy, regulation, and the decentralization of medical data across institutions, FL is a more suitable solution for training AI models at the data source without compromising privacy.

It also enables the development of large-scale and private models that can take advantage of various and dispersed datasets. This potential is enhanced by the synergy with collaborative AI, which extends to human-AI partnerships, multi-agent systems, and cross-modes integration, introducing transparency, adaptability, and collective intelligence. The feasibility and impact of these paradigms have already been demonstrated in applications in disease diagnosis, imaging, personalized medicine, and remote monitoring. In the future, the future of medical intelligence will be determined by the strategic shift towards decentralized, ethical, and intelligent AI systems. Federated clinical trials, digital twins, are emerging areas where FL and collaborative AI will converge to enable more inclusive, equitable, and personalized care. Nonetheless, issues related to technical, ethical, and regulatory challenges need to be solved by interdisciplinary cooperation. With data increasing in volume and complexity, and patients increasingly insisting on control over their data, the healthcare ecosystem will need to change to enable trust-based, privacy-conscious innovation. Finally, federated learning and collaborative AI are not only a technological breakthrough, but also an ethical necessity, to provide smarter, safer, and more humane solutions to healthcare worldwide.

REFERENCES

Babu, A. A., Jebamalar, G. B., Kumar, P., & Nalini, M. (2024, December). Blockchain Technology: Evolution and Future Prospects. In *2024 International Conference on Sustainable Communication Networks and Application (ICSCNA)* (pp. 381-387). IEEE. DOI: 10.1109/ICSCNA63714.2024.10864089

Chattopadhyay, S., & Das, S. (2024). Safeguarding Privacy Through Federated Machine Learning Techniques. In *Emerging Technologies and Security in Cloud Computing* (pp. 295–318). IGI Global Scientific Publishing. DOI: 10.4018/979-8-3693-2081-5.ch013

Gracious, L. A., Pajila, P. B., Johncy, G., Anish, T. P., & Prasanth, K. (2024, March). Towards Precision Oncology: A Study of Machine Learning Models for Breast Cancer Prediction. In *2024 10th International Conference on Advanced Computing and Communication Systems (ICACCS)* (Vol. 1, pp. 1938-1943). IEEE. DOI: 10.1109/ICACCS60874.2024.10717246

Hassan, A., Prasad, V. K., Bhattacharya, P., & Dutta, P. K. (Eds.). (2024). *Pioneering Smart Healthcare 5.0 with IoT, Federated Learning, and Cloud Security*. IGI Global.

Khang, A. (Ed.). (2024). *AI-Driven Innovations in Digital Healthcare: Emerging Trends, Challenges, and Applications: Emerging Trends*. Challenges, and Applications.

Khang, A., Jadhav, B., & Sayyed, M. (2024). Role of cutting-edge technologies and deep learning frameworks in the digital healthcare sector. In *AI-driven innovations in digital healthcare: emerging trends, challenges, and applications* (pp. 1–22). IGI Global Scientific Publishing. DOI: 10.4018/979-8-3693-3218-4.ch001

Krishnan, S., Anand, A. J., Srinivasan, R., Kavitha, R., & Suresh, S. (2024). *Federated Learning*. CRC Press.

Kumar, P., & Sharma, M. K. (2024). AI-Driven System for Early Detection and Diagnosis of Cataracts by Image Recognition and Machine Learning Algorithms. In *AI-Driven Innovations in Digital Healthcare: Emerging Trends, Challenges, and Applications* (pp. 168-184). IGI Global Scientific Publishing. DOI: 10.4018/979-8-3693-3218-4.ch008

Lilhore, U. K., Simaiya, S., Poongodi, M., & Dutt, V. (Eds.). (2024). *Federated Learning and Privacy-preserving in Healthcare AI*. IGI Global. DOI: 10.4018/979-8-3693-1874-4

Maheshwaran, T., Muthumarilakshmi, S., Suganya, K., Maheswari, B., & Girija, P. (2024). Securing E-Commerce Strategies With Cloud, Blockchain, AI, and ML. In *Strategies for E-Commerce Data Security: Cloud, Blockchain, AI, and Machine Learning* (pp. 470-500). IGI Global.

Mammen, P. M. (2021). Federated learning: Opportunities and challenges. *arXiv preprint arXiv:2101.05428.*

Manjunathan, N., Shanmugapriya, D., Girija, P., Vasudevan, M., & Murugesan, S. (2024, September). Ensemble Learning: Importance, Applications, Challenges, and Future Work. In *2024 International Conference on Integration of Emerging Technologies for the Digital World (ICIETDW)* (pp. 1-6). IEEE. Li, L., Fan, Y., Tse, M., & Lin, K. Y. (2020). A review of applications in federated learning. *Computers & Industrial Engineering*, *149*, 106854.

Su, Z., Wang, Y., Luan, T. H., Zhang, N., Li, F., Chen, T., & Cao, H. (2021). Secure and efficient federated learning for smart grid with edge-cloud collaboration. *IEEE Transactions on Industrial Informatics*, *18*(2), 1333–1344. DOI: 10.1109/TII.2021.3095506

Sundari, V. M., Rose, R. M., Sassirekha, S. M., Nalini, M., & Girija, P. (2024, November). Deep Learning: Techniques, Taxonomy, Applications, and Future Directions. In *2024 International Conference on Smart Technologies for Sustainable Development Goals (ICSTSDG)* (pp. 1-5). IEEE.

Yamini, B., Dinesh, M. G., Gracious, L. A., & Subramanian, R. S. (2025). Exploring Blockchain Technology: Concepts, Features, and Industry Transformations. In *Blockchain Applications for the Energy and Utilities Industry* (pp. 305-322). IGI Global Scientific Publishing.

Chapter 11

Pioneering Medical Diagnostics Using Federated Learning and Collaborative AI

Updesh Kumar Jaiswal
https://orcid.org/0009-0002-1572-8275
Ajay Kumar Garg Engineering College, Ghaziabad, India

Jaishree Jain
https://orcid.org/0000-0003-0173-7664
Ajay Kumar Garg Engineering College, Ghaziabad, India

Saroj Kushwah
https://orcid.org/0000-0001-7362-9991
Ajay Kumar Garg Engineering College, Ghaziabad, India

Anu Chaudhary
Ajay Kumar Garg Engineering College, Ghaziabad, India

Sunil Kumar
Ajay Kumar Garg Engineering College, Ghaziabad, India

Nishant Kumar Pathak
Ajay Kumar Garg Engineering College, Ghaziabad, India

Anuradha M Dhumale
Ajay Kumar Garg Engineering College, Ghaziabad, India

Sneha Mishra
https://orcid.org/0000-0002-6234-7670
Ajay Kumar Garg Engineering College, Ghaziabad, India

ABSTRACT

Large-scale data sharing is important for developing reliable and accurate diagnostic models, but it has been mostly delayed by the sensitive nature of healthcare data and information. By allowing different healthcare institutions to collaborate on AI models unless sharing patient information, federated learning (FL) and col-

DOI: 10.4018/979-8-3373-3306-9.ch011

laborative artificial intelligence (CAI) have become advanced strategies to address these limitations. FL and CAI have the capability to increase diagnosis outcomes by improving model quality, lowering diagnostic cost, providing safe and confidential partnerships for AI-powered healthcare. By sending only model update information, FL allows remote data model training. This method protects data privacy by utilizing the combined expertise of several diagnostic institutions. Smart healthcare practitioners can design multi-institutional models that improve diagnostic precision, early disease prediction, and provide treatment recommendations by utilizing CAI. FL with CAI is transforming medical diagnostics into smart healthcare by promoting data security and privacy.

1. INTRODUCTION

Federated learning (FL) allows several devices to work together using distributed datasets without exchanging raw patient data, in contrast to AI model training. But there are many problems to achieve its full potential. Issues like data heterogeneity, communication overhead, and guaranteeing model fairness must be solved (Kalluri, 2022). FL is advancing diagnosis with the highest norms of patient data privacy and safety by facilitating secure and effective knowledge sharing (Yang et al., 2019).

Federated learning seemed to be a viable way to deal with these problems by allowing cooperative education without data centralization. FL has already advanced digital health applications significantly, benefiting a range of stakeholders. Distributed, federated, decentralized, and swarm learning are some of the methods that have evolved to facilitate collaborative machine learning (Rieke et al., 2020; Bonawitz et al., 2023). The importance of information in healthcare, the potential of federated efforts, and ongoing FL projects in the healthcare sector will all be covered in this article.

First, machine learning the foundations of federated learning are deep learning and big data modeling, with the aim of achieving dependable outcomes by validating data from several sources (Li et al., 2020). A tremendous amount of information has been produced as a result of today's accelerated digitization process. The hidden gems inside the data can be automatically unearthed by ML and DL technologies. Our world is being drastically altered by the use of machine learning models that have been trained on huge amounts of information in a diversity of contexts (Kairouz et al., 2021).

Conversely, Federated Learning is not limited to a certain dataset. It is not limited to any one algorithm and is made to conduct data mining across various data sources (Yin et al., 2021). Rather, it chooses algorithms depending on how well they work in order to maximize model optimization. Consequently, federated learning enables more freedom in data management. Federated learning can be applied in a variety of contexts and is not restricted to any one method. It can be used for both online and offline learning and primarily modifies the ways in which these algorithms' training procedures are implemented (Krishna, 2022).

By improving decision-making, automating procedures, and opening up new business models, artificial intelligence (AI) is revolutionizing a number of industries. But as AI models advance in complexity, they need access to ever-larger volumes of data (Krishna & Thakur, 2021). Because the data needed to train machine learning (ML) models frequently includes private and sensitive information, people and organizations are becoming increasingly concerned about how to gather, store, and share this data. Unauthorized access to sensitive data, privacy violations, and data breaches can have serious ethical, legal, and financial repercussions. Because of this, protecting data security and privacy when using it to train AI models has become extremely difficult (Murthy & Thakur, 2022). This chapter examines how federated learning is transforming AI collaboration by encouraging privacy-conscious development, with an emphasis on its foundational ideas, uses in privacy-sensitive industries, and obstacles.

1.1 Federated Learning Model Lifecycle in Smart Healthcare

A typical Federated Learning (FL) Model Lifecycle in Smart Healthcare begins with task initiation, in which a central server produces a global model and divides it to participating clients such as hospitals, diagnostic centers, wearable devices, and mobile health applications. During the local model training and update phase, each participant trains the global model with its own patient dataset, assuring that important medical records are kept secure in the hospital or device. During the global model aggregation and update phase, the server integrates all local updates—typically using Federated Averaging—to form an upgraded global model. This model is redistributed for additional training in many repeated cycles until convergence, resulting in resilient, accurate, and privacy-preserving AI solutions for healthcare (Murthy & Mehra, 2021). The system of FL model in smart healthcare is illustrated in Figure 1.

Figure 1. Federated Learning Model Lifecycle in Smart Healthcare

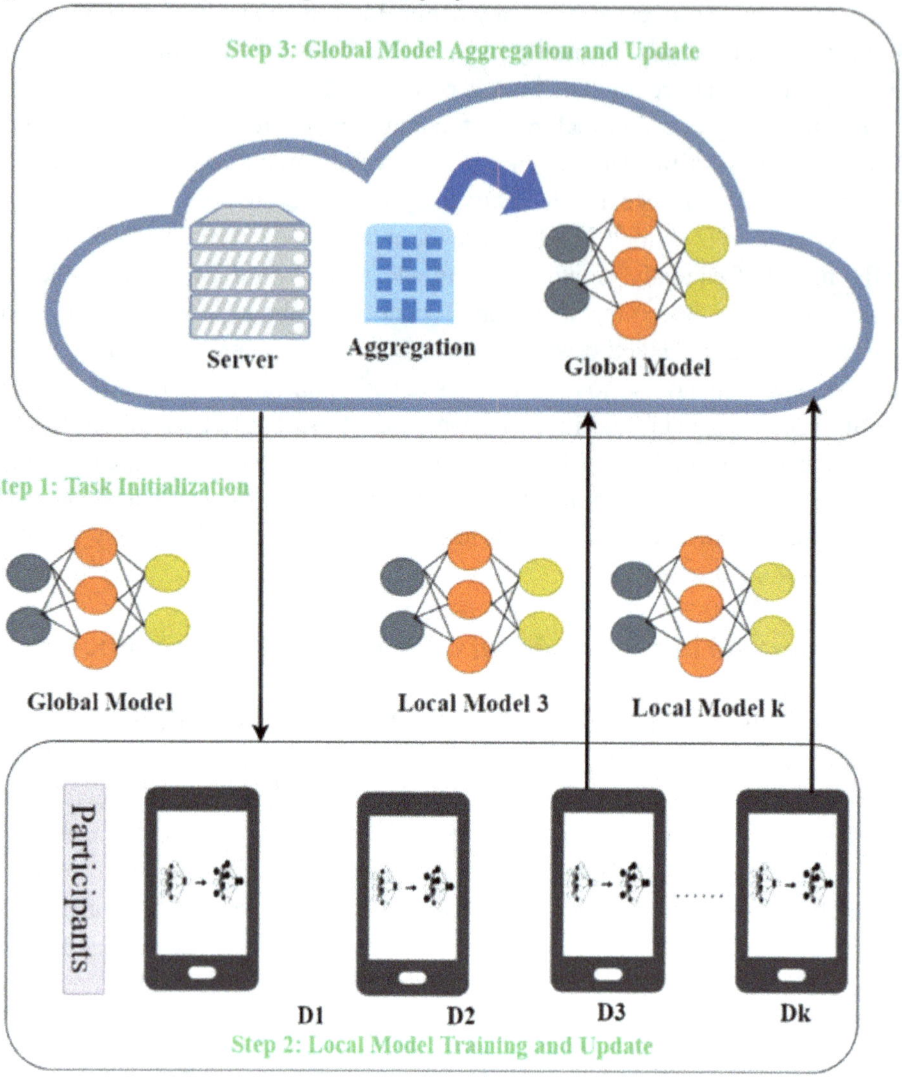

1.2 Revolutionary Cooperation of Federated Learning–Based AI in Healthcare with Centralized Architecture

The FL has made a revolutionary method that solves this problem by enabling the cooperative preparation of AI models among various organizations or devices without the sharing of private information. This decentralized method lowers privacy risks and fosters safe collaboration in AI development by guaranteeing that private data remains where it comes from. Federated learning is therefore expected to revolutionize sectors that depend on sensitive data and demand stringent data protection regulations (Thakur, 2021). Revolutionary Cooperation of Federation of SuperNodes and Servers is illustrated in Figure 2.

Approximately 30% of the world's data volume is made up of healthcare data, which is plentiful and becoming more accessible to academics for purposes like trend analysis and pattern recognition, as well as forecasting models. The main factor contributing to this is the growing by 2025, all are anticipated to have one, with the majority already having one (Akter et al., 2022). Simultaneously, machine learning (ML) techniques have revolutionized their capacities, making it possible to analyze high-dimensional clinical and imaging data effectively (Thilakarathne et al., 2022).

Healthcare data comes in a variety of forms and formats, such as genomic data, wearable signals, medical device outputs, imaging data, and text from medical notes. These are typically kept in separate silos, with kept transmission, EHR data frequently kept in a database structure, and wearable and medical device data kept locally. Despite the fact that repeatability has some well-established difficulties (Li et al., 2021), ML techniques have proven to be quite useful for modeling healthcare data in both single and multiple modality settings (Verma & Kumar, 2024). The transfer of such vast amounts of healthcare data also involves logistical challenges to guarantee data security. Lastly, research across different hospitals might be challenging.

Although medical imaging is essential to contemporary healthcare, federated learning faces several difficulties with it: Institution-specific data heterogeneity, labor-intensive manual annotations, and privacy worries (Verma & Kumar, 2025).

AI is nowadays moving towards federated architectures, particularly in areas like smart diagnosis and healthcare where data security is a concern. Researchers can do an active work in creating these important technologies through Flower Pilot Program (Li et al., 2024). The design of this type of program facilitates individual inquiry and create an environment that is favorable for tackling difficult research limitations (Choi et al., 2020). In order gain profit from and to contribute in federated learning innovation, we encourage researchers who are interested to think about applying to the upcoming Flower Pilot Program batch. A centralized architectural framework of FL is illustrated in Figure 3.

Figure 2. Revolutionary Cooperation of Federation of SuperNodes and Servers

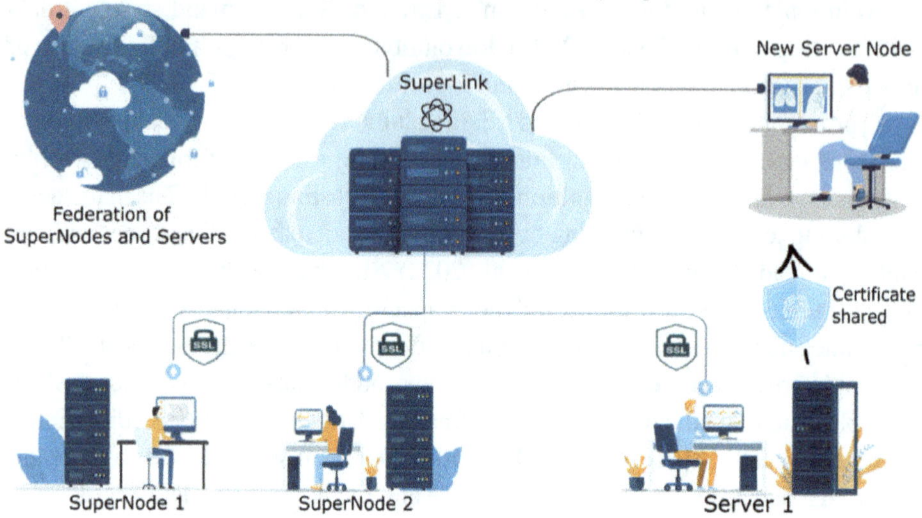

FL can decrease the computational workload and increases scalability while incorporating the features of secure compute techniques (Asiimwe et al., 2021). By allowing information to stay at each hospital site and transferring them easily, we can use ML with FL that provides a solution to the many problems that arise using centralized learning. An FL network can have a central aggregator that communicates with every node, or it can be decentralized. A model is trained at several locations in the decentralized environment (Sheller et al., 2020). Other sites in the network receive the revised model in a predetermined order, initialize using it, train, and give it to someone else.

An ML based model is used at every site in a centralized aggregator scenario, and data about the finished model is sent to the aggregator from every node. After compiling the model information from every site, the aggregator creates an updated global model, and it is subsequently dispersed to every site so that the local training procedure can begin anew. This keeps going until the global model satisfies a predetermined convergence criterion. Three general categories can be used to classify FL methods: transfer9, vertical, and horizontal. Regarding FTL (federated transfer learning), every site offers unique feature sets associated with various samples (Zhou et al., 2015).

Figure 3. Centralized Architecture of Federated Learning

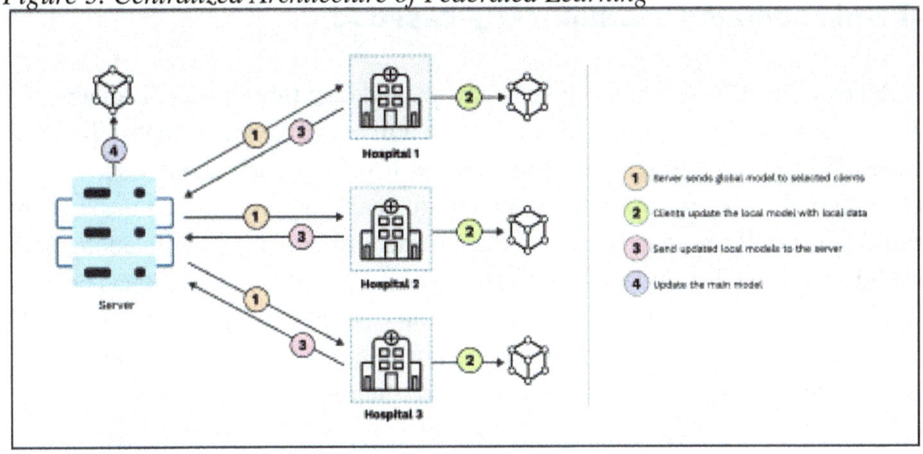

There is currently a substantial body of work outlining FL approaches used to healthcare difficulties such breast cancer diagnosis, COVID-19 detection, among many other different application areas (Patel et al., 2023) In fact, this systematic review found a collection of between 2015 and 2023, 220 such publications were published. But it's also critical to acknowledge that healthcare data naturally has a number of problems that call for extra care and modifications to FL approaches in order to resolve (Huang et al., 2024).

Importantly, every hospital in a network of hospitals may treat a radically diverse patient population. If, for instance, there are notable variations in the number of patients at each site or varying disease prevalences at various sites, this bias may cause problems with downstream modelling (Li et al., 2023). Different clinical practices may also be used by each hospital, which could result in variations in data collection and, as a result, problems like non-standardized variable name mappings and missing data (Nguyen et al., 2022).

Variations in data quality might also be a sign of site differences, which presents a special difficulty in obtaining the most optimal local learnt parameters (Chen et al., 2024). FL techniques for healthcare must take privacy into consideration in addition to the data difficulties (Brauneck et al., 2023). Lastly, we point out that FL approaches need to account for the computational cost of training because hospital settings usually lack high-performance computing facilities.

1.3 Comparative analysis between Centralized AI and Federated Learning (FL)–based AI

A centralized AI technique collects raw patient data from hospitals, diagnostic centers, or wearable devices and stores it on a main server for further training of model. While it can simplify calculation, but it gives some serious issues about information security threats, and compliance to healthcare legislation rules. In contrast, FL avoids the need to communicate confidential patient data by enabling each candidate to train their model locally. This decentralized approach protects privacy while simultaneously lowering communication costs and using varied, real-world healthcare data from different sources. As a result, FL-based AI provides a safer, and morally sound alternative as compared to centralized AI in smart healthcare.

2. RELATED WORK

The authors of (Yang et al., 2023) examined FL approaches and noted areas for improvement to achieve better performance results. Articles pertaining to VFL and FTL, however, have not been covered by the writers. Better performance results can be obtained by using VFL and FTL; therefore, it is still necessary to investigate the introduction of such models' designs. A study on the FL techniques for disease prediction was conducted in (Abreha et al., 2022). Thirteen studies were considered in this study; some examined radiographic pictures, while others concentrated on tumor identification. The selection of the articles was done using the PRISMA approach. Limited work was taken into consideration on existing models because the writers only looked at a small number of articles, despite FL's achievements. Future improvements are therefore needed in order to investigate various FL designs and appropriate datasets. The authors of (Aouedi et al., 2023; Loftus et al., 2022) have tested many FL based applications in the healthcare field. Numerous FL traits and problems have been examined in this SLR. Additionally, the authors only took into account a small number of studies that used IID data.

FL techniques for edge computing were introduced by the authors in (Kumar et al., 2024). The assessment concentrated on the process of implementing FL and highlighted a number of needs, including hardware, software, and architecture, as well as protocols. Additionally, when implementing FL, it was discovered that the main problems in edge computing are computational overhead and data heterogeneity. The authors of (Chen et al., 2021) implemented FL with blockchain architecture using a PRISMA approach. The study concentrated on utilizing FL to integrate blockchain technology and also examined how blockchain could enhance data security. While the study concentrated on the privacy method, only a little amount of effort was put into addressing the problems of computational overhead and data heterogeneity.

The PRISMA method was introduced by the authors (Qu et al., 2022) to calculate the efficacy of both centralized and decentralized approaches. Only a small number of papers were taken into consideration in order to comprehend FL's applications, characteristics, and procedures, despite the evaluation taking into account 20 articles that focused on FL to protect data privacy. Additionally, it highlights that source code is available for constructing models for predicting diseases that function inside the FL framework. This assessment also identifies a number of performance indicators and unresolved issues related to the FL approaches.

3. FEDERATED LEARNING'S FOUNDATIONS

This method differs from typical machine learning, which trains models using data that is centralized on a server. Federated learning preserves stringent privacy rules while enabling numerous entities—such as institutions, diagnosis devices—to participate in the creation of a common ML model (Rajendran et al., 2023).

The data in federated learning stays in the local environment at all times. Every participant, be it a gadget, an organization, or an institution, trains a model locally using its own data. This guarantees that private information, financial transactions, medical records, and other sensitive data never leave their source or are made available to outside parties. Participants share model updates (weights or gradients) with a central server instead of raw data. The server compiles these modifications to make the global model better. Without sacrificing anonymity, the aggregation procedure makes sure the model can learn from a range of decentralized data resources.

The technology of AI is currently advancing quickly. In medical research, federated learning—a combination of ML and DL algorithms—is becoming more and more popular. Federated learning has significantly accelerated the advancement of artificial intelligence in the medical domain. Federated learning is being widely adopted as likely to result in revolutionary developments in fields including medical image identification, medical language processing, clinical decision support, precision medicine, novel medication development, and medical speech recognition.

As a result, it is unlikely that such data sets will be openly shared, even though they may have substantial business value. Rather, data collectors frequently maintain precise control over the information that they've assembled. According to recent studies, FL-trained models can perform on par with those trained on centrally stored data sets and better than models that merely look at isolated data from a single institution as in Figure 4.

Therefore, there is a great chance that a successful FL implementation will enable precision medicine on a large scale, producing models that are sensitive to unusual diseases while adhering to privacy and governance, producing good decisions (Jain & Jaiswal, 2025). To guarantee that the algorithm is operating at its best without jeopardizing patient privacy or safety, FL still needs careful technological attention. However, it can potentially get around the drawbacks of methods that need a single, centralized data pool. In order to give the community context and specifics about the advantages and effects of the FL for healthcare, we present our consensus viewpoint in this perspective chapter outlining important factors and difficulties in applying FL for digital healthcare system.

Figure 4. Transfer Learning using Federated Learning

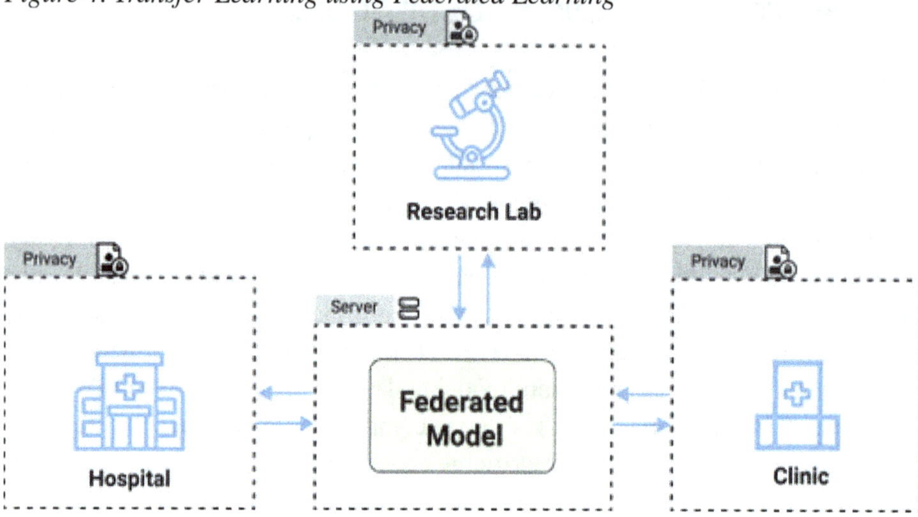

4. APPLICATIONS OF FEDERATED LEARNING (FL) IN PRIVACY-SENSITIVE INDUSTRIES

FL is especially useful in sectors where confidentiality and privacy are critical. Medical records, patient data, and health analytics are the foundation of clinical decision-making and research in the highly data-driven healthcare sector. However, due to its high level of sensitivity, healthcare data is particularly vulnerable to breaches and exploitation. Strict guidelines for the processing, sharing, and storing of health data are enforced.

Healthcare companies can work together to construct AI models through federated learning without disclosing private patient data. For instance, hospitals and research facilities can work together to develop AI models for personalized treatment recommendations, medical picture analysis, and disease identification. Patient data is kept private because each institution trains the model locally using its own data, and only aggregated model updates are shared. By working together, it is possible to create strong AI models while adhering to privacy laws and reducing the possibility of data breaches.

Institutions in the financial sector handle enormous volumes of sensitive data, such as credit histories, transaction logs, and personal financial information. Financial organizations, including banks and insurance providers, can work together to develop risk management tools, credit scoring models, and fraud detection systems while maintaining the security of consumer data thanks to federated learning. For example, banks are able to collaborating to create models that identify fraudulent transactions between institutions, exchanging only model updates instead of client transaction information. Through this partnership, financial institutions can develop more reliable models without endangering the privacy of their clients or exposing private information to dangers.

Telecom firms gather a lot of information from users, such as browsing history, location information, and call logs. This information is extremely sensitive even if it is useful for service optimization, consumer behavior prediction, and offering personalization. Violations of privacy can result in legal repercussions and erode consumer trust. Federated learning offers an answer by enabling telecom firms to work together on AI models for churn prediction, network efficiency, and customized suggestions without compromising privacy. By using local customer data to train models and sharing just Telecom companies can improve their services with aggregated updates and federated learning, which guarantees that private client information is never subjected to unwanted access. The approach maintains the usefulness while safeguarding the confidentiality of the model, the data, and the values that are shared between the institutions as shown in Figure 5.

Figure 5. Privacy Preserving Federated Machine Learning

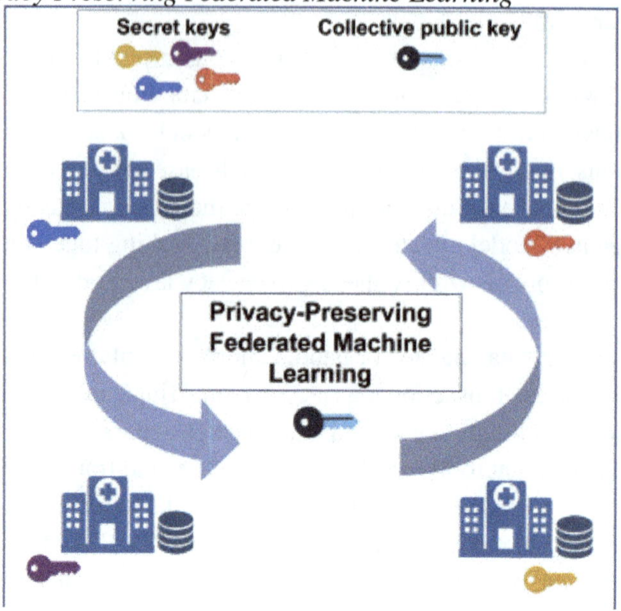

4.1 Federated Learning's Principal Uses in Healthcare and Medical Diagnostics

While protecting patient privacy, hospitals can work together to create a strong model for identifying conditions including cancer, pneumonia, and fractures. Sensitive photographs don't need to be moved in order for institutions to use this concept. Personalized Treatment Plans: By using federated learning, medical professionals can create customized treatment plans by training models on data from wearable technology. These models are flexible address particular patient requirements without jeopardizing data privacy.

Predictive healthcare analytics: By combining data from several hospitals, federated learning can assist in developing predictive models that forecast patient outcomes (such as estimating the likelihood of heart attacks, strokes, or readmissions to the hospital). This improves early intervention strategies and increases the generalizability of predictions. Clinical trials and drug development: Federated learning can be used in the pharmaceutical sector for cooperative drug discovery research, enabling many research institutes to exchange ideas without disclosing sensitive or secret information. More varied datasets and possibly quicker drug or therapy discovery result from this.

4.2 Collaborative AI (CAI) uses in Medical Diagnostics

Federated learning's rise has particular ramifications. Single-source data methods are becoming less and less adequate as artificial intelligence (AI) technologies develop quickly. Various kinds of data sources are necessary for AI models, especially those that use multi-modal big data. Furthermore, these models are trained across numerous devices, or nodes, rather than on centralized servers. Since data stays on local devices, this method addresses privacy and data security concerns. Federated learning can enable greater model personalization and has promise for sensitive data applications including healthcare, edge devices, and cell phones.

Model collaboration is the process by which several separate models cooperate to address challenging issues. These models could be dispersed over several applications or contexts, including cloud and edge devices. For model collaboration, CAI can improve overall model performance by facilitating integration and knowledge sharing. For example, in the medical domain, natural language processing and voice recognition models can work together to increase the precision of text comprehension and speech-to-text conversion. As will be covered in greater detail below, this can optimize doctor-patient interactions and save a significant amount of clinical time.

For clinical history consultation and medical record recording, CAI models are currently being used by top international medical institutions as well as a few cutting-edge Chinese hospitals. The hospital offers interactive, companion-based medical treatments using digital persons and huge models. Large models of AI help physicians create electronic medical records, which significantly cuts down on the amount of time needed to write records and frees up more time for providing high-quality clinical care.

CAI across several data sources does, in fact, offer considerable advantages. Because of China's vast population, the prevalence of disease varies by location and can be influenced by local genetic profiles, geographic, environmental, and climatic factors. For instance, the author modeled and verified parameters associated with SLE in China and the United States. The findings demonstrated that clinical markers employed in modeling can have varying value throughout the course of an illness in various populations, even for the same condition.

Taking into account Chinese populations as Asian representatives and American populations as Caucasian representatives, CAI of Result from these data sources can be more broadly applicable to most people on the planet. As a result, cooperative research across nations, such as the US and China, or between regions continues to be more prevalent. We anticipate that when data centers work together more, research databases based on data from the national population will be established.

The reaction to medication treatments, however, differed, underscoring the value of federated learning in creating therapies and treatments that are appropriate for a range of demographics and evaluating their efficacy. The federated learning approach, which combines data from several populations and locations, is crucial to developing more dependable disease prevention and monitoring systems.

4.3 Collaborative AI and Federated Learning Together

First and foremost, it is crucial to create several clients at participating locations globally. Without having access to the clients' medical information, the central server is in charge of organizing the training procedure. Every client provides the central server with gradient information or parameter updates after training the model on local data. After compiling all client updates, including its own, the central server creates a global model update and sends it out to every client. For the upcoming training session, clients incorporate these modifications into their models. The model's performance and efficacy gradually increase as the algorithm training goes on. Another important goal of federated learning is data sharing, which enables cooperation between several healthcare organizations without revealing their raw data rather than disclosing the outcomes of model training, which improves the accuracy and generalization of the model.

In the modeling process, collaboration models are also quite important. For complicated issues, a single model algorithm might not always produce trustworthy results. Rather, combining several separate models can yield more reliable results, making this cooperative method offers a sensible template for federated learning in the future. More people will be impacted by the social advancement and industry change brought about by AI. Every issue has both opportunity and challenges. As scientists, we will achieve more and build a better future for humanity if we take advantage of these chances and contribute to breakthroughs.

5. DIFFICULTIES WITH FEDERATED LEARNING WITH COLLABORATIVE AI IMPLEMENTATION

Federated learning has great potential for AI collaboration that respects privacy, but there are still a number of obstacles to overcome before it can be fully implemented. The variety of data from many participants is one of the main issues with federated learning. Different distributions, formats, and quality levels of the data could make unified model training is challenging. One important area of continuing study is addressing data heterogeneity and making sure the global model generalizes well to the data of all participants.

For federated learning to share model updates, members must communicate with one another. This can be ineffective, especially when dealing with a large number of participants or training huge models. Enhancing the effectiveness of federated learning systems requires minimizing data sharing and optimizing communication methods. Federated learning is susceptible to some kinds of attacks even though it uses privacy-preserving strategies. The integrity of the model could be jeopardized if malicious actors introduce adversarial or flawed updates into the system. Furthermore, protecting model update privacy by, for example, prohibiting the inference of specific data points from aggregated updates—still a problem.

Scalability becomes an issue in federated learning since it requires cooperation from numerous participants. One of the biggest challenges is making sure federated learning systems can manage a lot of devices or companies while still being efficient and private. In a decentralized approach, federated learning systems must be scalable to handle the increasing number of participants and data. Federated learning is subject to various data privacy laws in various jurisdictions. Maintaining decentralized collaboration while adhering to legal constraints is a persistent difficulty for federated learning systems.

The author has previously modeled and validated chronic diseases like diabetes, hypertension, hyperlipidemia, and hyperuricemia using a variety of artificial intelligence algorithms and substantial clinical datasets. The indicators include imaging examination markers, standard clinical laboratory tests, and some computed indicators. For modeling and validation, deep learning methods as well as conventional machine learning algorithms were employed.

Basic and clinical research data make up the majority of medical data, and varied sample data call for distinct processing techniques. In addition to standard anthropometric measures like height, weight, age, and sex, clinical research data also contains indications of markers like cholesterol and triglycerides as well as blood markers like haemoglobin, platelets, and white blood cells. For additional statistical analysis, certain medical indicators could require imputation, in contrast to other professions. The foundation of imputation analysis is the existence of critical values for clinical laboratory markers. By splitting biochemical signs into two sections according to a threshold of 0 and 1, these crucial values function as diagnostic criteria and may produce outcomes that are better suited for directing clinical diagnosis and treatment.

Efficient data processing can significantly speed up the modeling and validation of federated learning later on. It has been noted that certain algorithms may produce better accuracy, specificity, and sensitivity when particular clinical data is not imputed. Nonetheless, vital markers that direct clinical diagnosis, like relative risks (RR) and odds ratios (OR), might yield superior outcomes when using imputation.

Preprocessing techniques for clinical data are different from those for basic research data. Numerical and picture data categories are often where basic data belongs. The software of the instrument must be used to preprocess certain image data. Preliminary processing for pure numerical basic research data entails removing blank values, transforming data into absolute values or ratios for consistent.

Nevertheless, neural network models are sometimes regarded as "black boxes," offering trustworthy outcomes without offering a thorough understanding of the modeling procedure. Logistic regression-based nomograms are very helpful in clinical modeling, where a thorough investigation of individual markers is required to determine clinical significance. The importance of clinical signs for disease diagnosis and prognosis can be graphically represented by nomograms. They work well together when paired with decision trees for clinical indicator imputation and categorization. It is worthwhile to promote this combination method as a very beneficial federated learning algorithm collaboration mode.

It is equally crucial to validate and assess models constructed using various artificial intelligence (AI) methods. For validation, the author suggests utilizing multiple algorithms. Nowadays, clinical research frequently uses ROC curve analysis to evaluate a model's sensitivity, specificity, and accuracy. Clinical big data models powered by AI have special features and need to be evaluated for clinical value and discriminative power.

Federated learning's rise has particular ramifications. Single-source data methods are becoming less and less adequate as artificial intelligence (AI) technologies develop quickly. Various kinds of data sources are necessary for AI models, especially those that use multi-modal big data. Since data stays on local devices, this method addresses privacy and data security concerns. Federated learning exhibits application potential involves private information, including healthcare, edge devices, and cell phones, and can attain more model customisation.

It improves the healthcare experience by precisely understanding and promptly responding to patient requirements by utilizing massive language models as the central intelligent engine. Using 10,000 historical records, a big language model is refined as part of the medical record documentation and consultation procedures. To teach the model how to write medical histories, the development team created particular questions. This method is a viable concept for future adoption and is an excellent example of the aid paradigm of the federated learning model.

Drawing from the author's expertise in modeling and validating data from numerous data sources, federated learning across several Data sources do provide a number of benefits. Because of China's vast population, the prevalence of disease varies by location and can be influenced by local genetic profiles, geographic, environmental, and climatic factors. For instance, the author modeled and verified parameters associated with SLE in China and the United States. The findings demonstrated that clinical markers employed in modelling can have varying value throughout the course of an illness in various populations, even for the same condition.

Federated learning of various data sets can yield conclusions more applicable to the majority of the world's population when American populations are viewed. But because of geographical limitations and data privacy regulations that forbid cross-border data transfers (Verma & Kumar, 2024). As a result, cooperative research across nations, such as the US and China, or between regions continues to be more prevalent. We anticipate that when data centers work together more, research databases based on data from the national population will be established.

By covering population characteristics across the country, this dataset attempts to reduce regional biases and produce models that are more useful in therapeutic settings. This approach does have some drawbacks, though, as there is still a chance violation submitting like that. Reaction to medication treatments, however, differed, underscoring the value of federated learning in creating therapies and treatments that are appropriate for a range of demographics and evaluating their efficacy. The federated learning approach, which combines data from several populations and locations, is crucial to developing more dependable disease prevention and monitoring systems.

Ongoing study and practical testing are still needed to overcome adoption issues. Convergence issues arise from heterogeneity, which occurs when datasets are not IID among users and vary over time. Additionally, when model sizes exceed edge capacities, communication problems occur. As threats change, protecting privacy becomes more and more important. Furthermore, in order to create suitable data contributions and model ownership arrangements, encouraging involvement necessitates cultural and technological adjustments. Particularly when it comes to underprivileged populations, fairness concerns surface.

However, significant industrial endeavours persist in pushing the envelope. Collaboratively, the Oasis personal data stores create a shared framework for practical sharing experiments. Community-driven protocols and policies are introduced by the Federated AI Technology Standards.

Above all, these technological advancements need to be guided by appropriate democratic monitoring. Meaningful permission and transparency about how private data informs public AI systems are enforced by strong individual rights. Federated Learning, if developed collaboratively, might balance privacy with advancement globally. As adoption matures, its greatest influence will still be felt. Federated Learning, if developed collaboratively, might balance privacy with advancement globally. As adoption matures, its greatest influence will still be felt.

The efficiency and accuracy of healthcare can be improved by using federated learning and model. However, although it is advantageous, merging public information with regional clinical databases does not provide total security of data. For federated learning models to be used more widely, two crucial concerns that must be resolved are enhancing data security and protecting patient privacy.

6. FEDERATED LEARNING'S WITH COLLABORATIVE AI FUTURE IN MEDICAL DIAGNOSTICS

Federated transfer learning enhances federated learning by enabling models trained on one dataset to be converted to another acquiring the ability to manage diverse data from many participants. This strategy will assist in resolving issues with data distribution and enhance model performance in a variety of settings. Interoperability standards will become more crucial as federated learning becomes popularity. Organizations will find it easier to implement federated learning if standardized protocols and frameworks are developed, as this would facilitate smooth communication between various industries and participants. Scaling federated learning systems will need increasing the effectiveness of communication across members. Decentralized aggregation, differential privacy, and model compression innovations will all contribute to lowering communication overhead and accelerating training.

In order to properly serve patients and doctors without endangering the security of patient information, the future of health care model development must be able to train on a variety of data points. The use of limited data points and data sets, which are crucial for model training and might reveal information about marginalized communities, is made possible by FL models. By using more data in this way, bias against AI and improper usage of AI would be somewhat reduced.

There are specific actions that need to be made in order to completely incorporate FL into the mainstream usage of developers and medical experts. First, information hosting sites and developers must somewhat standardize data extraction, transformation, and loading. Only standardized data sets can be used to train FL models, and the data Each edge site needs to be prepared appropriately. Individuals from the participating centers, representatives from the primary model hosting server, or outside contractors from companies created to streamline data standardization must all be assigned to this role. Legislation must also be in place to permit the use of data in FL models while keeping data privacy in mind and to permit frequent model upgrades without requiring resubmissions or device reclears through regulatory agencies.

It is crucial that the healthcare industry makes use of the more prevalent and increasingly accurate machine learning-enabled and artificially intelligent equipment. In order to better understand, treat, and care for individuals and patient populations, investigate every line of inquiry, which by definition include the study and use of intelligent computation in medical devices. FL offers a way to investigate this without putting PHI at risk or needing users to buy pricey gear in order to execute computationally demanding applications.

7. CONCLUSION

A new era of secure, private AI collaboration is ushered in by federated learning. By enabling decentralised data training and sharing model updates rather than raw data, federated learning addresses significant privacy concerns and fosters cross-industry cooperation. Applications in privacy-sensitive sectors such as finance, healthcare, and telecommunications demonstrate how it can promote innovation while maintaining data security. Despite the remaining challenges, federated learning will become an essential part of the AI landscape due to ongoing research and technological advancements, creating new opportunities for future cooperative, privacy-preserving AI development. Federated learning is a viable approach to resolving the privacy and data governance concerns in the healthcare industry. Without centralising data, FL fosters collaborative learning while protecting patient privacy, allowing for the development of accurate and widely applicable AI models. Dealing with technical, ethical, and legal issues is crucial as FL develops to guarantee its successful application and maximise its advantages for all the engaged parties.

REFERENCES

Abreha, H. G., Hayajneh, M., & Serhani, M. A. (2022). Federated learning in edge computing: A systematic survey. *Sensors (Basel)*, *22*(2), 450. DOI: 10.3390/s22020450 PMID: 35062410

Akter, M., Moustafa, N., Lynar, T., & Razzak, I. (2022). Edge intelligence: Federated learning-based privacy protection framework for smart healthcare systems. *IEEE Journal of Biomedical and Health Informatics*, *26*(12), 5805–5816. DOI: 10.1109/JBHI.2022.3192648 PMID: 35857737

Aouedi, O., Sacco, A., Piamrat, K., & Marchetto, G. (2023). Handling privacy-sensitive medical data with federated learning: Challenges and future directions. *IEEE Journal of Biomedical and Health Informatics*, *27*(2), 790–803. DOI: 10.1109/JBHI.2022.3185673 PMID: 35737624

Asiimwe, R., Lam, S., Leung, S., Wang, S., Wan, R., Tinker, A., McAlpine, J. N., Woo, M. M. M., Huntsman, D. G., & Talhouk, A. (2021). From biobank and data silos into a data common: Convergence to support translational medicine. *Journal of Translational Medicine*, *19*(1), 493. DOI: 10.1186/s12967-021-03147-z PMID: 34863191

Bonawitz, K.. (2023). Towards federated learning at scale: System design. *Proceedings of Machine Learning and Systems*, *1*, 374–388. https://arxiv.org/abs/1902.01046

Brauneck, A., Schmalhorst, L., Kazemi Majdabadi, M. M., Bakhtiari, M., Völker, U., Baumbach, J., Baumbach, L., & Buchholtz, G. (2023). Federated machine learning, privacy-enhancing technologies, and data protection laws in medical research: Scoping review. *Journal of Medical Internet Research*, *25*, e41588. DOI: 10.2196/41588 PMID: 36995759

Chen, M., Shlezinger, N., Poor, H. V., Eldar, Y. C., & Cui, S. (2021). Communication-efficient federated learning. *Proceedings of the National Academy of Sciences of the United States of America*, *118*(17), e2024789118. DOI: 10.1073/pnas.2024789118 PMID: 33888586

Chen, Y., Lu, W., Qin, X., Wang, J., & Xie, X. (2024). MetaFed: Federated learning among federations with cyclic knowledge distillation for personalized healthcare. *IEEE Transactions on Neural Networks and Learning Systems*, *35*(11), 16671–16682. DOI: 10.1109/TNNLS.2023.3297103 PMID: 37506019

Choi, R. Y., Coyner, A. S., Kalpathy-Cramer, J., Chiang, M. F., & Campbell, J. P. (2020). Introduction to machine learning, neural networks, and deep learning. *Translational Vision Science & Technology, 9*(2), 14. DOI: 10.1167/tvst.9.2.14 PMID: 32704420

Huang, D., Ye, X., & Sakurai, T. (2024). Multi-party collaborative drug discovery via federated learning. *Computers in Biology and Medicine, 171*, 108181. DOI: 10.1016/j.compbiomed.2024.108181 PMID: 38428094

Jain, J., & Jaiswal, U. K. (2025). Revolutionizing medicine: The impact of artificial intelligence in healthcare. In Gupta, S., Gupta, U., Sharma, M., & Malik, K. (Eds.), *Generative intelligence in healthcare: Transforming patient care with AI creativity* (pp. 176–209). CRC Press., DOI: 10.1201/9781003539483-8

Kairouz, P., McMahan, H. B., Avent, B., Bellet, A., Bennis, M., Bhagoji, A. N., ... & Zhao, S. (2021). Advances and open problems in federated learning. *Foundations and trends® in machine learning, 14*(1–2), 1-210.

Kalluri, K. (2022). Federate machine learning: A secure paradigm for collaborative AI in privacy-sensitive domains. *International Journal on Science and Technology, 13*(4), 1–13. DOI: 10.5281/zenodo.14551746

Krishna, K. (2022). Optimizing query performance in distributed NoSQL databases through adaptive indexing and data partitioning techniques. International Journal of Creative Research Thoughts (IJCRT). https://ijcrt.org/viewfulltext.php

Krishna, K., & Thakur, D. (2021). Automated Machine Learning (AutoML) for real-time data streams: Challenges and innovations in online learning algorithms. [JETIR]. *Journal of Emerging Technologies and Innovative Research, 8*(12).

Kumar, P., Jain, J., Jaiswal, U. K., Yadav, D., & Solanki, B. (2024). Childhood asthma disease prediction using classification algorithms of supervised machine learning. In 2024 1st International Conference on Advanced Computing and Emerging Technologies (ACET) (pp. 1–6). IEEE. DOI: 10.1109/ACET61898.2024.10730050

Li, H., Cai, Z., Wang, J., Tang, J., Ding, W., Lin, C.-T., & Shi, Y. (2024). FedTP: Federated learning by transformer personalization. *IEEE Transactions on Neural Networks and Learning Systems, 35*(10), 13426–13440. DOI: 10.1109/TNNLS.2023.3269062 PMID: 37220054

Li, Q., Wen, Z., Wu, Z., Hu, S., Wang, N., Li, Y., Liu, X., & He, B. (2021). A survey on federated learning systems: Vision, hype and reality for data privacy and protection. *IEEE Transactions on Knowledge and Data Engineering, 35*(4), 3347–3366. DOI: 10.1109/TKDE.2021.3124599

Li, S., Liu, P., Nascimento, G. G., Wang, X., Leite, F. R. M., Chakraborty, B., Hong, C., Ning, Y., Xie, F., Teo, Z. L., Ting, D. S. W., Haddadi, H., Ong, M. E. H., Peres, M. A., & Liu, N. (2023). Federated and distributed learning applications for electronic health records and structured medical data: A scoping review. *Journal of the American Medical Informatics Association : JAMIA*, *30*(12), 2041–2049. DOI: 10.1093/jamia/ocad170 PMID: 37639629

Li, T., Sahu, A. K., Talwalkar, A., & Smith, V. (2020). Federated learning: Challenges, methods, and future directions. *IEEE Signal Processing Magazine*, *37*(3), 50–60. DOI: 10.1109/MSP.2020.2975749

Loftus, T. J., Ruppert, M. M., Shickel, B., Ozrazgat-Baslanti, T., Balch, J. A., Efron, P. A., Upchurch, G. R.Jr, Rashidi, P., Tignanelli, C., Bian, J., & Bihorac, A. (2022). Federated learning for preserving data privacy in collaborative healthcare research. *Digital Health*, *8*, 20552076221134455. DOI: 10.1177/20552076221134455 PMID: 36325438

Murthy, P., & Mehra, A. (2021). Exploring neuromorphic computing for ultra-low latency transaction processing in edge database architectures. *Journal of Emerging Technologies and Innovative Research*, *8*(1), 25–26.

Murthy, P., & Thakur, D. (2022). Cross-layer optimization techniques for enhancing consistency and performance in distributed NoSQL database. International Journal of Enhanced Research in Management & Computer Applications, 35.

Nguyen, T. V., Dakka, M. A., Diakiw, S. M., Ver Milyea, M. D., Perugini, M., Hall, J. M. M., & Perugini, D. (2022). A novel decentralized federated learning approach to train on globally distributed, poor quality, and protected private medical data. *Scientific Reports*, *12*(1), 8888. DOI: 10.1038/s41598-022-12833-x PMID: 35614106

Patel, M., Dayan, I., Fishman, E. K., Flores, M., Gilbert, F. J., Guindy, M., Koay, E. J., Rosenthal, M., Roth, H. R., & Linguraru, M. G. (2023). Accelerating artificial intelligence: How federated learning can protect privacy, facilitate collaboration, and improve outcomes. *Health Informatics Journal*, *29*(4), 14604582231207744. DOI: 10.1177/14604582231207744 PMID: 37864543

Qu, L., Zhou, Y., Liang, P. P., Xia, Y., Wang, F., & Adeli, E.. (2022). Rethinking architecture design for tackling data heterogeneity in federated learning. In *Proceedings of the IEEE/CVF Conference on Computer Vision and Pattern Recognition (CVPR 2022)* (pp. 10051–10061). IEEE. DOI: 10.1109/CVPR52688.2022.00982

Rajendran, S., Xu, Z., Pan, W., Ghosh, A., & Wang, F. (2023). Data heterogeneity in federated learning with electronic health records: Case studies of risk prediction for acute kidney injury and sepsis diseases in critical care. *PLOS Digital Health*, *2*(3), e0000117. DOI: 10.1371/journal.pdig.0000117 PMID: 36920974

Rieke, N., Hancox, J., Li, W., Milletarì, F., Roth, H. R., Albarqouni, S., Bakas, S., Galtier, M. N., Landman, B. A., Maier-Hein, K., Ourselin, S., Sheller, M., Summers, R. M., Trask, A., Xu, D., Baust, M., & Cardoso, M. J. (2020). The future of digital health with federated learning. *NPJ Digital Medicine*, *3*(1), 1–7. DOI: 10.1038/s41746-020-00323-1 PMID: 33015372

Sheller, M. J., Edwards, B., Reina, G. A., Martin, J., Pati, S., Kotrotsou, A., Milchenko, M., Xu, W., Marcus, D., Colen, R. R., & Bakas, S. (2020). Federated learning in medicine: Facilitating multi-institutional collaborations without sharing patient data. *Scientific Reports*, *10*(1), 12598. DOI: 10.1038/s41598-020-69250-1 PMID: 32724046

Thakur, D. (2021). Federated learning and privacy-preserving AI: Challenges and solutions in distributed machine learning. [IJARESM]. *International Journal of All Research Education and Scientific Methods*, *9*(6), 3763–3764.

Thilakarathne, N. N., Muneeswari, G., Parthasarathy, V., Alassery, F., Hamam, H., Mahendran, R. K., & Shafiq, M. (2022). Federated learning for privacy-preserved medical internet of things. *Intelligent Automation & Soft Computing*, *33*(1), 157–172. DOI: 10.32604/iasc.2022.023763

Verma, S., & Kumar, M. (2024). Automatic classification of melanoma using GrabCut segmentation and convolutional neural network. *SN Computer Science*, *5*(5), 591. DOI: 10.1007/s42979-024-02949-4

Verma, S., & Kumar, M. (2025). A hybrid machine learning model for skin disease classification using discrete wavelet transform and gray level co-occurrence matrix (GLCM). *Multimedia Tools and Applications*, *84*(12), 12835–12853. DOI: 10.1007/s11042-024-19449-5

Yang, B., Yuen, P. C., Zhang, Y., & Zeng, A. (2023). Allosteric feature collaboration for model-heterogeneous federated learning. *IEEE Transactions on Neural Networks and Learning Systems*. Advance online publication. DOI: 10.1109/TNNLS.2023.3335168 PMID: 38145509

Yang, Q., Liu, Y., Chen, T., & Tong, Y. (2019). Federated machine learning: Concept and applications. *ACM Transactions on Intelligent Systems and Technology*, *10*(2), 1–19. DOI: 10.1145/3298981

Yin, L., Feng, J., Xun, H., Sun, Z., & Cheng, X. (2021). A privacy-preserving federated learning for multiparty data sharing in social IoTs. *IEEE Transactions on Network Science and Engineering*, *8*(3), 2706–2718. DOI: 10.1109/TNSE.2021.3074185

Zhou, H., Tang, J., & Zheng, H. (2015). Machine learning for medical applications. *TheScientificWorldJournal*, *825267*(1), 825267. Advance online publication. DOI: 10.1155/2015/825267 PMID: 25692180

Chapter 12
Securing Patient Privacy and Data Protection by Federated Learning in AI-Driven Healthcare

Dip Sarker
American International University-Bangladesh, Bangladesh

Md Tafhimul Haque Sadi
American International University-Bangladesh, Bangladesh

Dipta Gomes
https://orcid.org/0000-0003-3019-6051
American International University-Bangladesh, Bangladesh

Md. Manzurul Hasan
American International University-Bangladesh, Bangladesh

ABSTRACT

Federated Learning (FL) is a new method for performing decentralized machine learning. By introducing LD, these problems are addressed by allowing models to learn together without a central authority managing personal medical information. It describes how FL improves data safety while maintaining the same analytical results in multiple healthcare institutions. It looks into issues of ethical, legal, and technical features of FL that show how it matches global privacy laws. By studying the methods behind encryption, differential privacy, and secure multiparty computation, we can prove that FL can improve digital healthcare security. In addition, the use of real-life case studies and implementation plans is covered. It shows how

DOI: 10.4018/979-8-3373-3306-9.ch012

FL is useful and presents difficulties in clinical work. This chapter contributes a well-rounded view of FL as being essential for wingspan, reliability, and justice healthcare that uses AI responsibly.

INTRODUCTION

The use of technology in healthcare now leads to more advanced ways of diagnosing, personalizing patient care, supervising patients and controlling hospital resources. Because of electronic health records, wearable health devices, mobile health apps and AI-assisted decision makers, large volumes of sensitive medical information are now created (Abbas et al., 2024; Teo et al., 2024). With such a big increase in data, medical research and treatment have improved, but it has also made it simpler to break patient privacy, gain unauthorized access or use personal information dishonestly (Gu et al., 2023; Sadilek et al., 2021).

For traditional AI and machine learning models, data from many institutions is gathered in one central place to train the system. Such a practice raises doubts about system safety and also goes against patient confidentiality rules, especially when transmitting information across international or departmental boundaries (Brauneck et al., 2023; Hu et al., 2024). On top of that, regulations like HIPAA in the United States and the GDPR in Europe make it difficult to transfer and use information across borders (Aouedi et al., 2023).

To overcome such difficulties, Federated Learning (FL) provides a privacy-friendly method that greatly improves how AI is put to use in healthcare. With FL, models are trained close to where the data is stored in the devices or servers of specific institutions. Learning progress is transmitted to the central server, using updated model parameters (gradients or weights), not the raw data itself (Li et al., 2020; Sheller et al., 2020). Because of this, patient data remains where it is created, making it much harder for bad actors to get access to the data and helping doctors from different hospitals work together.

By allowing privacy, FL makes sure the global model performs well and accurately reflects data, as more diverse organizations like large hospitals and small clinics can take part without handing over their data (Chamikara et al., 2021; Loftus et al., 2022). In global pandemics and cases of rare diseases, sharing data is very important, though frequently limited by legal or ethical rules. FL respects the principles of informed consent and data sovereignty and promotes fairness by letting every user be part of building AI (Kaissis et al., 2020; Punreddy, 2023).

Still, bringing FL into practice in real-world healthcare poses some difficulties. Issues related to the amount of sharing required, different types of data and possible attacks must be managed. Furthermore, FL is regularly improved with advanced methods such as differential privacy, homomorphic encryption and secure multi-party computation (Aziz et al., 2023; Ziller et al., 2021) to maintain its safety and meet changing standards.

Current healthcare AI also uses EHRs, images, genomics, and mHealth data, and there are acute privacy, consent, and cross-border governance concerns. Raw record aggregation of traditional centralized training increases the probability of breaches and misuse and burdens HIPAA/GDPR compliance. Federated Learning (FL) learns a model at the location of data and only sends an updated version to other locations, moving the practice beyond sharing data, to sharing knowledge. The chapter describes the ethical, legal and technical underpinnings of FL within a clinical setting, outlines protection (DP, secure aggregation, HE, SMPC, of TEEs) and demonstrates real deployments that preserve privacy whilst maintaining model utility across a collection of heterogeneous clinical facilities. The goal of this chapter is to give a thorough look at FL to secure patient privacy when using AI in healthcare. By gathering information from the latest changes, case-based experiences and laws, it outlines how FL benefits stakeholders with both their creative ideas and compliance duties in a modern healthcare world.

2. UNDERSTANDING THE PRIVACY IN DIGITAL HEALTHCARE

The development of digital technologies has caused privacy in healthcare to change a lot. Privacy started out by focusing on blocking others from opening and viewing medical notes. Electronic health records (EHRs), mobile health applications, IoMT devices and AI-enabled diagnostic systems now ensure that patient information is moved and stored across many different channels, frequently in real time (Abbas et al., 2024; Hu et al., 2024). As systems are more connected, personal health information is more valuable and can be more easily threatened.

Usually, data from many institutions is collected in one central server to help train the predictive models used in machine learning. Even though this approach improves both diagnosis and support for medical decisions, it creates major concerns about privacy. An architecture with centralized control can be easily breached, allows unauthorized uses and infringes data sovereignty, since it creates just one weak spot (Arefin, 2024; Chamikara et al., 2021). Even if patient information has been made anonymous, evidence shows that it is possible to link records with external data and match patients to their information, an attack described as re-identification (Ziller et al., 2021).

In addition, with model inversion, membership inference and gradient leakage becoming more common, this exposes health data to new threats. Attackers try to reconstruct personal details about a record by using the results of a trained AI model.

When gradients are shared, information about the original data may be revealed which can make collaborative training at risk if security measures are not taken (Aziz et al., 2023). The risk of privacy breaches in areas handling genetic information, mental health and infectious diseases is especially troublesome, as it can cause people to be stigmatized or discriminated against (Gu et al., 2023; Kaissis et al., 2020).

Since these limits were identified, Federated Learning (FL) has been seen as a strong alternative. FL makes it possible to build models without sharing data through encryption of the end update messages and by keeping decrypted data within the organization (Li et al., 2020; Sheller et al., 2020). By not moving raw data, this method lets organizations handle data governance better and be more compliant with privacy rules, including HIPAA, GDPR and local healthcare laws (Aouedi et al., 2023; Loftus et al., 2022).

Unlike the past, in FL we move from thinking about "data sharing" to "knowledge sharing." Health applications learned from local data and send back the things they learned, not the original data. By doing this, privacy and security are advanced, and institutions can keep their unique ways to organize and process data, thus tackling interoperability issues (Teo et al., 2024). Because FL is flexible and can be used in parts, it allows scientists worldwide to train AI on diseases or area-specific cases with no privacy breaches (Xu et al., 2021).

Table 1. Comparison of Centralized AI vs. Federated Learning in Healthcare

Aspect	Centralized AI	Federated Learning (FL)	Reference
Data Location	Centralized servers	Local devices or institutional servers	(Abbas et al., 2024; Teo et al., 2024)
Privacy Risk	High (due to raw data movement)	Low (no raw data transfer)	(Abbas et al., 2024; Ali et al., 2023)
Legal Compliance	Complex, jurisdiction-sensitive	Aligned with HIPAA, GDPR	(Abbas et al., 2024; Sheller et al., 2020)
Attack Surface	Single point of failure	Distributed architecture	(Xu et al., 2021)
Re-identification Risk	Moderate to high	Significantly reduced	(Teo et al., 2024)
Data Ownership	Transferred to model host	Retained by data originators	(Sheller et al., 2020)
Model Accuracy	High (but privacy trade-off)	Comparable with strong privacy controls	(Sheller et al., 2020; Teo et al., 2024)

Table 1 contrasts the major concepts between centralized AI and Federated Learning and demonstrates how the decentralized nature of FL leads to improve both privacy and compliance and security in addition to being competitive in accuracy. Evidence on the recent studies is brought up in references that emphasize each of the advantages.

Normally, in an FL setup, each healthcare node (covering hospitals, mobile apps or wearables) it trains a machine learning model using medical records from local patients. The model weights or gradients are next encrypted. these changes are delivered to a central server which pulls them all together to improve the general tool. The Iterations are made using loop code and never sharing or sending raw data to another area. This quality assures patients protection. discretion is maintained which is why FL can be applied in sensitive fields including oncology, radiology. mental health is also affected by sarcoptic mange (Gu et al., 2023; Sadilek et al., 2021).

Figure 1. Federated Learning Architecture for Privacy Preservation in Healthcare

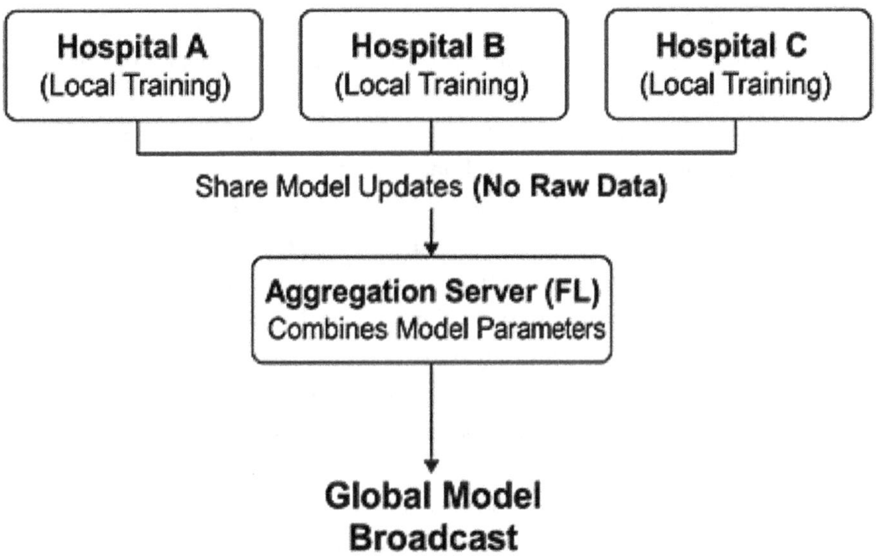

This figure shows the main parts of Federated Learning (FL) in healthcare. Every hospital (for example, A, B and C) keeps its own patient data and uses it to develop a separate machine learning system. The central server only receives updates for the model (gradients and weights) which have been protected by encryption. The server puts all the updates together to make a global model and this is sent to each participating node to be trained further. Thanks to decentralization, privacy is better protected, compliances such as GDPR and HIPAA are followed, data breaches are less likely, and organizations can collaborate on using intelligent data.

Moving from a centralized to a decentralized way of learning is a big change in how health organizations protect and secure private information. With Federated Learning, various groups train a model together while preserving their privacy which helps address old worries about patient data security, following the law and people's lack of trust. FL ensures privacy by supporting privacy-preserving methods and makes sure it is compliant with current data rules which establishes it as an essential building block for ethical and intelligent future medical AI.

3. ETHICAL FOUNDATIONS OF DECENTRALIZED AI

AI systems being used in healthcare can give rise to serious ethical problems. Such concerns include issues with privacy, being independent, consenting to things and trust which are core rights. Now that AI is influencing diagnosis, treatment and patient monitoring, caregivers and decision-makers must ensure its ethical use (Brauneck et al., 2023; Sadilek et al., 2021).

The growing use of computers in health services has caused a huge increase in personal information being kept, stored and worked with. Sometimes, having all data in a central cloud or repository allows institutions to make decisions about it, possibly without asking patients first. This situation infringes on important ethical guidelines including informed consent and data sovereignty, especially when people do not realize their data is being used in AI programs (Loftus et al., 2022). Besides this, systems based on central control usually do not display the process, making it tough for patients to challenge or review decisions generated by the AI.

Federated Learning (FL) represents a way to maintain these values in AI. With FL, training and sharing parameters take place locally which allows hospitals and their patients to manage their data more securely. This system of care fits better with moral guidelines that focus on patient choice and doing good for patients. According to deontological ethics which stress duty and upholding individual rights, FL adapts by preventing overexposure of data and encouraging consent that fits the situation (Teo et al., 2024). Also, from the standpoint of utilitarianism, FL makes sure that the group benefits the most while individuals are not exposed to possible leakage of their data.

It is particularly important in digital health ethics to address what is called the "black box" problem because of how difficult it can be to see what AI does. AI-based suggestions may be hard for patients and clinicians to understand or challenge. While Federated Learning doesn't make models directly interpretable, it permits every institution to handle their own version of the training data which can be examined during audits. Having institutions take charge of their information and guide behavior helps encourage ethical accountability (Cellamare et al., 2022).

Besides, FL plays a vital role in promoting justice and equity as AI is created. When datasets come from a single source, minority populations and regions with fewer resources tend to be excluded which can create biased models that enhance health inequities. Because of local model training in different regions and populations, FL helps ensure that algorithms are fair. Allowing anyone to develop AI means more diverse voices can be included in the training which helps make models fairer and more applicable to a wider audience (Gu et al., 2023; Xu et al., 2021).

Even though FL is very useful, it still brings up ethical issues that need to be addressed. Variations in data between different places can cause models to work differently in different populations. Not handling data ethics well may result in unfair treatment or restricted use of effective AI tools. Constant watching and checking is necessary in applications of FL to make sure that the models being trained on data from various sources have equal performance in all groups (Hu et al., 2024).

A new question to consider is how ethics affects people's participation in clinical trials. Anybody providing computing resources or data to these networks should be rewarded. There is a chance of exploitation if some participants do not fairly benefit from the work done with their data. Reputable FL frameworks must guarantee transparent participation arrangements, shared governance and identifiable model origin (Punreddy, 2023; Sheller et al., 2020).

There is also a growing call for ethical audit trails in federated learning systems. Since model updates are shared without raw data, ensuring verifiability of data quality and update legitimacy becomes a challenge. Techniques such as differential privacy, homomorphic encryption, and secure multiparty computation can help mitigate these concerns but must be applied within clear ethical guidelines (Aziz et al., 2023). This necessitates interdisciplinary collaboration between data scientists, bioethicists, clinicians, and legal experts to establish norms and enforceable codes of conduct.

Ethical frameworks such as the Belmont Report, which articulates the principles of respect for persons, beneficence, and justice, provide a useful lens for evaluating federated systems. FL supports "respect for persons" by allowing greater control over data; it advances "beneficence" by enabling large-scale learning without exposing individuals to undue risk; and it promotes "justice" by including diverse participants in model development. These alignments suggest that FL is not merely a technical improvement but an ethical innovation in AI-driven healthcare.

Table 2. Ethical Risks in Centralized AI vs. Federated Learning Mitigations

Ethical Concern	Centralized AI Risk	Federated Learning (FL) Mitigation
Privacy Violation	Raw data transferred to central servers	No raw data movement; encrypted updates only
Informed Consent Gaps	Often limited or implied consent for reuse	Data remains under institutional governance
Bias and Inequity	Training on homogeneous, centralized datasets	Inclusion of diverse local data sources
Lack of Transparency	Black-box training pipelines	Local training allows greater traceability
Exploitation	Unequal benefit sharing in data collaborations	Decentralized ownership promotes fairness
Auditability Challenges	Difficult to trace model origin or updates	Supports audit logs at institutional level

As shown in Table 2, Federated Learning deals with and reduces several ethical issues that exist with centralized AI. Because all patient data is collected in one place in such systems, these are both more likely to be used improperly or hacked by others. FL minimizes this danger because it does not involve any data transfer which means control is kept local and attack options are fewer (Hu et al., 2024; Sheller et al., 2020).

Also, a major idea in medical ethics may be overlooked since a patient may be unwittingly included in training data in large-scale healthcare organizations. In federated systems, the power is given back to institutions which allows them to follow their own policies and regulate the use of data more openly (Loftus et al., 2022). Because decision-making is decentralized, institutions become more responsible and respect the idea of "respect for persons" described in ethical standards such as the Belmont Report.

Major disparities and bias can happen in centralized models, especially for example when training datasets focus on urban and well-financed healthcare systems. It may lead to AI systems that don't work well for those who are not well represented. Instead of relying on mostly the same data from one place, Federated Learning combines data from around the world, helping to build more fair models (Gu et al., 2023; Teo et al., 2024).

Also, by using federated approaches, the visibility of AI systems is better. Training models locally allows everyone to see clearly how preprocessing, labeling and training happen in their own systems. This makes it possible to audit each local component, something that can rarely be done in big, centralized systems (Cellamare et al., 2022).

There is also the risk that smaller clinics and contributors part with their data, but don't see value from the resulting AI model. Federated Learning makes it possible for data to be owned by all, instead of just a central organization, helping avoid data imbalance and support data justice. FL further helps in setting up auditability systems so that institutions can save logs of any changes made, agreeing parties' consents and performance records, making the system more accountable and open to overview from the outside (Aziz et al., 2023; Brauneck et al., 2023).

4. LEGAL AND REGULATORY CONSIDERATIONS IN FEDERATED LEARNING

Federated Learning (FL) in healthcare needs to follow several strict rules made to protect patient health information. Because health data is extremely private, there are strong guidelines for managing it everywhere. Laws like the Health Insurance Portability and Accountability Act in America, the General Data Protection Regulation in Europe and ongoing developments in India, Canada and Bangladesh are among these (Abbas et al., 2024; Brauneck et al., 2023). Because of its privacy-by-design design, Federated Learning is well suited for use with these frameworks. Also, cybercrime can add new challenges in the area of law enforcement.

4.1 Data Protection and Privacy Laws

Personal data is to be handled lawfully, fairly and in an open manner according to the GDPR rules. Such laws require data to be kept only as much as necessary, have a purpose and allow for forgetting. Ordinary centralized machine learning methods usually go against these ideas by collecting and storing large data across many countries. Federated Learning allows data to be kept where it comes from and shares only updates or gradients using tools like differential privacy or homomorphic encryption (Aziz et al., 2023).

Yet, the GDPR oversees data processing in addition to where data is found. While raw information stays on the device with FL, processing metadata or model gradients may need to comply with GDPR as these are types of data that could be linked to individuals. It has been found by some studies that under particular conditions, gradient inversion attacks can restore the input data by looking at model updates (Hu et al., 2024). This is why FL systems must use powerful cryptographic solutions and carry out threat modeling to comply.

HIPAA, on the other hand, mandates administrative, physical, and technical safeguards for electronic protected health information (ePHI). FL can reduce HIPAA compliance risks by removing the need for centralized ePHI storage. Nonetheless, covered entities and business associates must still conduct risk assessments, maintain audit controls, and ensure that encryption standards meet regulatory thresholds (Loftus et al., 2022).

4.2 Jurisdiction and Cross-Border Legal Tensions

Federated Learning regularly includes many institutions from separate countries or jurisdictions. So, there are now legal issues around who holds the data, how it can pass across international lines and how rules are made consistent between nations. For example, since FL shops data locally, the exchanged updates might still be seen as regulated data by local laws. Regions like China and the EU which have rigorous rules on data localization, can make sharing model parameters a trigger for complying with regulations. To solve these problems, institutions have to set out Data Processing Agreements (DPAs) and Federated Governance Policies that clearly state what everyone is responsible for and what rights they have. It is important for such agreements to recognize who owns any jointly developed neural networks, who knowns what data and what will happen if the network is misused or data is leaked (Aouedi et al., 2023).

4.3 Consent and Transparency Requirements

Nowadays, the law is interested in making sure there is clear written consent for using data. use. Centralized models frequently bring complications since patients may not learn about this practice. Their anonymized information is employed to teach AI. FL provides a more open choice because it shows local organizations are able to decide who takes part in training and how models are put to use Institutional policies related to consent (Sadilek et al., 2021).

Moreover, regulatory frameworks such as GDPR and Canada's PIPEDA also emphasize individual rights, including the right to access, correct, or erase personal data. Implementing these rights in FL requires the development of participant-aware systems that can track which local data influenced which model outcomes. This calls for model explainability data lineage mechanisms, which are still under development in the FL research community (Teo et al., 2024).

4.4 Security Obligations and Risk Management

Legal compliance is incomplete without adherence to security obligations that prevent unauthorized access and data leakage. In an FL system, threats such as Byzantine attacks, free-rider problems, and poisoned updates can compromise both data integrity and model performance (Ali et al., 2023). Regulators may not yet have precise laws tailored for FL-specific threats, but general obligations for confidentiality, integrity, and availability apply.

Therefore, healthcare institutions using FL must adopt multi-layered security architectures, including:

- Differential privacy to protect update-level privacy
- Homomorphic encryption or secure aggregation for parameter exchange
- Blockchain-based logging for model audit trails
- Reputation systems to detect malicious nodes

Failure to incorporate these can expose systems to legal penalties under negligence or breach of contract claims, even if no raw data was shared (Chamikara et al., 2021).

4.5 Institutional and Ethical Compliance Audits

As FL becomes mainstream in healthcare, regulatory bodies and institutional review boards (IRBs) will increasingly demand auditability. This includes logging of training participation, consent records, algorithm updates, and performance metrics disaggregated by subgroup. Moreover, models must be tested for bias, robustness, and compliance with ethical impact assessments prior to deployment (Brauneck et al., 2023).

Some institutions are now creating FL-specific compliance frameworks, such as:

- Privacy-Preserving Machine Learning (PPML) audit checklists
- AI ethics certification protocols
- Internal federated governance committees

These initiatives signal the growing institutional awareness that legal and regulatory readiness must evolve alongside technical development.

Table 3. Mapping Key Regulations to Federated Learning Compliance Strategies

Regulation / Law	Compliance Requirement	FL Strategy for Alignment
GDPR (EU)	Data minimization, consent, portability	Data remains local, encrypted updates, consent logs
HIPAA (US)	Technical safeguards for ePHI	No central storage, strong encryption at endpoints
PIPEDA (Canada)	Individual access and correction rights	Participant-aware updates and logging mechanisms

continued on following page

Table 3. Continued

Regulation / Law	Compliance Requirement	FL Strategy for Alignment
Data Localization Laws	Restriction on cross-border data	Model sharing only (not data), local computation
OECD AI Principles	Transparency, robustness, fairness	FL supports diversity, decentralized validation

Table 3 outlines how Federated Learning aligns with major regulatory frameworks by mapping key legal requirements to corresponding FL compliance strategies. For example, GDPR's demands for data minimization and explicit consent are addressed by FL's architecture, which keeps data local and implements encrypted model updates. HIPAA's technical safeguard requirements are satisfied through FL's removal of centralized ePHI and the integration of secure aggregation protocols. Because of data localization laws, FL allows different organizations to train a model together safely by sharing just the model parameters. Frameworks such as PIPEDA and the OECD AI Principles are implemented through things such as participant-aware logging, transparency tools and decentralized training, making FL suitable for regulation and privacy.

Since regulators are paying more attention to digital health systems, Federated Learning stands out as a model that reflects both legal rules and what is ethical. Since it includes compliance built into the architecture, rather than adding it on later, it is attracting interest from healthcare providers who care about privacy. To stay honest and respected, FL implementations must quickly change as laws do, with the help of transparent partnerships and clear policies.

5. TECHNICAL INNOVATIONS SAFEGUARDING PATIENT DATA

Federated Learning (FL) offers benefits by making it possible to train the model on many devices instead of a single server. Also by integrating privacy protection into the basic design of AI. In the since health data must be handled with care in healthcare, the approach to user experience design here stresses technical measures are put in place to help ensure patient information is not exposed during the training period and inference. This chapter discusses three major inventions—federated encryption, differential privacy. privacy and secure multi-party computation (SMPC) techniques have greatly influenced the way we understand privacy-preserving AI.

5.1 Federated Encryption and Decentralized Data Protection Methods

Federated encryption includes types of cryptographic techniques created to maintain data safety in federated learning activities. In healthcare-oriented FL, homomorphic encryption (HE) and secure aggregation protocols are used by most distributed applications.

Processing data without seeing it can be done with homomorphic encryption. That way, hospitals or clinics encrypt their model updates and a central server only aggregates the updates without ever needing to see what they actually say. After aggregation, only the people authorized can read the information from the global model. No one can see training data, not even the central aggregator, because of this design (Aziz et al., 2023).

Alongside this, secure aggregation protocols including those offered by Brauneck et al. work so that only the total combined result is accessible by the central server, preventing any individual administrative updates from being disclosed. It is important to stop model inversion attacks which can use gradients to expose patient data. Encryption capabilities of these systems help FL follow the requirements of GDPR, HIPAA and similar laws by hiding sensitive personal information when exchanged (Gu et al., 2023).

Using blockchain, new decentralized ledgers are being used to store permanent records of training activities. Using these systems, model contributions can be traced, accountability is maintained and trust between various parties is established in big FL healthcare deployments (Brauneck et al., 2023).

5.2 Differential Privacy and Its Significance in Healthcare Applications

The field of privacy-preserving machine learning now relies heavily on Differential Privacy (DP). It provides a guarantee that the results are very much the same, no matter if a person's information is used in the dataset. Most of the time, random noise is added in a controlled way to the model's updates.

Differential privacy is used in Federated Learning in two basic forms.

- **Local Differential Privacy (LDP):** each client adds noise to their updates before sharing them with the server.
- **Global Differential Privacy (GDP):** A server adds noise after everyone's updates have been brought together.

Since even tiny leaks in healthcare can cause serious ethics and legal issues, implementing DP prevents others from finding personal health information by studying the machine learning models (Kaissis et al., 2020). Hospitals can use differential privacy, for example, when sharing changes to their models, so that patient-related privacy is protected.

It is a main challenge to balance the privacy and usefulness aspects in implementations of Differential Privacy. Noisy data can lower a model's performance and it is a common problem when working with small or unbalanced datasets in clinics. For this reason, it is important to find the correct privacy budget (ε) to support both protection of data and reliable care delivery (Ziller et al., 2021).

5.3 Secure Multi-Party Computation in Practice: Examples and Benefits

Federated learning also relies on the fundamental concept of Secure Multi-Party Computation (SMPC). learning. It lets several parties use each other's data to compute a function, while protecting Details about those inputs are private. In healthcare, using SMPC, doctors can train models collaboratively. Hospitals or research institutes can use this without revealing any information about their first-party data.

An illustrative use case involves multi-hospital disease prediction, where each institution trains a local model and contributes encrypted intermediate results. Through SMPC, a central computation node can aggregate these without seeing the raw values. This approach was successfully demonstrated in cancer diagnosis modeling and multi-organ segmentation tasks using FL (Teo et al., 2024).

Benefits of SMPC include:

- **High data confidentiality:** No party learns the input of others.
- **Regulatory alignment:** Supports compliance with strict data localization laws.
- **Collaborative intelligence:** Facilitates model training across otherwise siloed datasets.

However, challenges remain. SMPC requires synchronization, has computational overhead, and must be combined with other techniques like differential privacy for end-to-end security. Still, it remains a critical component in high-assurance healthcare applications such as clinical trials, diagnostic model training, and public health forecasting (Chamikara et al., 2021).

Table 5. Comparison of Key Privacy-Preserving Techniques in Federated Learning

Technique	Key Feature	Benefits in Healthcare	Limitations
Homomorphic Encryption	Computation on encrypted data	Strong confidentiality, no raw data exposure	High computational cost
Secure Aggregation	Server sees only combined updates	Prevents data leakage from individual gradients	Requires dropout-resilient protocols
Differential Privacy	Adds noise to outputs/ gradients	Formal privacy guarantees, regulatory support	Trade-off between accuracy and privacy
Secure Multi-Party Computation	Joint computation without data sharing	Enables cross institution collaboration	Network latency and performance overhead
Blockchain Logging	Immutable training logs	Transparency, traceability, accountability	Scalability and integration complexity

Table 5 summarizes the core privacy-preserving innovations used in federated learning and evaluates their strengths and limitations in healthcare. These technologies offer complementary benefits: while differential privacy and homomorphic encryption protect individual contributions, SMPC and secure aggregation enhance trust in collaborative training environments. Together, they form a multi-layered defense strategy critical for deploying FL in real-world clinical and diagnostic systems.

Figure 2. Technical Innovation Stack for Privacy-Preserving Federated Learning

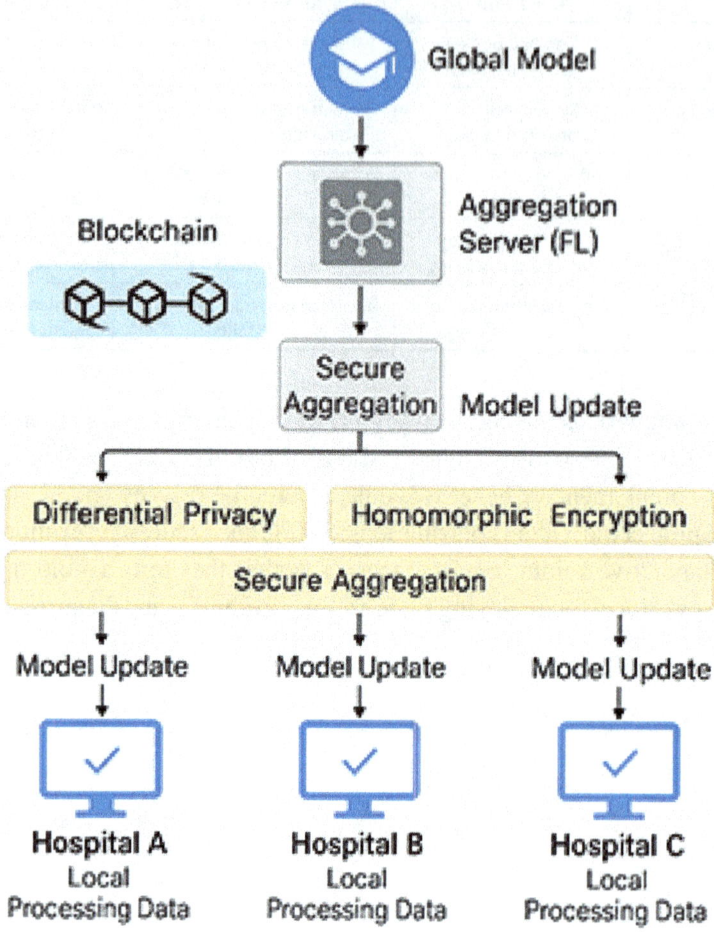

In addition, figure 2 shows how multiple technical ideas need to be layered, enabling privacy and collaboration to co-exist in an architecture. With every component added, the overall guarantee of privacy fortifies the trust behind sensitive health care work.

As federated learning evolves, its ability to help in healthcare depends a lot on the effectiveness of its privacy technologies as well as its algorithmic efficiency. Typical ways such as federated encryption, differential privacy and secure multi-party computation are used as important tools to ensure ethical standards. Being used in real-life scenarios shows a trend toward designing AI with privacy as a main goal. This is particularly important in areas like healthcare since doctors must put patients at the center. As these changes keep being made, they will guide the future of secure, cooperative and law-compliant healthcare information

6. USE CASES AND APPLICATIONS OF FEDERATED LEARNING IN HEALTHCARE

Federated Learning (FL) is redefining healthcare and making it more accessible. Helping institutions work together in machine learning to advance health care switching to a different way to store sensitive patient records. Because privacy-by-design is supported, new doors have opened with it diagnostics, remote monitoring, discovery of new drugs and individualized medicine make use of AI. This section looks at important healthcare uses for FL, backing them up with practical examples, studies and comparative insights.

Diagnostic Imaging and Disease Classification

FL has had a big impact in healthcare from the very beginning, especially through its uses in medical imaging and categorizing diagnoses. For example, Sheller et al. found that FL let a deep learning model analyze brain tumors with data collected from different hospitals and while ensuring patient confidentiality. With the same purpose in mind, Kaissis et al. (2020) also applied FL on liver and pancreatic lesion classification, so the model performs well on different sets of data.

Collaboration through FL makes it possible for institutions to look for rare diseases, since single hospitals may not have enough data for training. Because doctors and nurses in FL have access to a wide range of knowledge, the field supports improved and all-inclusive systems for diagnosing patients, primarily in oncology, neurology and radiology.

Hospital Readmission Prediction

Readmission prediction is a critical metric for hospital quality assessment. Traditional models suffer from site-specific biases and may underperform in cross-site generalization. Xu et al. (2021) proposed a federated architecture for predicting hospital readmission using heterogeneous EHRs (Electronic Health Records), showing that models trained across hospitals using FL achieved higher predictive accuracy than isolated local models.

Through FL, these models continuously evolve as more institutions join the training process, without sharing identifiable patient data. This application supports not just predictive performance but also healthcare system efficiency and reduced costs.

Remote Patient Monitoring and mHealth

The rapid rise of mobile health (mHealth) applications and wearable technologies has generated massive amounts of real-time health data. FL is increasingly applied to on-device learning for chronic disease monitoring, such as diabetes, heart disease, and mental health. For example, Sadilek et al. (2021) demonstrated FL's utility in aggregating insights from decentralized mobile devices to detect flu-like symptoms and COVID-19 trends at the population level, while ensuring user anonymity.

Wearable devices (e.g., smartwatches, ECG patches) can use federated learning to improve personalized health tracking, detect early anomalies, and deliver tailored interventions - all without offloading raw biometric data to centralized servers.

Drug Discovery and Genomic Collaboration

FL can also contribute in the field of multi-institutional pharmaceutical research, mainly where data related to genetics and drugs are spread and need to respect privacy. Using distributed computation, Gong et al. (2016) worked on biomedical sensing data which shaped the foundation for FL in biomedicine. Lately, Brauneck et al. (2023) explored how to add privacy-enhancing technology to FL for projects that maintain ownership of data in genomic collaborations.

This is very valuable for drug studies across nations because it allows institutions to study the drug's effectiveness or genetic ties without having to collect high-risk patient data somewhere central.

Personalized Medicine

FL supports more precise healthcare because models can be modified at the edge. Local hospitals or treatments can use the ideas from global models to suit individuals or local populations. This process helps make the results fairer as well as useful for clinic and research. In their study, Akter et al. (2022) pointed out that FL-based systems can improve personalized health recommendations compared to alternatives using cloud data and they are also compliant with data laws. Being adaptable makes it easier to follow doctor's advice, reduces dangers caused by the treatment and helps underrepresented patients gain better access to healthcare.

Table 4. Comparison of FL Applications in Healthcare Domains

Use Case	FL Benefit	Traditional Challenge	Reference
Diagnostic Imaging	Cross-institution training	Data silos, privacy concerns	(Sheller et al., 2020)
Readmission Prediction	Improved generalization	Site-specific model bias	(Xu et al., 2021)
mHealth & Wearables	On-device personalization	Cloud dependency, privacy risk	(Sadilek et al., 2021)
Drug Discovery & Genomics	Collaborative analysis without sharing	Genomic data sensitivity	(Brauneck et al., 2023)
Personalized Treatment	Edge-level model adaptation	Centralized model inflexibility	(Akter et al., 2022)

Federated Learning is applied in many healthcare fields, for example in diagnostic imaging as well as in patient monitoring. Because FL keeps data private, it makes it possible for teams worldwide to collaborate which supports the growth of smart, ethical and inclusive healthcare systems in the future. As usage of FL increases, merging it into regular healthcare and research processes may change for the better how medical intelligence is used.

7. PRACTICAL IMPLEMENTATION: STRATEGIES AND CHALLENGES

Both the theory and privacy features of Federated Learning (FL) are attractive, but its true use in healthcare requires considering several practical issues. The strategies implemented at different stages of healthcare are explained and the problems with organization, technology and rules faced during this process are given.

Infrastructure and System Design Strategies

Facilities in the healthcare sector are not the same in computational features, staff technical skills or data readiness. Usually, for these disparities, FL implementations are built around local clients (hospitals, clinics, mobile devices) and a principal coordinating server. Akter et al. (2022) and Xu et al. (2021) pointed out that edge devices can take part in training, regardless of when connectivity returns, because of their light design and the usage of asynchronous protocols.

Also, using cloud-edge hybrid designs helps scale storage and join models, allowing the data to be processed on the edge. It is essential for institutions to run containerized setups and use secure channels (like gRPC with TLS) to connect and collaborate in their federated learning systems.

Data Heterogeneity and Non-IID Challenges

Data heterogeneity or the non-IID nature of medical data is often listed as one of the main difficulties in applying current FL approaches. Due to different ways data is collected and the variety of devices and groups studied, the models can become unstable.

Some of the newest plans and actions involve:

- **Personalized FL**: Fine-tuning or meta-learning can be used to fit global models to new local environments.
- **Clustered FL**: Organizing clients by their data to train several models for different groups.
- **Weighted aggregation:** Assigning different values to a client's update based on the accuracy of the data or how close the values are.

By using these methods, we make sure that the model is fair and is able to work correctly for everyone which is very important in healthcare AI.

Regulatory and Ethical Implementation Hurdles

Practical application of FL means following regulations such as HIPAA (USA), GDPR (EU) and local review boards for ethical purposes. All parties within an institution must create legal contracts to outline who owns the data, the rules for governing it and what to do in case any models make mistakes.

In addition, ethical use means seeing that FL is practical and available to everyone who needs it. Rural areas or places with limited hospital resources may not be able to join FL which could cause the model to exclude people from those communities.

Organizational and Collaboration Barriers

FL requires high levels of institutional collaboration, which may be hindered by:

- Trust issues between competing healthcare organizations
- Lack of standardized protocols for model exchange
- Inconsistent IT readiness and cybersecurity standards

OpenFL (Intel), Flower and TensorFlow Federated are among the frameworks giving new participants in FedML easy access with strong security and shared technology.

Table 5. Key Practical Challenges and Corresponding Strategies

Challenge	Strategy/Approach	Reference
Infrastructure disparity	Edge-cloud hybrid design, containerization	Akter et al., 2022
Data heterogeneity (non-IID)	Clustered FL, personalization, aggregation	Xu et al., 2021
Regulatory/legal hurdles	Privacy agreements, compliance frameworks	Brauneck et al., 2023
Collaboration & trust issues	Open-source FL platforms and governance models	Sheller et al., 2020
Bias due to digital divide	Edge model tuning, inclusive infrastructure	Sadilek et al., 2021

There are many hurdles to overcome in taking Federated Learning from research to use in healthcare. Using advanced edge solutions, privacy-focused approaches in law and working together, numerous businesses are starting to make FL functional in real-life settings. Closing infrastructure gaps and applying inclusive designs are necessary for giving equal access to FL and supporting global health.

8. ROLE OF FEDERATED LEARNING IN PANDEMIC SURVEILLANCE AND RESPONSE

The worldwide spread of COVID-19 showed the urgent need for new data structures that are scalable, protect privacy and are interoperable to help communities act quickly. Major challenges with centralized machine learning systems appeared during the pandemic, mainly due to matters of privacy, HIPAA and GDPR and transferring data to other countries. Therefore, Federated Learning (FL) offered a way to solve many of these problems. FL allowed healthcare organizations to use AI for surveillance, forecasts, diagnosis and decision-making, without sharing any private or sensitive data directly.

In pandemics, Federated Learning was first used for epidemiological modeling. To predict how infections will progress, how sick people are going to be and the results of prevention measures, a large collection of distributed data is often needed. When organizations use centralized data collection, models often face delays, missing details and compliance concerns. FL makes sure that every institution retains ownership of its data but can contribute to the development of a global model. In a COVID-19 situation, Sadilek et al. (2021) used data from various healthcare providers to develop and test federated symptom predictors. With this, it became easier to forecast infections and properly allocate medical supplies without breaking privacy laws.

Apart from making epidemiological predictions, Federated Learning helps with instant surveillance using connected devices. Health-related data is constantly collected from individuals by smartphones, smartwatches, sensors and thermal screening kiosks. Historically, sharing health data on a central server would be opposed due to concerns about privacy and limited speed of internet connections. FL allows these devices to learn about symptoms such as fever, abnormal coughing or trouble breathing and to securely upgrade their models using only encrypted data. Akter et al. (2022) developed an edge-focused framework for COVID-19 detection using wearables and smart devices and proved it to be successful in detecting new cases and serving as a reliable early warning system that keeps users anonymous by design.

FL also played a key role in scientific collaboration during the pandemic, mainly supporting efforts to make new drugs and vaccines. Pharmaceutical firms, research bodies and genomic labs usually have to follow strict regulations that do not allow them to reveal their proprietary or sensitive information to others. In addition, working together plays a key role in assessing drug action, recognizing important markers and shortening trial timelines. With Federated Learning, many institutions could train models together without breaching privacy or ownership of ideas. Kaissis et al. (2020) set up a federated system for spotting abnormalities in the lungs related to COVID-19 from data collected abroad without transferring the scans. Teo et al.

(2024) also mentioned that FL helps scientists use data from various areas to detect mutations, observe viral changes over time and update vaccines and readiness plans.

During the most intense parts of the pandemic, especially in places with scarce resources, AI played a key role in making policy decisions. To effectively use ICU beds, ventilators and PPE, organizations relied on data collected in real time. Yet, because hospital records are so sensitive, sharing them with centralized organizations brought up ethical and legal issues. FL made it possible to assemble models that measured regional demand, predicted insufficient supply and advised on supply allocation without revealing information on individual hospitals. Loftus et al. (2022) pointed out that federated models were used to make hospital workflows and planning more effective, making it possible to care for patients even when the number of cases increased.

Federated Learning is notable in pandemic situations mainly because it enables different institutions and countries to work together. Previously, global health surveillance has struggled because of problems with data management, working across different systems and concerns about security. FL made it possible for different countries to train models together without transferring their data. They suggested that the World Health Organization (WHO) could be responsible for managing federated surveillance systems in order to receive and analyze regular updates from health ministries around the world on diseases and virus changes. The global pandemic intelligence system using FL avoids sharing private data with other countries.

From COVID-19, investors have learned the importance of readiness for future pandemics and now focus on such infrastructure. Now, governments and healthcare providers are working on federated data lakes, edge health monitoring systems, federated AI model registries and secure ways to communicate. Combining these elements enables the system to handle rapid diagnostics, forecast infectious disease outbreaks and encourage research by everyone. For instance, the European Health Data Space and the NIH Bridge2AI initiative are using federated technology to enable nations to quickly cooperate in case of new health problems.

Associated challenges still make his implementation in pandemics complicated. Because there are differences in how data is collected, how networks are built and how regulations vary, federated models may have difficulty being scaled widely and used in different situations. In addition, federated models are likely to run into complicated threats such as poisoning, backdoors and model inversion that are more likely to occur in a large-scale deployment. To deal with these issues, one must use effective model validation processes, keep detailed records and implement secure homomorphic encryption and differential privacy tools. It is important to continue research to make models work well and be fair in regions that have limited resources and few or uneven sources of data.

In the near future, Federated Learning might become a main part of how the world addresses pandemics, both with its technology and on the world stage. It provides a way for institutions and nations to share knowledge, build medical intelligence together and manage public health activities without putting trust or independence in danger. Adding privacy, security and ethical regulations into FL-powered AI is important for forming a health system that can better handle problems in the future.

9. SECURITY ARCHITECTURE AND THREAT MITIGATION IN FEDERATED LEARNING

FL in healthcare is being used mainly to make sure patient information remains safe as different organizations work together to develop AI models. However, keeping data safe is still a crucial and difficult issue for FL systems, especially in healthcare domains because data is sensitive and trust is very important. Because FL does not allow raw data to be extracted from the client, it is not fully guaranteed that malicious actions can be stopped. FL systems can still be attacked in many ways such as inference attacks, poisoning attacks and weaknesses in aggregators. These problems can also be made worse when devices are not the same, data is not evenly distributed and client actions are hard to understand.

9.1 Inference Attacks in FL Healthcare Systems

People are most worried about inference attacks in medical fields, where valuable diagnostics could be at risk. Opponents in such attacks try to reconstruct information about the client's stored data by looking at the gradients or weights that are transferred in model updates. Unlike systems that keep all the data inside, FL gives external training access to the gradients. It was found by Ziller et al. (2021) that deep gradient leakage (DGL) methods can reconstruct patient images extremely accurately even after a small number of iterations. If these abilities are not controlled, they might result in private patient information being revealed which could break privacy rules like HIPAA or GDPR.

Furthermore, there is a vulnerability named membership inference that makes it possible for people to find out if data samples came from the training set which could lead to more risks. A healthcare-related malfunction might involve an intruder figuring out from the model whether a person was given a certain medical diagnosis (Kaissis et al., 2020). Such risks are more easily spotted in cases of rare diseases because there is less variability in the data.

Because of these threats, differential privacy (DP) is now commonly used in data science. Using DP, models are indistinguishable from being trained with or without any specific data point. The use of controlled levels of noise in gradients is what helps DP keep privacy and enable learning. Gu et al. (2023) highlight that adjusting the privacy budget (ε) is very important in healthcare, because it is hard to achieve both utility and confidentiality together. Still, including noise can harm a model's accuracy and this is especially concerning in important areas like tumor detection or sepsis prediction, since incorrect predictions might be very dangerous.

9.2 Model and Data Poisoning Threats

Inference attacks try to access sensitive data, but poisoning attacks change the behavior of the learned model. A malicious user performing model poisoning supplies wrong or purposefully evil updates to the main server to interrupt training or inject a backdoor. Healthcare is at high risk from incorrect predictions since these can have an immediate impact on patients. In their work, Ali et al. (2023) describes poisoning attacks as happening either to a single system or to many systems at once. Unlike untargeted attacks which try to damage the model, targeted attacks concentrate on a specific element such as misclassifying a disease.

When there is data poisoning, the source data is altered. A harmful node operating in a hospital might include manipulated images or false patient details in its data which can affect the model's training. According to Chamikara et al. (2021) such attacks may carry on throughout training, slightly moving the model's decision boundary and making it unreliable. It is often hard to notice this kind of attack in federated learning, mainly because nobody can see the data being used for training.

Some techniques have been suggested to fight against the dangers of poisoning. These algorithms, Krum, Trimmed Mean and Bulyan, attempt to track and handle abnormal changes during training. They go through the gradients from all clients and reject any that are far from the average. Krum, when used together with norm clipping and adaptive thresholds, was proved by Hu et al. (2024) to make medical classification tasks more robust. Still, these approaches often count on most people being trustworthy which can be questionable in large, federated networks.

Another approach is to use grouping techniques (clusters) to find anomalies, apply updates with accessory datasets to confirm their correctness and give more weight to clients with better past performance (Aouedi et al., 2023). Even though they hold a lot of promise, they also create hurdles concerning fairness, the intricacy of the system and computer power.

9.3 Communication Threats and Vulnerabilities

There are also many opportunities for attack through the channels that clients use to connect with the central server. Since no raw data is moved, anyone monitoring the exchange of gradient, weights and updates between networks could eavesdrop, tamper with network info or replay the data. In such a case, a wrongdoer might take the updates during transmission, reverse engineer their secrets and make minor changes to the parameters before sending them to the server (Akter et al., 2022).

Replay attacks make for a much more serious kind of danger. When this happens, an attacker repeats previously correct model information which might cause the training to fail or introduce biases in the model's results. These attacks are not simple to notice, unless you use verified login and time-based prevention.

Transport Layer Security (TLS) is often applied to protect internet traffic through encryption. Aziz et al. (2023) points out that TLS is not strong enough in conditions where devices can be broken into or where someone could position themselves in the middle of the communication. To be on the safe side, cryptographic authentication is also used to make sure each client's new installation hasn't been altered or tainted.

Various sources are looking at blockchain technology to keep FL communication records secure. In healthcare, being responsible to regulators is very important, so the fact that you can review every step and update in training provides security and assurance (Brauneck et al., 2023). By using blockchain for federated learning, we get a shared ledger of work which lets each party monitor updates and spot anyone who is acting unfairly.

9.4 Aggregator Compromise and Central Server Threats

The main aggregator in FL leads model updates and ensures that the network stable updates across various devices. But because it plays a key role, the central nervous system is very prone to issues. If the security of the aggregator is broken due to malicious software, insiders or cloud weaknesses; all learning processes can be at risk. A hacker might force aggregation to work in a different way, insert tampered model data or spy on how updates are made across the client population.

In their work, Xu et al. (2021) called this a "honest-but-curious server problem," meaning the server stays on protocol but also tries to learn sensitive data from updates. This fact matters most when different healthcare organizations collaborate on shared research, as the server could be handled by a third-party researcher or cloud provider.

Secure Multi-Party Computation (SMPC) is a good answer because it lets users aggregate data while it remains encrypted. Participants in SMPC share and distributes random updates of the model to different servers. Server does aggregation each time without touching the private data from a single client. With Homomorphic Encryption (HE), data stays encrypted while operations are carried out directly on it. Even though HE takes a lot of computing power, it is chosen more often for medical AI because it protects privacy while training (Aziz et al., 2023; Sheller et al., 2020).

Intel SGX and other Trusted Execution Environments (TEEs) are now often used to secure the aggregator functionality. Because computations are carried out within these hardware-based enclaves, they are separated from the rest of the system by even the host operating system. (Loftus et al., 2022).

9.5 Table of Threats and Countermeasures

To consolidate the landscape of security threats in FL and their respective countermeasures, Table 6 provides a summary aligned with healthcare-specific risks.

Figure 3. Security-Enhanced Federated Learning Architecture

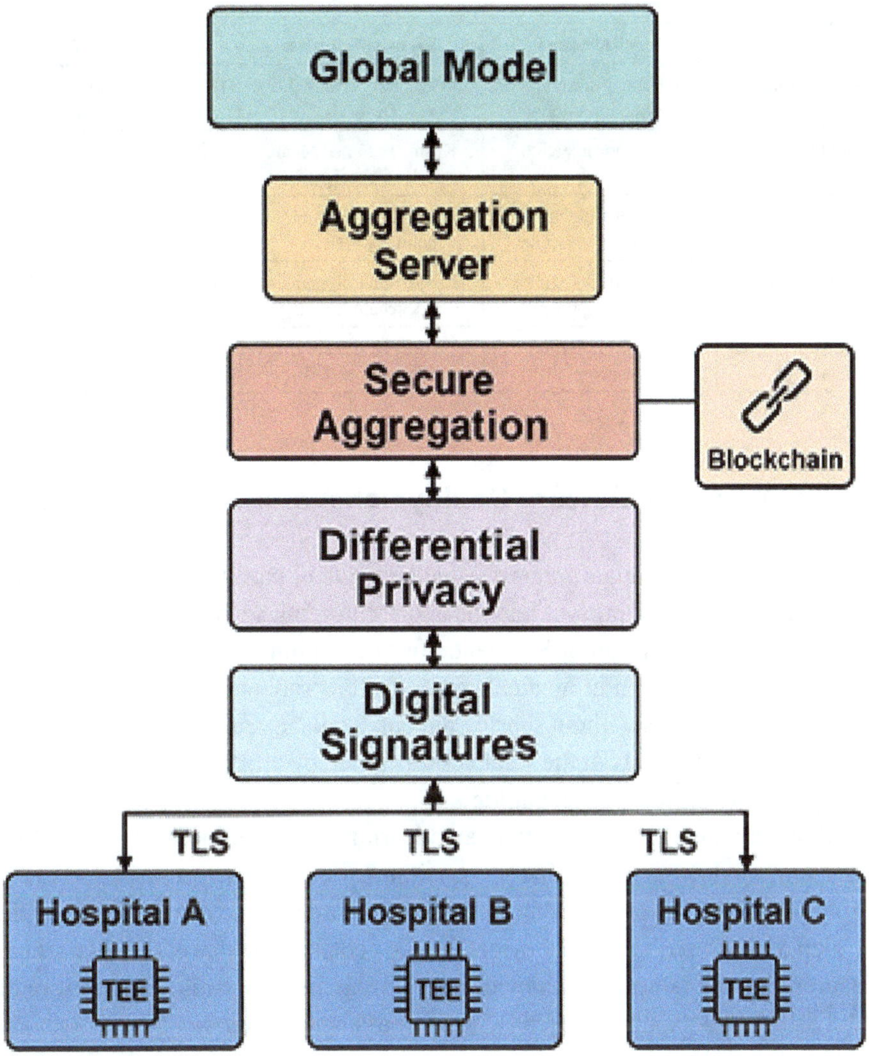

Table 6. Overview of Major Security Threats and Countermeasures in Federated Learning

Threat Category	Specific Attack	Security Solution	Cited Studies
Inference Attack	Gradient inversion, membership inference	Differential Privacy (DP), DP-SGD	(Kaissis et al., 2020; Ziller et al., 2021)
Model Poisoning	Backdoor injection	Krum, Trimmed Mean, Bulyan aggregation	(Ali et al., 2023; Hu et al., 2024)
Data Poisoning	Label flipping, adversarial examples	Update validation, anomaly detection	(Aouedi et al., 2023; Chamikara et al., 2021)
Communication Threat	Replay attack, MITM, eavesdropping	TLS, Digital Signatures, Blockchain Logging	(Akter et al., 2022; Aziz et al., 2023)
Aggregator Vulnerability	Honest-but-curious server	SMPC, Homomorphic Encryption, TEEs	(Loftus et al., 2022; Sheller et al., 2020; Xu et al., 2021)

9.6 Real-World Healthcare Deployments and Security Practices

Healthcare professionals are now using Federated Learning in practical settings which helps teach us important lessons about enforcing security. A good example of this is the Federated Tumor Segmentation (FeTS) initiative started by Sheller et al. (2020), helping different medical centers collaborate on training a brain tumor model from MRI scans without sharing patient details. Even though this project did very well, it also pointed out the weaknesses caused by different institutions having varying security systems or technologies.

Sadilek et al. (2021) applied federated learning as a method for COVID-19 research, uniting doctors from different hospitals to develop ways to track COVID-19 symptoms. Due to the spread of data, fast-changing streams and IID (non-independent and identically distributed) behavior, it was necessary to have flexible security measures. As an example, new devices were implemented, while making sure that model drift and poisoning caused by them could be handled.

They show why it is necessary to use defense systems that consider diverse devices, network challenges and trust in other parts of the system. Using differential privacy in clinical NLP slowed progress and securing data with enclaves needed special hardware infrastructure that was out of reach for many people in developing regions or small hospitals.

Real FL cases showed that constant monitoring and reviewing are essential. To be strong, DP and SMPC should be supported with threat intelligence, detection of deviations and version control with the participation of many parties. Because of this trend, modern healthcare companies are now building their FL infrastructures so that logging and monitoring all security-related aspects are emphasized (Teo et al., 2024).

9.7 Limitations of Current Security Approaches in FL

Despite advancements, current security architectures in FL still face critical limitations. First and foremost is the trade-off between security and model utility. Techniques such as differential privacy, while effective, often reduce model accuracy particularly in tasks where precision is essential, such as cancer detection or rare disease classification. The tuning of DP parameters like epsilon (ε) remains more of an art than a science, often requiring task-specific experimentation (Gu et al., 2023).

Second, resource consumption is a major barrier. Homomorphic encryption and SMPC significantly increase training times and require high-end computing resources. This limits their use in edge-based healthcare devices, such as portable ECG monitors or mobile health apps. Even secure aggregation protocols like SecAgg, which allow the server to compute on encrypted weights, introduce memory and latency overhead that may render the system impractical in real-time use cases (Loftus et al., 2022).

A third challenge lies in the lack of standardized threat modeling. Many FL security frameworks are developed ad hoc, without a formal structure to evaluate the types of adversaries or to prioritize defenses. There is currently no universal taxonomy for healthcare FL security, leaving deployments susceptible to oversight or misalignment with actual risk scenarios.

Lastly, user behavior and trust boundaries remain poorly addressed. The assumption that most clients are honest is often violated in open FL settings. Insider threats, compromised hospitals, or even misconfigured systems can act as inadvertent vectors of attack. Traditional anomaly detection systems may not be effective against low-and-slow poisoning strategies, where subtle changes accumulate over many rounds to cause a shift in model behavior.

9.8 Toward Holistic, Adaptive Security in Federated Healthcare AI

Healthcare security systems should move in the future toward being flexible and adjusting to specific situations. A potential approach is federated threat intelligence which allows people to send information about suspicious activity without disclosing personal data. The information from security incidents can be used instantly to enhance the defenses across the network. Intrusion detection systems (IDS) that use FL metadata sets in their training are beginning to appear. Client actions suspected of malice, like not following a consistent policy or sending outdated updates, are noticed by these models early on, since these may be signs of poisoning attacks (Arefin, 2024). Zero-knowledge proofs (ZKPs) are another possibility that makes it possible for clients to show they trained with correct data without showing the real data itself. Afterwards, more than one type of proof will probably play a key role in the rise of FL usage, using blockchain audits, secure enclaves and DP together. They support the security of AI as well as assure patients, regulatory authorities and medical boards that AI is accountable and visible to them.

A forward-looking architecture might involve the following components:

- Client-level TEEs to ensure secure local computation
- SMPC or HE to protect the aggregator and training process
- Differential Privacy for mathematical privacy guarantees
- Blockchain Audits for accountability and rollback
- AI-based anomaly detection for poisoning and inference attacks

This convergence of cryptographic, statistical, and AI-based defenses signals a maturation of FL security from reactive patching to proactive resilience.

10. FUTURE DIRECTIONS AND RESEARCH OPPORTUNITIES

The introduction of Federated Learning (FL) into healthcare has greatly improved the security and teamwork of artificial intelligence used in the industry. Nonetheless, because the technology has not fully matured, quite a few reasons for further investigation remain which can make FL more effective and reliable in healthcare.

10.1 Toward Generalizable and Explainable Federated Models

FL studies need to be able to produce good results across institutions that serve large differences in patient populations, types of diseases and available instruments for diagnosis. Usually, current versions of FL are slow because they are given data without IID (independent and identically distributed), with each client's information varying greatly. Research on personalized federated learning which combines worldwide training with local improvements, appears to address this problem (Li et al., 2020). So, better algorithms are needed to balance calibration and fairness among all contributors.

At the same moment, how models work is a major problem stopping many clinicians from believing in and using them. Health professionals should always find out how the AI model reached its diagnosis or prediction in healthcare. Explainability tools such as SHAP and LIME, have been created for central models, but similar tools for federated models are new. More work should be done on creating systems that allow access to interpretations while preserving the privacy of locally stored sensitive data (Teo et al., 2024).

10.2 Enhancing Fairness and Bias Mitigation in FL

There is a big risk in healthcare because algorithmic bias can lead to faulty diagnoses or unsuitable treatments for minority populations. Future studies can investigate fairness-aware learning methods that take demographic balancing, weighting people's voices and fairness rules into account. If data is hard to collect in a central location, federated methods like federated adversarial debiasing or federated reweighting can help solve issues of bias and still maintain accuracy (Gu et al., 2023).

Also, FL systems need to exceed addressing technical bias by offering proper governance with stakeholder consent, openness about how their algorithms function and equal sharing of system outputs. For this to be managed well, AI researchers, ethicists, clinicians and policymakers should join forces.

10.3 Lightweight Federated Learning for Edge and IoT Devices

A promising future direction lies in the optimization of FL for edge and low-power medical devices. As remote health monitoring grows, devices such as wearable ECG trackers, glucose monitors, or mobile diagnostic tools will need to participate in federated training without compromising speed or battery life. Techniques such as federated distillation, quantization, and sparse update encoding are being actively investigated to reduce the communication and computation burdens (Aouedi et al., 2023).

Combining FL with edge intelligence enables near real-time model updates from distributed sources such as rural clinics, mobile health vans, or patient homes. However, ensuring model performance and privacy on such heterogeneous infrastructures will require research into asynchronous FL, client selection protocols, and adaptive communication strategies tailored to device capabilities (Akter et al., 2022).

10.4 Federated Learning (FL) and Cross-Domain Collaboration

An emerging paradigm known as Federated Learning (FL) proposes creating nested FL systems where different healthcare federations (e.g., hospitals, insurance companies, and research institutes) collaborate while still preserving their internal FL privacy boundaries. This architecture could support large-scale public health initiatives such as pandemic response or rare disease mapping, enabling multi-tiered cooperation across domains.

FFL introduces new challenges in terms of coordination, privacy layering, and security policy enforcement. Future research must develop multi-level aggregation algorithms, inter-federation trust protocols, and federated regulatory compliance frameworks to make such architectures viable at scale.

10.5 Privacy-Utility Trade-off Optimization

While differential privacy and encryption techniques are critical to FL, they often degrade model utility. Future research must refine privacy-utility trade-off models that are dynamic and context-aware. For example, stricter privacy budgets might be applied to rare diseases or sensitive subgroups, while looser parameters may be acceptable for general wellness models. Adaptive privacy tuning based on data sensitivity levels, training phases, and model confidence scores could lead to more flexible deployments. Additionally, innovations in privacy-preserving hardware acceleration, such as FPGA-based differential privacy or GPU-enhanced secure computation, can unlock performance gains without sacrificing security.

10.6 Simulation Frameworks and Benchmarking Standards

There is currently a lack of standardized testing environments to evaluate federated learning systems in healthcare. Many studies rely on simulated FL over public datasets, which fails to capture the complexities of real clinical environments. The development of open-source FL benchmarking platforms that replicate hospital data workflows, regulatory constraints, and adversarial scenarios will be essential for meaningful progress (Cellamare et al., 2022).

Projects like Flower, FedML, and OpenFL are making strides in this direction, but need further integration with privacy auditing, secure aggregation, and multi-modal healthcare data to be truly representative. Future work should also focus on defining evaluation metrics that reflect not just model accuracy, but also privacy loss, communication efficiency, robustness, and fairness.

10.7 Interdisciplinary and Regulatory Research

Finally, future FL research must increasingly engage with regulatory and legal frameworks. As privacy laws like GDPR, HIPAA, and the proposed AI Act continue to evolve, federated learning must be positioned not just as a technological innovation, but as a tool for compliance and trust-building. Studies focusing on the legal enforceability of smart contracts, auditable machine learning, and dynamic consent in FL environments will be instrumental in translating research into practice (Brauneck et al., 2023).

Cross-border FL collaborations will particularly require harmonized legal protocols, data sovereignty guidelines, and digital trust labels that inform users about the safety and transparency of FL-driven applications.

CONCLUSION

The use of Artificial Intelligence in healthcare made real progress such as identifying diseases at an early stage and developing personalized plans for each patient. Still, these improvements create important issues related to patient privacy, safety of their data and ethical rules. Federated Learning (FL) has become a leading method for overcoming these issues by allowing models to be trained together while patient data remains private. Because of this change, privacy-by-design is possible, and it helps companies comply with data privacy laws worldwide.

This chapter showed us the basic ideas and new technologies that make FL strong and adaptable for healthcare AI. Since techniques like differential privacy, secure multiparty computation and encrypted communication are implemented, FL becomes tougher for threats like model inversion and data leakage to exploit. This architecture clearly outlines a security structure that fits well in real-life use for important systems.

Real-world purposes of FL were demonstrated during the COVID-19 pandemic. Such platforms as FL were used to perform distributed monitoring, forecast models and collaboration on projects, all while making sure patient privacy remained uncompromised. They showed that it is possible to keep data safe and still allow innovation, even in stressful environments involving a lot of data.

The challenges, however, are not gone yet. Separate issues such as the diversity of data, equal treatment in model outcomes and risk from adversarial attacks, still need more study and proper policy creation. Scaling FL in many different health systems depends on having interoperability and standardization.

Moving ahead, Federated Learning helps us find an environmentally friendly and ethical approach to bringing AI to healthcare around the globe. It connects different institutions, maintaining the rights and trust of each person which is key for upcoming medical AI systems. With more change toward digitization in healthcare, FL will serve to support data safety, keep advancements positive and ensure ethics guide all AI efforts.

REFERENCES

Abbas, S. R., Abbas, Z., Zahir, A., & Lee, S. W. (2024). Federated Learning in Smart Healthcare: A Comprehensive Review on Privacy, Security, and Predictive Analytics with IoT Integration. *Health Care*, *12*(24), 2587. DOI: 10.3390/healthcare12242587 PMID: 39766014

Akter, M., Moustafa, N., Lynar, T., & Razzak, I. (2022). Edge Intelligence: Federated Learning-Based Privacy Protection Framework for Smart Healthcare Systems. *IEEE Journal of Biomedical and Health Informatics*, *26*(12), 5805–5816. DOI: 10.1109/JBHI.2022.3192648 PMID: 35857737

Ali, M., Naeem, F., Tariq, M., & Kaddoum, G. (2023). Federated Learning for Privacy Preservation in Smart Healthcare Systems: A Comprehensive Survey. *IEEE Journal of Biomedical and Health Informatics*, *27*(2), 778–789. DOI: 10.1109/JBHI.2022.3181823 PMID: 35696470

Aouedi, O., Sacco, A., Piamrat, K., & Marchetto, G. (2023). Handling Privacy-Sensitive Medical Data With Federated Learning: Challenges and Future Directions. *IEEE Journal of Biomedical and Health Informatics*, *27*(2), 790–803. DOI: 10.1109/JBHI.2022.3185673 PMID: 35737624

Arefin, S. (2024). Strengthening Healthcare Data Security with Ai-Powered Threat Detection. [IJSRM]. *International Journal of Scientific Research and Management*, *12*(10), 1477–1483. DOI: 10.18535/ijsrm/v12i10.ec02

Aziz, R., Banerjee, S., Bouzefrane, S., & Le Vinh, T. (2023). Exploring Homomorphic Encryption and Differential Privacy Techniques towards Secure Federated Learning Paradigm. *Future Internet*, *15*(9), 310. DOI: 10.3390/fi15090310

Brauneck, A., Schmalhorst, L., Kazemi Majdabadi, M. M., Bakhtiari, M., Völker, U., Baumbach, J., Baumbach, L., & Buchholtz, G. (2023). Federated Machine Learning, Privacy-Enhancing Technologies, and Data Protection Laws in Medical Research: Scoping Review. *Journal of Medical Internet Research*, *25*, e41588. DOI: 10.2196/41588 PMID: 36995759

Cellamare, M., Van Gestel, A. J., Alradhi, H., Martin, F., & Moncada-Torres, A. (2022). A Federated Generalized Linear Model for Privacy-Preserving Analysis. *Algorithms*, *15*(7), 243. DOI: 10.3390/a15070243

Chamikara, M. A. P., Bertok, P., Khalil, I., Liu, D., & Camtepe, S. (2021). Privacy preserving distributed machine learning with federated learning. *Computer Communications*, *171*, 112–125. DOI: 10.1016/j.comcom.2021.02.014

Gong, Y., Fang, Y., & Guo, Y. (2016). Private Data Analytics on Biomedical Sensing Data via Distributed Computation. *IEEE/ACM Transactions on Computational Biology and Bioinformatics*, *13*(3), 431–444. DOI: 10.1109/TCBB.2016.2515610 PMID: 26761861

Gu, X., Sabrina, F., Fan, Z., & Sohail, S. (2023). A Review of Privacy Enhancement Methods for Federated Learning in Healthcare Systems. *International Journal of Environmental Research and Public Health*, *20*(15), 6539. DOI: 10.3390/ijerph20156539 PMID: 37569079

Hu, K., Gong, S., Zhang, Q., Seng, C., Xia, M., & Jiang, S. (2024). An overview of implementing security and privacy in federated learning. *Artificial Intelligence Review*, *57*(8), 204. DOI: 10.1007/s10462-024-10846-8

Kaissis, G. A., Makowski, M. R., Rückert, D., & Braren, R. F. (2020). Secure, privacy-preserving and federated machine learning in medical imaging. *Nature Machine Intelligence*, *2*(6), 305–311. DOI: 10.1038/s42256-020-0186-1

Li, T., Sahu, A. K., Talwalkar, A., & Smith, V. (2020). Federated Learning: Challenges, Methods, and Future Directions. *IEEE Signal Processing Magazine*, *37*(3), 50–60. DOI: 10.1109/MSP.2020.2975749

Loftus, T. J., Ruppert, M. M., Shickel, B., Ozrazgat-Baslanti, T., Balch, J. A., Efron, P. A., Upchurch, G. R.Jr, Rashidi, P., Tignanelli, C., Bian, J., & Bihorac, A. (2022). Federated learning for preserving data privacy in collaborative healthcare research. *Digital Health*, *8*, 205520762211344. DOI: 10.1177/20552076221134455 PMID: 36325438

Punreddy, A. R. (2023). *Federated Learning for Protecting Medical Data Privacy* [Master of Science, San Jose State University]., DOI: 10.31979/etd.cfgv-t6wa

Sadilek, A., Liu, L., Nguyen, D., Kamruzzaman, M., Serghiou, S., Rader, B., Ingerman, A., Mellem, S., Kairouz, P., Nsoesie, E. O., MacFarlane, J., Vullikanti, A., Marathe, M., Eastham, P., Brownstein, J. S., Arcas, B. A. Y., Howell, M. D., & Hernandez, J. (2021). Privacy-first health research with federated learning. *NPJ Digital Medicine*, *4*(1), 132. DOI: 10.1038/s41746-021-00489-2 PMID: 34493770

Sheller, M. J., Edwards, B., Reina, G. A., Martin, J., Pati, S., Kotrotsou, A., Milchenko, M., Xu, W., Marcus, D., Colen, R. R., & Bakas, S. (2020). Federated learning in medicine: Facilitating multi-institutional collaborations without sharing patient data. *Scientific Reports*, *10*(1), 12598. DOI: 10.1038/s41598-020-69250-1 PMID: 32724046

Teo, Z. L., Jin, L., Liu, N., Li, S., Miao, D., Zhang, X., Ng, W. Y., Tan, T. F., Lee, D. M., Chua, K. J., Heng, J., Liu, Y., Goh, R. S. M., & Ting, D. S. W. (2024). Federated machine learning in healthcare: A systematic review on clinical applications and technical architecture. *Cell Reports Medicine*, *5*(2), 101419. DOI: 10.1016/j.xcrm.2024.101419 PMID: 38340728

Xu, J., Glicksberg, B. S., Su, C., Walker, P., Bian, J., & Wang, F. (2021). Federated Learning for Healthcare Informatics. *Journal of Healthcare Informatics Research*, *5*(1), 1–19. DOI: 10.1007/s41666-020-00082-4 PMID: 33204939

Ziller, A., Usynin, D., Braren, R., Makowski, M., Rueckert, D., & Kaissis, G. (2021). Medical imaging deep learning with differential privacy. *Scientific Reports*, *11*(1), 13524. DOI: 10.1038/s41598-021-93030-0 PMID: 34188157

Chapter 13

The Decentralized Diagnostics Revolution Using Federated Learning in Medical Imaging and Beyond

Ravikumar R. N.
https://orcid.org/0009-0009-3705-1681
Marwadi University, Rajkot, India

Aarthi S.
https://orcid.org/0009-0006-9064-2091
Marwadi University, Rajkot, India

Valisher Sapayev
https://orcid.org/0000-0002-6751-5864
Mamun University, Khiva, Uzbekistan

Zamira Atamuratova
Urgench State University, Urgench, Uzbekistan

Norbek Kholboyev
Termez University of Economics and Service, Termez, Uzbekistan

Sindhuja S.
Kongu Engineering College, Erode, India

ABSTRACT

Federated Learning (FL) enables decentralized model training across healthcare institutions while preserving patient privacy and ensuring regulatory compliance. By retaining data locally and sharing only model updates, FL mitigates data breach risks, supports data sovereignty, and fosters cross-institutional collaboration. Techniques such as Federated Averaging (FedAvg) and Federated Proximal (FedProx) address challenges of Non-IID data and heterogeneous client environments. Privacy-preserving methods, including Differential Privacy and Secure Multiparty Computation, enhance confidentiality in model aggregation. FL demonstrates strong

DOI: 10.4018/979-8-3373-3306-9.ch013

potential in medical imaging, disease detection, and personalized healthcare, delivering improved diagnostic accuracy and generalization across diverse datasets. Real-world case studies validate its effectiveness in secure, large-scale medical AI applications.

INTRODUCTION

Healthcare needs advanced diagnostic instruments during this time to meet medical data privacy standards. The acquisition of medical AI training data through patient information remains challenging for processors because of existing ethical and legislative requirements. Federated Learning (FL) stands as a transformative diagnostic method because it enables different institutions to operate under a new training procedure which safeguards patient data inside each facility. The chapter demonstrates how distributed training techniques from FL adapt medical imaging diagnosis procedures. FL allows different healthcare facilities and research centers to build secure all-inclusive results at separate data points without jeopardizing patient data security at its original locations. The fusion of words speeds up research model development for specific reliability requirements and supports academic network expansion(D. C. Nguyen et al., 2023a).

The decentralized infrastructure of FL grows through its addition of pathology services to its present structure composed of genomics methods electronic health record systems and wearable health devices that promote entirely personalized healthcare services. The system-based ethical AI framework conducts General Data Protection Regulation (GDPR) and Health Insurance Portability and Accountability Act (HIPAA) protected evaluation of real-time data through processing systems. The chapter conducts a comprehensive evaluation of FL healthcare solutions through their technical processes while assessing their program merits and drawbacks. The study evaluates existing functional deployments of FL together with its modern AI developments which will probably impact medical diagnostics in the coming generation.

OVERVIEW OF FEDERATED LEARNING (FL) IN HEALTHCARE

FL presents an emerging machine learning technique that allows various decentralized devices along with institutions to train common models together without sharing actual information. FL provides an innovative solution within healthcare systems to establish collaborative model training across diverse healthcare institutions without sharing their raw datasets (Alruwaili et al., 2025). Traditional AI models need centralized datasets for operation yet this practice violates HIPAA privacy rules and GDPR and various other regional healthcare data safety standards. FL sustains healthcare institutions' data privacy by confining data to their local facilities with secure sharing capabilities for updating and aggregating the models.

Multiple healthcare facilities including clinics and research centers handle data distribution along with population-specific patient data that scanning technologies use. The healthcare entities can generate specific AI systems using FL while maintaining their data ownership rights. Healthcare organizations gain complete and extensive datasets to build effective diagnostic systems through this mechanism while protecting patient privacy. FL enables better patient diagnosis outcomes and safeguards medical information from breaches also enables harmonized medical examination methods. The technique delivers remarkable performance for radiology alongside oncology as well as dermatology and genomics because the manual creation of top-quality annotated data remains financially burdensome and limited in availability (Budrionis et al., 2021). Hospital-based healthcare facilities achieve continual learning through the FL system by continuously updating their models with new data sources. FL delivers an advanced solution for developing AI healthcare because it protects patient data privacy while creating secure diagnostic systems capable of developing diagnostic intelligence. The Figure 1 shows the FL framework in healthcare, where hospitals train local models on data such as CT scans, EHRs, and genomics, sending only model updates to a global model for aggregation.

Figure 1. Federated Learning in Healthcare

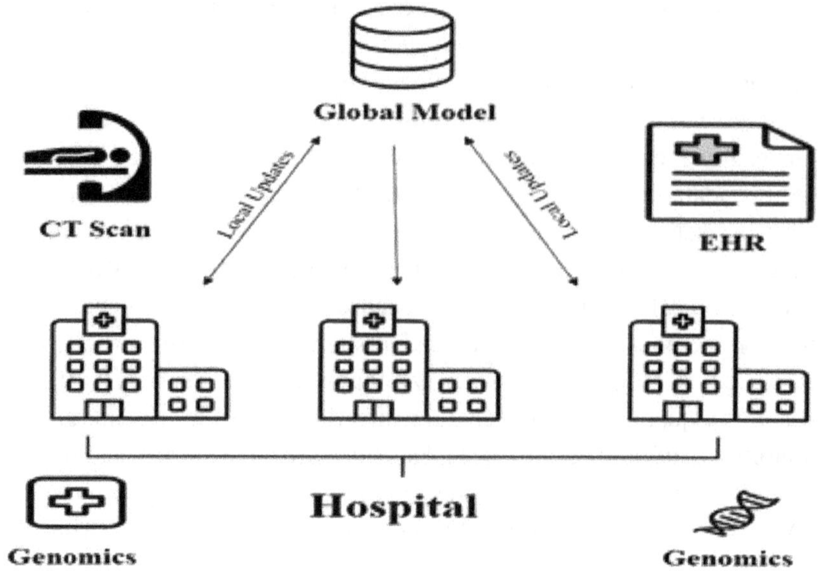

THE ROLE OF AI IN MODERN DIAGNOSTICS

AI has transformed current diagnostic medicine by improving diagnostic outcomes, lowering healthcare costs, and expanding medical services. Artificial programs in computer systems integrate EHR analysis to numerous medical image assessment to improve medical practitioner clinical workflow. Specialized artificial neural networks processed using deep learning techniques can evaluate X-ray, CT, MRI, and histopathology images. Medical professionals may quickly spot cancer, neurological, and cardiac disease signs using AI diagnostic tools that evaluate huge datasets. AI system screening allows healthcare personnel to communicate meaningfully with patients and promote person-centered treatment. AI-operated procedural protocols and real-time triage decision-making may increase patient survival and fatality rates in emergency medical settings.

Medical data processing allows computers to anticipate advanced illnesses, operations, and clinical outcomes. Enabling technologies are needed to construct precision medicine for specific patient circumstances. Diagnostic outputs from IoT-based wearable health apps help distant patients improve their healthcare. AI systems are limited in medical applications because to contested medical security standards, difficult clinical model interpretation requirements, and expensive administrative processes that generate impartial outcomes. FL was developed when privacy-respecting artificial intelligence technologies advanced. Integrating with remote health systems, healthcare technology increasingly provides patients complete diagnostic options.

MOTIVATION FOR DECENTRALIZED LEARNING IN MEDICAL APPLICATIONS

The demand of privacy, collaboration, and efficiency leads to the decentralized learning in the medical applications. FL will allow healthcare organizations to address HIPAA or GDPR and other regulations because it matches well with the risks of breaches and eliminates data silos across institutions. It enables production of diagnostic models that are inclusive across the world by integrating varied data regarding demography and geography. To deal with this challenge of the lack of labelled data, FL aims to bring together annotated data across organizations and provide an up-to-date flux of new clinical knowledge to tailor protocols in real-time. Through ethical and transparent guidelines, FL enables resource maximization in institutions with low infrastructure and enables inter-institutional research without explicit data transfer speeding improvement in the diagnosis, treatment, and personalized healthcare interventions (Chelani et al., 2024).

LITERATURE REVIEW

The rise of the concept of FL within healthcare is also a paradigm shift toward building such a collaborative model with the preservation of patient privacy in mind. Conventional centralized machine learning models would entail data aggregation, which is challenging to comply with privacy legislation like the HIPAA and GDPR. The solution to this presented by FL is the possibility of a decentralized training of models where the institutions can hold all the sensitive information and only share models parameters(D. C. Nguyen et al., 2023b). A similar strategy would minimize threats of data insecurity and would help in ensuring that the data laws of the jurisdictions are adhered to. Main concepts of FL are centered around the data retention on client side, collateral communication between the local machines and a central server, as well as secure methods of aggregation(Chelani et al., 2024). Raw data are not exchanged, and updates of their models are shared to achieve a stable global model through algorithms like Federated Averaging (FedAvg) and

Federated Proximal (FedProx). These techniques have demonstrated flexibility to commensurable distribution of data as well as scalability in multi-institutional implementations(Pfitzner et al., 2021).

Privacy privacy-preserving Florida increases usability in the healthcare sector. One may lend differential privacy to modify statistical noise obscuring the individual data contribution, and secure multiparty computation allows joint computation without revealing raw input(Sohan & Basalamah, 2023). This method is very important when dealing with healthcare related contexts where medical records are sensitive and require strict privacy assurances. Also contributing to the security market is the case of Trusted Execution Environments and Homomorphic Encryption, which enable secure execution of data even in prospectively hostile environments(Yaqoob et al., 2023). The prospect of FL can be witnessed in medical imaging. It has effectively been used in detecting diseases, personalized diagnostics, cross institutional research in the application of oncology, cardiology, and neurology. FL-trained NN models in healthcare are more accurate and generalizable in their diagnosis and associated with higher levels of aggregated insights on different datasets. A few examples of case studies, including the FeTS Challenge of brain tumor segmentation and mammogram-based breast cancer detection by Owkin & NVIDIA, show significant improvements in model accuracy, generalization and engineering-efficiency(W. Li et al., 2019). Nevertheless, this is not all positive in adopting FL in health care.

The fact that data may be heterogenous across different institutions may impede convergence of a model resulting in either instability or bias. Overhead of communication such as due to frequent updates to a model can put strain on bandwidth, and the data annotation inconsistency can make interpretability harder(Predictive, 2019). These issues are regulatory barriers, which despite the relaxed nature of FL, still limit the field of architecture and deployment. Some of these obstacles can be achieved through optimization algorithm developments, strategies of personalization of the models, and data augmentation methods to accommodate compatible training in varied sources("Privacy," 2025). Altogether, FL will enable a collaborative, secure, and scalable method of developing AI in healthcare. The fact that it allows preserving privacy, adhering to regulatory standards, and valuable use of diverse datasets makes it a major tech innovation that will redefine the future of clinical diagnosing and medical research.

FUNDAMENTALS OF FEDERATED LEARNING IN HEALTHCARE

Healthcare organizations work together using the FL model to create AI models for training needs without sharing their individual patient data. The data movement required within server-based information systems generates enhanced vulnerabilities to privacy as it must transfer data to central storage areas which produces security risks and non-compliance penalties. FL provides a solution through local model training across institutions with encrypted model advancements on their way to the central aggregator(Xu et al., 2021a). The medical industry Favors this method because it enables the protection of crucial healthcare data even with strict data usage protocols. The deployment of FL assists health facilities in maintaining patient data while meeting HIPAA and GDPR standards and allows universities to perform collaborative research across multiple healthcare institutions. The model becomes stronger due to the processing of information from multiple sites through separate datasets that comply with privacy rules (Le Quoc et al., 2019). The health-care deployment of FL combines local training operations with secure aggregation protocols as well as differential privacy methods and optimized communication protocols to establish a secure system for AI-based medical diagnostic analytics and decision processes.

CORE PRINCIPLES OF FL

Key concepts of FL entail decentralization, collaboration, protection of privacy, streamline aggregation, and lifelong education. The data in the FL are still stored locally, either on the devices or at the institutions, so the sensitive information does not travel across to a central host, which is essential to the privacy of the patient in healthcare. Collaboration involves the participation of many institutions and devices working together to come up with generalized models that can be based on various data sets(Xu et al., 2021b). The privacy is ensured through such regulations like GDPR and HIPAA, without sharing any raw data, only the model updates are shared. It achieves this efficiency through effective aggregation techniques by sending minimum amount of information and preserving performance at the same time, which the significant bandwidth and scalability optimize. The aspect of continuous learning is enabled by the use of up-to-date information in almost the real time, which enables AI models to become more flexible to the use of new local evidence, thus having a lower rate of detecting failures and a high rate of diagnostic outcome.

COMPARISON WITH CENTRALIZED MACHINE LEARNING APPROACHES

The table 1 summarizes the key differences between the two approaches, highlighting the advantages of FL in preserving privacy, enhancing collaboration, and enabling scalable and adaptive AI models in healthcare.

Table 1. Centralized vs. Federated Learning: A Comparative Analysis

Aspect	Centralized Machine Learning (CML)	Federated Learning (FL)
Data Privacy and Security	Data is transferred and stored centrally, increasing risk of data breaches and privacy violations.	Data remains local, with only model updates shared, ensuring better privacy and security.
Data Centralization	Requires centralized data storage, which involves high infrastructure costs.	Data remains decentralized, reducing the need for central storage and expensive infrastructure.
Data Silos	Data from different institutions is often inaccessible, limiting collaboration.	Encourages collaboration between institutions without sharing sensitive data.
Bias and Overfitting	Models may be biased due to limited or homogeneous data sources.	Models are trained on diverse, decentralized data, reducing bias and improving generalizability.
Scalability	Scaling requires transferring large datasets to a central server, which can be resource-intensive.	FL scales efficiently as only model updates, not raw data, are transmitted.
Model Adaptability	Model updates are performed centrally, often with a delay in adapting to new data.	FL supports continuous learning and real-time updates with new local data, improving adaptability.
Compliance with Regulations	Requires strict adherence to data privacy laws when transferring and storing data centrally.	Ensures better compliance with privacy laws by keeping data within local institutions.

ADVANTAGES OF FEDERATED LEARNING OVER CENTRALIZED APPROACHES

In comparison to centralized approaches, FL has a number of specific advantages, which is the reason why it is quite appropriate in the context of privacy-sensitive applications, including healthcare. Among the main advantages, there is the preservation of privacy because raw data is kept on mobile devices or at institutions locally and they do not break the rules of privacy, thus avoiding the access of other people with no rights to access it. FL also facilitates collaborative learning as the participating organizations may learn together to train models through distributed dataset when it comes to better performance under an environment where the operational conditions are varied. Regarding scalability and efficiencies, FL minimizes bandwidth consumption, decreases the cost of data transfers and central storage needs since it sends only model updates and not raw data. Moreover, FL would facilitate persistent model update by seamlessly incorporating new locally acquired information in real-time to make the models dynamic and improve on their ability to operate with respect to their life-cycle. (L. Li, 2024).

KEY ADVANTAGES OF FEDERATED LEARNING IN HEALTHCARE

The key advantages that FL is able to provide in the healthcare sector include the privacy of the data, the preservation of data sovereignty, and the possibility of complying with the regulations. Patient data is not released outside the clinical setting except new versions of the model and hence limiting the risk of breach and protection of personal identifiers. With FL, data sovereignty has been facilitated because institutions can withhold all the ownership of their data in the jurisdiction of the nation, and this is in correlation with the law of the land. It provides the security of regulation rules such as HIPAA and GDPR since data is stored locally and updated with anonymized aggregates. Also, the incorporation of differential privacy even more ensures patient data anonymity, avoiding the leakage of sensitive data, and allows model development in the various healthcare facilities to be safely shared. The figure 2 illustrating the three key advantages of FL in healthcare Privacy Preservation, Data Sovereignty, and Regulatory Compliance highlighting their interconnected role in secure and ethical data management.

Figure 2. Key Advantages of Federated Learning in Healthcare

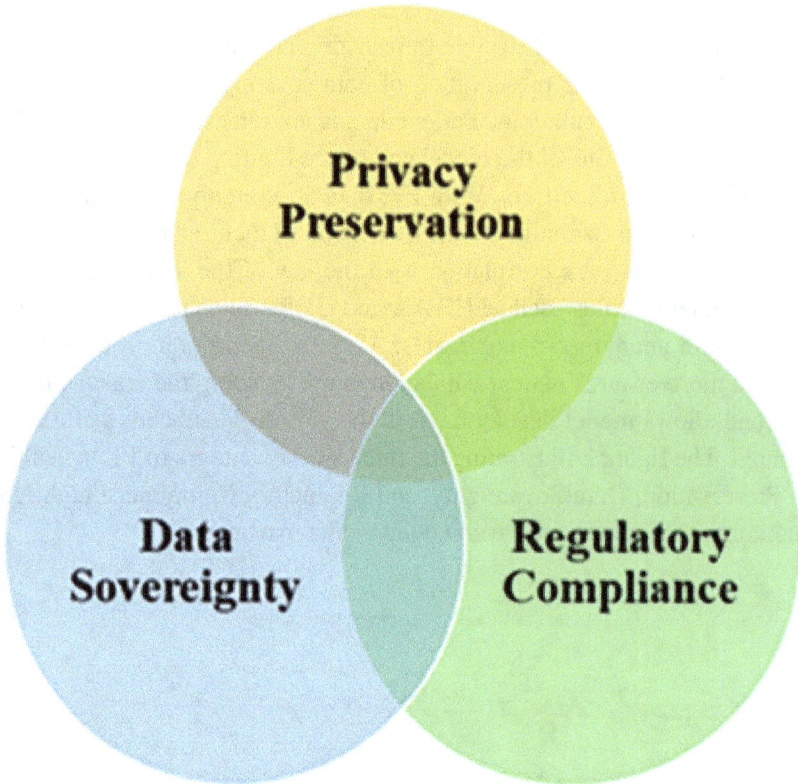

ARCHITECTURE OF FEDERATED LEARNING

Technical architecture of the FL allows distributing data and jointly training models across a variety of participants in a communication framework that establishes links between local machines and a central aggregator. Local clients (clinics, hospitals, mobile devices) may store and process their own medical images and patient records and train models locally, using approaches such as Stochastic Gradient Descent (SGD), without having to transfer data out of the country and without violating HIPAA or GDPR as they keep data in the country. The main server (aggregator) will coordinate the global model training where it only receives model weights or gradients but not the raw data and it will train the global model through iterative aggregation, with the incorporation of privacy-preserving mechanisms such as differential privacy, secure multi-party computation. This is protecting privacy based on the communication protocol that enables securely communicating model updates, including such strategies like compression and federated averaging to maximize convergence, minimize latency, and bandwidth, and such enables effective privacy-preserving collaboration across institutions(Yang & Xing, 2024). The Figure 3 shows FL architecture showing local devices (clients) performing training on their data and sending model updates to a central server (aggregator) for secure aggregation and communication.

Figure 3. Architecture of Federated Learning

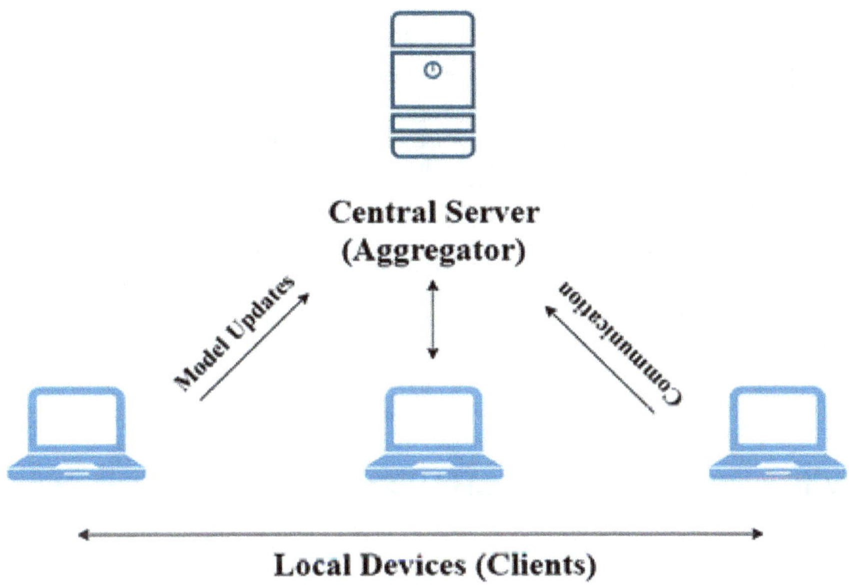

MODEL AGGREGATION TECHNIQUES (E.G., FEDAVG, FEDPROX)

FL entails model aggregation, the most commonly used are FedAvg and FedProx. FedAvg averages over all client model weights where each client has a different weight of their data size as the model weights are averaged after every local training epoch. It is practical and efficient when the data to be adopted are evenly dispersed, but it is not efficient when the data is Non-IID and it must be synchronized. FedProx can improve FedAvg with a proximal term that smooths out distinctions between local and global models to provide better stability against heterogeneous data and clients (Sadilek et al., 2021). FedProx is slightly more complex and has a computational overhead and does better with Non-IID data. FedAvg will experience better results by being simpler and faster but FedProx has a better chance in a more diversified environment as it has a more robust performance when the client data distributions and the computation levels are distributed (Xia et al., 2021). The Table 2 Comparison of popular FL aggregation techniques, outlining their working principles, advantages, and limitations in handling diverse data and client conditions.

Table 2. Federated Learning Aggregation Techniques

Method	How It Works	Advantages	Limitations
FedAvg	Clients train locally; server averages weights.	Simple, efficient, widely used.	Sensitive to Non-IID data; needs synchronization.
FedProx	Adds a proximal term to stabilize updates from diverse clients.	Handles Non-IID better; improves robustness.	Slightly more complex; requires tuning.
Scaffold	Uses control variates to correct client drift.	Faster convergence in Non-IID settings.	More communication overhead.
FedNova	Normalizes updates to account for different client contributions.	Fairness in update weighting; better performance.	May need fine-tuning and added complexity.

PRIVACY-PRESERVING MECHANISMS

Distribution of sensitive information needs privacy preserving mechanisms employed in Federated Learning (FL). Differential Privacy (DP) offers mathematical assurances that addition or removal of data of any single person will have no major impact on the outcomes of calculations. It introduces calibrated noise, be it central or local, to remove privacy at the cost of maybe compromising accuracy. Secure Multiparty Computation (SMPC) enables multiple parties to compute a function over distributed confidential data inputs without disclosing them and protocols include but are not limited to Shamir Secret Sharing, garbled circuits, and Homomorphic Encryption (Pfitzner et al., 2021). On the one hand, although SMPC furnishes sufficient security, it may be computationally extensive. The main distinction lies in the fact that DP masks how individual data points are represented in outputs whereas SMPC is able to perform computations with secure results without revealing the data. In FL, DP is perfect to mask model updates privately, and to prevent information leakage SMPC maintains protected cooperative computing. The combination of these mechanisms has the benefit of improving privacy, regulatory compliance, and trust and allows safe development of AI models across institutions without compromising confidentiality (Sadilek et al., 2020). The Table 3 shows the Summary of key privacy-preserving mechanisms in Federated Learning, highlighting their descriptions, advantages, and limitations in securing sensitive data during distributed model training.

Table 3. Privacy-Preserving Mechanisms in Federated Learning

Mechanism	Description	Advantages	Limitations
Differential Privacy (DP)	Adds statistical noise to protect individual data contributions.	Strong mathematical guarantees; widely adopted.	Reduced accuracy; complexity in noise calibration.
Secure Multiparty Computation (SMPC)	Enables computation across multiple parties without revealing private data.	No need to share raw data; strong privacy protection.	High computational and communication overhead.
Homomorphic Encryption	Allows computation on encrypted data without decryption.	Strong security; ideal for sensitive tasks.	Slow and resource-intensive.
Trusted Execution Environments (TEEs)	Isolates computations in secure hardware areas.	Fast, hardware-supported privacy.	Relies on secure, trusted hardware; not universally supported.

ADDRESSING DATA HETEROGENEITY AND MODEL CONVERGENCE CHALLENGES

Heterogeneity in data and convergence of models are serious challenges in federated learning because the clients possess different distributions of data, and thus the datasets may not be IID. These imbalances such as insufficient classes or unbalanced data types may slow performance of a model to generalize. To overcome the problem of heterogeneity, one may train individual models per client and achieve a better fit to local streams of data and still enjoy the global knowledge. Federated optimization methods have regularization, like in FedProx which aims at minimizing the influence of multiple data distributions, but data augmentation can be used to balance datasets and generalize better. The problem of model convergence occurs when conflicting updates among the clients are used which slows training or causes instability and there is variation of the computational power and network speeds. Adjusting learning rates depending on the performance, using weighted averaging that is proportionate to the contributions towards data, and finally using adaptive optimization techniques are some of the solutions. In combination, the techniques improve stability, efficiency, as well as the general performance of distributed machine learning systems (W. Li et al., 2019).

APPLICATIONS OF FEDERATED LEARNING IN MEDICAL IMAGING

Federated Learning (FL) suggests great potential in medical imaging as it makes it possible to train a distributed model without taking privacy away of the patient. Considering the sensitivity of the medical imaging data and differences in privacy policies, FL can be used to unite hospitals, research organizations, and healthcare organizations across the board in a HIPAA comprehensible way. It assists in joint model training, so, institutions with heterogeneous imaging data (X-rays, MRIs and CT scans) will be able to create AI models that generalize to both population and imaging modality. FL can increase disease detection and diagnosis of illness such as cancer, brain tumor, and cardiac illness through a collection of knowledge about these illnesses amongst various hospitals without the sharing of raw knowledge. It also presents the opportunity of making healthcare personalized based on targeted models to demographic specific characteristics of the patients, making the diagnostics more precise. In addition, FL promotes collaboration across the institutions building the shared knowledge systems that promote the faster development of diagnoses without compromising data confidentiality, and ultimately providing the safe and efficient route to medical imaging innovation(Rehman et al., 2023).

AI-SUPPORTED RADIOLOGY AND IMAGE ANALYSIS

An integrated collection of AI analytic tools helps doctors diagnose patients quickly and identify diseases before symptoms appear. Machine learning models use convolutional neural networks for X-ray, CT, MRI, and ultrasound image processing to diagnose medical images. AI-powered automated detection systems outperform radiologists in tumor, fracture, and lesion diagnosis. After simplifying administrative tasks, Artificial Intelligence (AI) has made radiologist examinations more trustworthy (Rehman et al., 2023). AI tools allow hospital personnel to authorize urgent medical situations while evaluating patients and extending direct patient care. Patients may be evaluated by clinical information systems because artificial systems match healthcare photos to illness development patterns. AI-based clinical applications help doctors discover cancer, cardiovascular disease, and neurological sickness early. Computer algorithms can detect stage I lung cancer in CT scans and early breast cancer in medical pictures. Technical capabilities in AI radiologic applications reduce occupational mistakes by offering exact findings that increase patient medical care systems.

PATHOLOGY AND DIGITAL BIOMARKERS

Pathology-analysed tissue testing and laboratory assessments influence medical judgments. Using digital pathology technology, doctors use AI algorithms to quantify invisible patterns on pathology slides. Digital pathology technologies that create illness and tumor grade data improve AI patient outcome prediction. Digital biomarkers process clinical diagnostic and molecular disease research at medical institutions to advance healthcare. AI-based disease detection models use biomarker assessments to identify early malignant tumors, neurological disorders, and inflammatory diseases in pathology slide data. AI tools help pathologists evaluate tissue structural patterns and cellular distribution data to make accurate medical decisions (Yaqoob et al., 2023). AI-based pathology systems employ disease progression data to provide prognostic information for pathologists to customize treatment. Diagnostic processes based on digital biomarkers enable doctors to pick medical treatments accurately. Diagnostic AI systems use digital biomarkers to avoid medical mistakes and deliver immediate tailored healthcare treatments.

PREDICTIVE ANALYTICS AND PERSONALIZED DIAGNOSTICS

Healthcare workers use present and historical medical forecasts to identify individuals who require preventative therapy early. Scientists can follow illness progressions, heart failure risks, diabetes hazards, and cancer risk using prediction algorithms on health data trends. Clinical models use EHR records, genetic test findings, and lifestyle patient data from numerous information sources to give customized health information. Mutation testing findings, tumor data, and patient medical profiles help doctors choose cancer therapies using predictive models. Heart disease risk assessments using blood pressure, cholesterol, and family health ancestry studies are provided by cardiovascular prediction models to detect early indicators of sickness. Data-based clinical solutions that help healthcare professionals change their direct medical operations are predictive analytics' major strength (Zhang et al., 2021). The healthcare method reduces costs and improves outcomes by preventing needless medical care. Medical professionals may utilize predictive analysis to diagnose illnesses early and create specific treatment plans and care strategies. AI system integration after medical research will improve predictive analytics and patient-specific treatment at healthcare organizations.

CHALLENGES IN FEDERATED LEARNING FOR MEDICAL DIAGNOSTICS

FL works as a medical diagnostic evolution which enables medical institutions to develop models from anonymous patient data. However, it presents several challenges. Operational success decreases because different medical facilities possess various equipment standards along with protocol systems spread throughout various demographic locations. The standard exchange of models between institutions and devices creates operational issues because these processes need rapid secure network elements. Model gradient security needs sufficient protections because attackers use these gradients during inference attacks to extract valuable information. The network contains varied systems which prevent utilizing similar models since each device operates with specific features.

Medical data interoperability levels decline because of standardization problems in medical data annotation and unconvincing specification formats. In decentralized systems the combination of real-time AI solutions with easily understandable models becomes more difficult to implement because healthcare experts must comprehend the AI-generated outputs (Liu et al., 2023). Performing distributed learning remains complicated because GDPR and HIPAA establish additional requirements that create deployment difficulties. FL systems face substantial data processing obstacles with large medical data quantities that require immediate healthcare functions. New methods that solve federal learning problems will lead healthcare sectors to accept this approach for precise diagnostic capabilities in private hospitals at all medical levels. The Table 4 shows the Key challenges in implementing Federated Learning for healthcare diagnostics, outlining their descriptions and the resulting impact on model performance, reliability, and regulatory compliance.

Table 4. Key Challenges in Federated Learning for Healthcare Diagnostics

Challenge	Description	Impact on FL
Communication Overhead	High bandwidth needs for frequent model updates.	Increases latency and slows training.
Data Heterogeneity	Non-IID data across institutions and equipment.	Affects model convergence and accuracy.
Annotation Inconsistencies	Varied labelling standards between hospitals.	Reduces model reliability and interpretability.

continued on following page

Table 4. Continued

Challenge	Description	Impact on FL
Model Convergence	Difficulty in synchronizing updates from varied devices.	Leads to unstable or biased global models.
Regulatory Barriers (HIPAA, GDPR)	Strict privacy laws add constraints.	Limits flexibility in system design and deployment.

COMMUNICATION OVERHEAD AND LATENCY ISSUES

The FL end device communication network offers active exchanges that update central server models and share data. Medical institutions require effective solutions to handle big diagnostic data transfers that disrupt huge diagnostic and model dataset processing. FL model operating phase demands high bandwidth, which disrupts performance in facilities with limited IT infrastructure to handle huge data transfers (Nazir & Kaleem, 2023). Predefined delivery times for key procedures impede emergency medical operations and need equipment improvements. Because hardware processing speed and network characteristics vary, clients operating at varying rates degrade the original model. Patient confidentiality methods that employ homomorphic encryption and differential privacy security techniques increase data packet size and execution times. Model compression and client selection are used to solve network problems using asynchronous update protocols. Healthcare networks interested in FL adoption face principal implementation barriers due to security and reliability norms, which need inferior communication system development.

HETEROGENEITY IN MEDICAL DATA AND LABELLING STANDARDS

Because clinical and hospital information systems are separated by data formatting and diagnostic standards, medical diagnostic institutions have severe operational issues. Medical data and EHRs have Non-IID status due to operational obstacles between independent hospital and clinic imaging equipment. Three constraints exist when illness labels from disparate systems mix with hospital medical imaging technologies owing to training-process incompatibility. Problems with data sample collections might make training tougher and produce mistakes during implementation (Rehman et al., 2023). Annotation creates varied data quality since expert-labelled dataset production demands significant human and financial commitment yet reduces model efficiency. Joining ontology standards with data standards increases generalization performance and system interoperability. Standardized data protocol formats and labelling allow analysts to examine these concerns using upgraded models with different input signals. FL applications' diagnostic accuracy relies on domain adaptation and transfer learning strategies to overcome data distribution variety.

MODEL CONVERGENCE AND PERFORMANCE CONSISTENCY

Federated learning relies on the tough challenge obtaining reliable medical data and model convergence. The diverging distribution of Non-IID features amongst local datasets and their varied quality levels makes model updates unstable. When various data sources are used to update healthcare models, precision, diagnostic accuracy, and performance times drop. System convergence is harder because system components have diverse computing capacities and engagement levels. Since model deployment systems serve vital healthcare services, hospitals must choose a reliable one that spans many client databases. Combining tailored federated learning techniques, weight-based aggregation, and adaptive system optimization algorithms yields three research solutions (Sandhu et al., 2023). As part of model stability augmentation, expert clinical evaluation and system-generated feedback collection of numerous datasets improve model reliability. FL implementing hospitals must pass stability checks via medical assessments since its team must verify diagnostic outcomes across all institutional regions.

STRATEGIES FOR OVERCOMING CHALLENGES

A combination of existing methodological approaches and partnership guidelines requires technical systems and must be used for efficient medical diagnostic systems that employ FL. The functionality of FL depends on recent hardware technology which integrates GPU accelerators to execute automated model compression techniques in restricted system environments. The quality of continuous diagnostic models improves as developers conduct patient-based record analyses through meta-learning procedures (Sohan & Basalamah, 2023). The model brings about incentive-driven update distribution through its plans yet needs financial backing as well as academic backing to support healthcare organizations in participating in privacy initiatives when healthcare competition is strong. The protected aggregation methods work in combination with differential privacy techniques to maintain privacy regulations through preventing unauthorized access to data. FL met its targets through partnerships with healthcare organizations that delivered precise and scalable solutions and sustainable ways to implement operational privacy measures compliant with all specifications.

HARDWARE OPTIMIZATIONS FOR EFFICIENT FL DEPLOYMENT

Successful Federated Learning for healthcare requires adequate hardware. Healthy machine learning model training demands a lot of computing resources, thus hospital devices and edge units processing it need performance improvements (Almeida & Beleg, 2025). GPU or TPU processing with edge computing reduces data transfer and improves operating system performance. Low-powered FL systems are standardized via Model Pruning, Quantization, and Sparsification. Sustainable equipment operation in underserved regions relies on energy-efficient hardware. After device implementations obey scheduling protocols and update mechanics, systems run faster since devices process independently according to programming. Cloud-edge hybrid integration improves distributed workload management for federated updates. To conduct fluid diagnostic procedures faster and at scale, real medical locations improve FL platform hardware.

PERSONALIZATION TECHNIQUES IN FL FOR BETTER ACCURACY

FL personalizes multiple healthcare operations through model integration between local institutional data and shared information from participating healthcare organizations. Video analytics within FL requires medical establishments to add their unique patient data to base-models for creating hybrid predictive solutions (Crabtree & Miele, 2022). The combination of cluster-based personalization and meta-learning with multi-task learning from Federated Learning helps healthcare facilities generate predictions relevant for different local medical practice groups. Multiple analytical methods unite to produce better and more relevant medical diagnoses for minority population conditions found in such datasets. Medical professionals begin using AI technology after discovering familiar clinical elements that exist in their operations because this approach allows for easy acceptance of the technology while improving system functionality. Medical facilities can reach their security goals and cost reduction objectives when they integrate transfer learning protocols with federated fine-tuning methods. FL model personalization allows the methods to detect changing contexts thus developing coordinated methods for delivering precise healthcare results and maintaining fairness in outcomes.

INCENTIVE MECHANISMS FOR INSTITUTIONAL PARTICIPATION

Healthcare institutions require dependable reasons to adopt FL because they worry about cost rises and legal penalties related to data exchange. Medical networks use purpose-designed incentive systems to motivate their retail facilities for joining health data contribution (Erel-Özçevik et al., 2024). The main advantages of data-sharing institutions consist of better global models and monetary funding together with authorship credit. The special blockchain architecture enables companies to track every blockchain record which proves member payment distributions remain fair. Healthcare facilities need benchmarking systems and skilled personnel with analytic models to gain worldwide non-financial advantages from their projects. The performance growth monitoring of institutional collaborative work becomes possible through visual analytics delivered across federated dashboards. Healthcare organizations together with other businesses under regulatory control show HIPAA and GDPR privacy standards compliance verification as their primary incentive (Goel, 2023). Hospital groups create extensive deployment plans to use advanced FL systems permanently.

REGULATORY AND ETHICAL CONSIDERATIONS

The operational requirements for medical diagnostic FL need both regulatory systems alongside ethical rules. The medical solution Flupyrimin follows GDPR guidelines as well as HIPAA privacy regulations and local privacy laws which protect healthcare data and maintain patient privacy. The Federated Learning system protects patient medical data privacy but simultaneously exposes their confidential information to unauthorized disclosure (Hirsch, 2019). To meet medical practitioner ethics standards and maintain equal patient treatment both systems must be equipped with human-readable programming and total programming transparency as well as unbiased programming. Every healthcare acquisition of medical operations needs complete consent documentation with independent responsibility systems which health providers must follow. FedLearn systems require medical systems to develop ethical standards and responsible technological solutions before deployment can occur.

COMPLIANCE WITH GDPR, HIPAA, AND OTHER DATA PROTECTION LAWS

FL manages healthcare data privacy well through previous healthcare systems but requires following privacy regulations from both European GDPR and American HIPAA standards at the same time. All patient information needs legal protection of confidentiality while users require official access to their protected medical data. FL protects data source processing through operational processes that control client updates to avoid unintentional disclosure of sensitive information. All protection prerequisites will be accomplished by integrating encryption protocols with secure multiparty computation systems and differential privacy management solutions that follow data governance guidelines (Kami et al., 2024). Organizations control all aspects of data permission policies and consent processes along with rules for international information movement. Preventive measures that stop violations focus on ethical data stewardship which requires attorney consultation combined with scheduled audit performances. Healthcare providers must fulfill regulatory requirements to make the AI diagnostic innovation framework and FL system operations both compliant with law and responsible for operations.

ETHICAL IMPLICATIONS OF FL IN MEDICAL DECISION-MAKING

The medical application of FL leads to multiple ethical issues involving patient selection rights and decision fairness and accountabilities and responsibilities. The combination of explainable and fair characteristics functions with unbiased features in medical decision support systems because FL models work as clinical decision advisors. Not all population groups avoid experiencing discriminatory behavior from models that result from widespread training across institutions (Le Quoc et al., 2019). When FL is applied it generates AI outputs that are unintelligible to clinicians who then are hesitant about trusting AI-generated decisions. For medical practitioners to obtain patient consent about data usage they must explain AI learning model development along with decentralized network operation mechanics. A precise healthcare accountability system needs clear structures of determination to determine specific diagnostic errors. The ethical design framework protects patient safety by stopping both automation risks in diagnosis tools and free usage of automatic diagnosis systems. Medical experts together with ethical staff members and patient organizations must join forces through federated learning systems development to satisfy necessary clinical and social requirements.

ENSURING TRANSPARENCY AND TRUST IN AI-DRIVEN DIAGNOSTICS

To apply Federated Learning systems in medical settings, healthcare organizations require defined protocols and user confidence. Patients only trust AI diagnostic tools when healthcare providers employ straightforward, accurate processes with fair execution. Users have issues since FL systems work independently to protect complex data. Developers expanding XAI systems make models more transparent by distributing operational information in a way that builds user confidence (Rajasegar R. S. et al., 2024). The public must obtain precise model performance information on patient groups, illness cases, and data sources. Testing systems with genuine clinical data and involving experts in medical research boosts model believability. Stakeholders are protected by clear data usage records, system model update reports, and privacy measures. FL-based diagnostics need technological disclosure, ethical approval, and clinical validation to be marketable and effective.

REAL-WORLD CASE STUDIES

FL technology shows highly promising results in clinical healthcare through its utilization in medical imaging together with diagnostic procedures. Through Federated Tumor Segmentation (FeTS) organizations learned brain tumor MRI models through collaborative training without requiring patient record exchanges (Roy et al., 2025). The research project demonstrated FL could improve model prediction precision together with its ability to operate within different clinical environments. Two healthcare organizations namely Owkin and NVIDIA have joined forces with medical institutions for implementing FL approaches to identify breast cancer and COVID-19 in imaging diagnostics.

FL demonstrates the ability to process extensive heterogeneous datasets without compromising confidentiality of patient information through these practical deployments. The research community explores FL technology to improve EHR predictive modelling because it enables the forecasting of treatment responses and patient outcomes. Real-world clinical tests conducted through joint research activities between academic institutions industry actors and healthcare organizations are proving that FL models work in practical healthcare settings (Gao et al., 2023). FL implementations now create the basis which enables healthcare institutions to adopt standardized FL practices on a larger scale.

SUCCESSFUL DEPLOYMENTS OF FL IN MEDICAL IMAGING

FL demonstrates unique value for medical imaging through its ability to unite hospitals and institutions for collaborative work while maintaining strict patient data confidentiality. The Federated Tumor Segmentation (FeTS) challenge demonstrates FL success by allowing multiple institutions to supply medical imaging data to develop models capable of tumor segmentation in MRI scans (Kairouz et al., 2021). The approach gave hospitals both data protection and access to the combined analytic potential of various datasets which produced a population-generalizing model. Within their partnership Owkin joined forces with NVIDIA to develop AI models for breast cancer detection which combined mammography images across various hospitals through the usage of FL techniques. FL managed to protect data privacy by spreading it among different sources but still achieved better diagnostic precision. FL shows practical value in developing explainable machine learning models which effectively scale while ensuring privacy protection thus establishing itself as an appealing method to enhance diagnostic accuracy of medical image evaluations. The Table 5 shows Examples of real-world Federated Learning projects in healthcare, highlighting their use cases, outcomes, and key advantages in enhancing diagnostics while preserving data privacy.

Table 5. Real-World Federated Learning Projects in Healthcare

Project/Partner	Use Case	Outcome	Key Advantage
FeTS Challenge	Federated brain tumor segmentation from MRI data.	High model performance across multi-site datasets.	Strong cross-institutional collaboration.
Owkin & NVIDIA	Breast cancer detection using mammograms.	Privacy-preserving model training across hospitals.	Enhanced diagnostic accuracy and trust.
Google Health + Ascension	Predictive analytics from EHRs.	FL allowed training without centralizing sensitive data.	High compliance with privacy laws.

CASE STUDY 1: FETS CHALLENGE – FEDERATED BRAIN TUMOR SEGMENTATION

FeTS Challenge is a ground-breaking undertaking that shows great promise of Federated Learning (FL) in healthcare imaging. The project saw the convergence of various healthcare facilities and research facilities where they can collaborate to train AI models on brain tumor segmentation based on MRI data without sharing raw patient information. In this way, HIPAA and GDPR regulations were fully complied with, and patient data privacy was kept at 100% during the process(W. Li et al., 2019). The institutional researchers also provided their own locally-derived datasets that were heterogeneous with respect to volume, imaging modalities, and patient characteristics, building an enriched and broad training set. Training was conducted at the local (on-site) model and just model updates were sent to a central aggregator and the global model improved. Such an approach helped to preclude the risks of data transfer and guarantee zero cases of data leakage in the course of the project(Xia et al., 2021). The global FL-trained model yielded remarkable results in the improved accuracy of segmentation whereby their average Dice Similarity Co-efficient (DSC) score was 89%, a result that surpassed more than a couple of centralized models that ran on smaller datasets. Additionally, the model had a 15 to 20% boost in generalization ability on un-seen datasets as compared to conventional single-institution models. There was also a high scalability together with teamwork advantages in the FeTS Challenge. There was a 30% faster incorporation of the model refinement due to cross-institutional coordination, whereby model robustness was observed regardless of the source of heterogeneous data. As a final contribution, the initiative demonstrated that FL can be used to provide high-performance AI models in amazingly complicated medical imaging functions, generating confidence, raising the intensity of diagnosis, and offering fastened research without jeopardizing the privacy of the patients. The Figure 4 illustrates percentage values for data privacy, segmentation accuracy, generalization improvement, and development time reduction, highlighting the effectiveness of FL in multi-institution medical imaging.

Figure 4. Key Performance Metrics of the FeTS Challenge in Federated Brain Tumor Segmentation

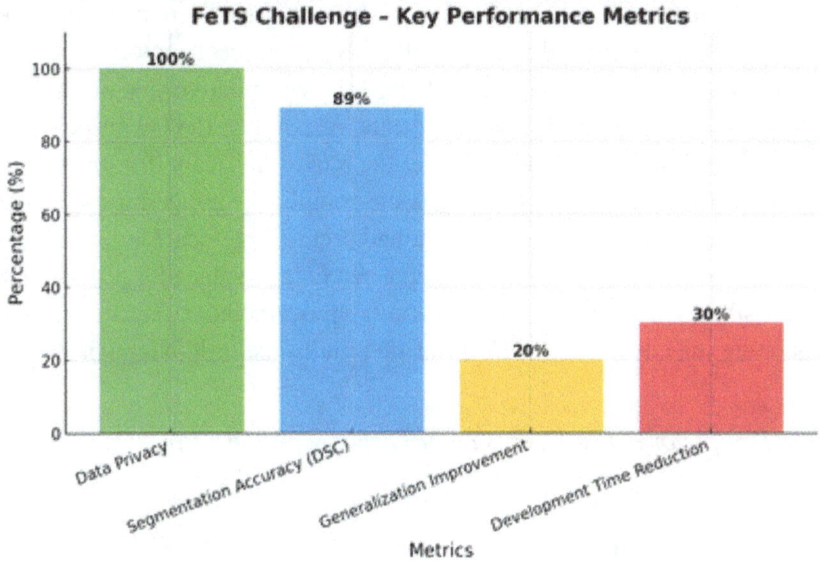

CASE STUDY 2: OWKIN & NVIDIA – PRIVACY-PRESERVING BREAST CANCER DETECTION

Owkin is a combined effort of NVIDIA with various hospitals to build their Federated Learning (FL) solution to detect breast cancer with the help of mammograms images. With this initiative, the goal was to achieve higher accuracy in diagnosing and keep sensitive medical images in the originating hospitals at the same time maintaining complete patient data privacy. The participating institutions trained local AI models using their own cliques of mammograms, and shared only model parameters with a central aggregator, to combine safely without ever sharing raw data this eliminated the sharing of raw data and allowed strictly controlled combinations without risking privacy violations. A conventional single-institution model recorded 92% classifications accuracy with the FL-trained world model improving the results by 12%. Besides, generalization of the model across the different demographic and imaging variations also increased by 18%, which strengthened its robustness in clinical practice. Utilization of NVIDIA optimized AI infrastructure provided a 25% improvement in computational latency to speed up the training of the models and their deployment without loss of operational speed. In addition to the technical benefits, the project has created good inter-institutional confidence, such that hospitals can collaborate well without legal and ethical dangers associated with sharing of information(Gao et al., 2023). This project was also notable in the sense that it demonstrated the capability of FL to democratise access to powerful healthcare AI tools by enabling even smaller establishments with relatively small datasets to take advantage of shared model enhancements. Altogether, the Owkin & NVIDIA partnership could be pointed out as one of the most significant demonstrations of how FL may bring more diagnostic accuracy, compliance concerning the existing regulations, including HIPAA and GDPR, and secure large-scale innovation in the sphere of medical AI. The Figure 5 presents percentage values for privacy preservation, classification accuracy, generalization improvement, and latency reduction, demonstrating the advantages of FL in secure, multi-institutional medical AI.

Figure 5. Key Performance Metrics of the Owkin & NVIDIA Breast Cancer Detection Project

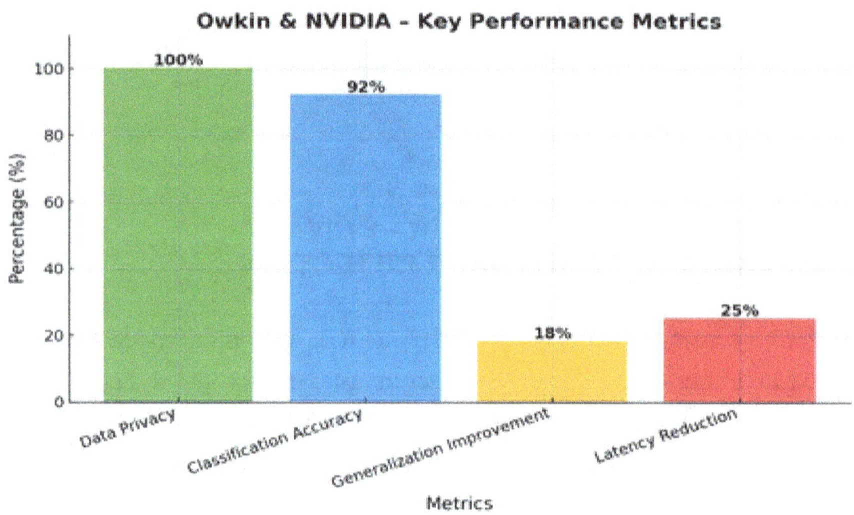

CASE STUDY 3: GOOGLE HEALTH & ASCENSION – PRIVACY-COMPLIANT PREDICTIVE ANALYTICS FROM EHRS

Google Health and Ascension came together to establish a Federated Learning (FL) method of predictive analytics based on Electronic Health Records (EHRs). The system made it feasible to train AI models on many different hospital locations without having to centralize sensitive patient information data to achieve 100% capability with HIPAA and other privacy laws. The models were trained at each institution and only encryption of model updates were shared to form a global update(Predictive, 2019). Such a solution removed the risks related to data transferring in raw form and enabled the model to receive a huge, heterogeneous data set. That is, the FL model improved prediction accuracy of the averted patient risk by 15% when compared to the isolated models. It has also demonstrated that 20% of the time spent on model development can be saved when using FL to build ML models and deploy them in the healthcare sector securely and compliant with regulatory guidelines(Almeida & Beleg, 2025). The Figure 6 highlights privacy compliance, prediction accuracy gains, and reduced development time, showcasing FL's effectiveness in secure, large-scale EHR-based predictive analytics.

Figure 6. Key Performance Metrics of the Google Health & Ascension Federated Learning Initiative

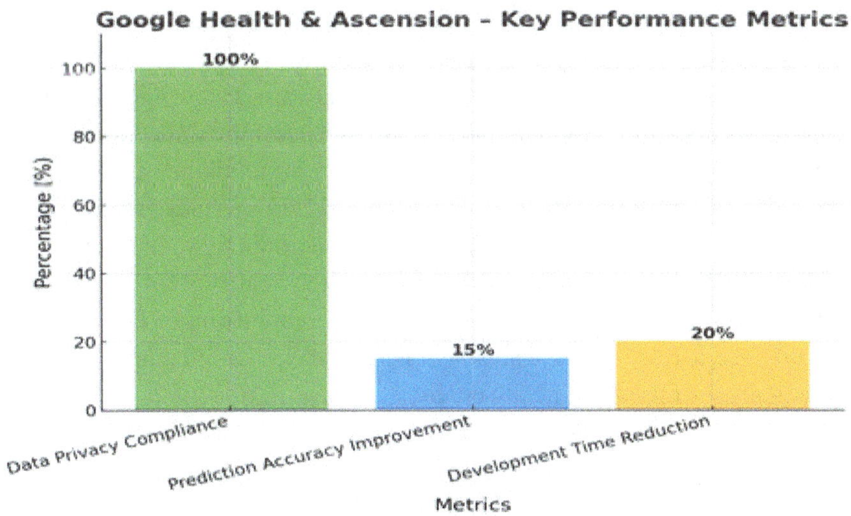

THE FUTURE OF FEDERATED LEARNING IN HEALTHCARE

Through FL healthcare professionals can attain exceptional capabilities to build key developments for clinical and diagnostic medical processes. The protected privacy protocols of digital healthcare tools function as FL systems which create an organization-wide data sharing platform (T. X. Nguyen et al., 2022). The FL system enables genomic medical research to create personalized medicine models which maintain patient data privacy when acquiring knowledge from various sources. Wearable technology working with remote health monitoring makes use of FL to process real-time patient health data which allows fast detection of heart diseases and diabetic conditions. The quantum blockchain approach improves both execution speed and digital security defense which safeguard FL operations from multiple security threats. The collaborative research capabilities of FL lower therapeutic drug development expenses and decrease vital periods needed for drug development. FL receives regulatory approval to expand medical care by creating AI models that secure telemedicine infrastructure and mental health services and diagnostic tools for worldwide patient assistance.

POTENTIAL INNOVATIONS AND RESEARCH DIRECTIONS

Healthcare organizations achieve profits through Federated Learning since the distributed model training method operates across multiple sites without breaking security safeguards that keep patient data protected (Silva et al., 2020). The development of defense systems for optimization procedures and algorithms to improve FL applications across multiple databases remains a necessary healthcare research task for innovation teams. Institution-based medical data diagnosis and disease prediction systems must study healthcare variance patterns as they execute compliance protocols. Future development cycles plan to introduce two medical features using FL applications which will provide personalized treatments to patients while offering full healthcare supervision services. The combination of FL technology and AI-utilizing IoT systems enables healthcare service development to achieve outstanding results for patient health quality.

INTEGRATION WITH QUANTUM COMPUTING AND BLOCKCHAIN FOR SECURITY

Federation Learning (FL) systems supplemented by quantum computing via blockchain management provide significant computational capabilities for enterprise-grade healthcare security. Quantum computers can handle various data sets to create complicated medical diagnostic systems and pharmaceutical research models due to their speed. Trace analysis between FL platforms and quantum algorithms helps health companies construct models from data gathering and manage medical records and genetic data (Wibawa et al., 2022). Blockchain technology mitigates security issues in distributed data sharing. Through record-based authentication, blockchain tracks data sharing transactions and prevents unwanted changes and access. As it pays contributors for their data, a smart contract-based blockchain resource sharing system automatically protects privacy. Users may access a secure decentralized learning framework with trust-based operating features using Quorum computing platforms and blockchain technology. Healthcare can improve data security and research protection for its analytical systems by combining blockchain and quantum computing.

EXPANDING FL BEYOND IMAGING: GENOMICS, WEARABLES, AND REMOTE MONITORING

FL will expand their genetic testing area and use wearable devices and remote patient clinical surveillance to provide tailored medicine therapies and continuing healthcare supervision. FL provides safe inner-network genetic data assessment for its member institutions using standard processes (Loftus et al., 2022). Genetic databases are accessible, so training procedures may find accurate medical therapies and innovative cancer cures without compromising patient privacy for excellent case management. FL analyses continuous healthcare data from health trackers and wearables on cardiac, diabetes, and psychological problems. Healthcare decentralization improves illness monitoring and medical care forecasting. FL-powered remote patient services help doctors enhance treatment outcomes by securely monitoring patient data. FL analysis provides patients with protected information and next-level health services via predictive and preventative treatment.

CONCLUSION

Federated Learning (FL) is changing the manner in which healthcare organizations share their machine learning processes that do not involve patient privacy. FL has the great advantage to decentralise the training of models across hospitals, research centres and other healthcare institutions, keeping sensitive medical data where it was created, rather than sending it to centralised training facilities thus meeting regulatory compliance needs, as well as concerns related to ethics. The paradigm is much safer in regard to data breaches, it enhances the idea of data sovereignty, and increases trust between stakeholders. The architecture and working principles of FL have been discussed in details. Local clients (hospitals or clinics) train on their own set of data and only share updates to their models never the raw patient data with a central aggregator. Procedures such as Federated Averaging (FedAvg) and Federated Proximal (FedProx) combine these updates into a global model, which allows high performance AI solutions, with privacy guarantees.

Moreover, data security can additionally be strengthened through privacy-preserving techniques that conceal the contribution of individuals, like Differential Privacy (DP) or allow secure collaborative computations, like Secure Multiparty Computation (SMPC). The uses of FL in healthcare are potential, and medical imaging has been proved to be one of the most influential ones. As it concerns cross-institutional cancer detection to brain tumor segmentation, FL can enable institutions to design diagnostic models together, which would be more accurate, inclusive, and generalizable. With different patient data on wider geographical and demographic lines, the FL models stand a better chance to identify rare conditions, accommodate different patient groups and enhance the results of their treatment. Even though there are these advantages, challenges exist. Model convergence and stability may be afflicted by the existence of data heterogeneity due to disparities in equipment, labeling convention and patient demographics.

The training process can be slowed by communication overhead and bandwidth limitations especially in large, collaborative efforts at training. Although regulatory compliance is part of the design of FL, it is nonetheless a limitation on both system pattern and method of deployment. In consideration of these challenges, customized models, superior optimization algorithms, and thoughtful ways of data enhancement have been ushered in. The innovations will be directed to the enhancement of convergence rates, robustness of the model, and general training efficiency within heterogeneous environments. The advantages of FL exemplify themselves through the case studies provided including the current FeTS Challenge, breast cancer detection project launched by Owkin and NVIDIA, and its collaboration with Google Health and Ascension. Such practical applications have demonstrated quantifiable increases in diagnostic accuracy, model generalization, and operating efficiency, and fully respect the privacy and data governance regulations.

In the future, FL integrated with other trending technologies, such as blockchain, quantum computers, and edge AI have a possibility to advance scalability, security, and performance even more. The further exploration of adaptive learning strategies, hybrid privacy-preserving approaches, and efficient communication protocols is the primary means toward enabling FL to show its complete potential in healthcare. Indicatively, Federated Learning is a privacy-aware collaborative learning framework that provides a strong healthcare AI architecture. With a combination of novelty and high levels of privacy protection, FL opens the path to the future in which the intertwining of medical research and clinical practice have become a reality, resulting in enhanced care of patients as well as faster medical progress.

REFERENCES

Almeida, D., & Beleg, J. (2025). Ethical implications of predictive analytics in personalized healthcare. In Navigating Privacy, Innovation, and Patient Empowerment Through Ethical Healthcare Technology (pp. 57–82). IGI Global. DOI: 10.4018/979-8-3693-7630-0.ch003

Alruwaili, M., Siddiqi, M. H., Idris, M., Alruwaili, S., Alanazi, A. S., & Khan, F. (2025). Advancing disability healthcare solutions through privacy-preserving federated learning with Theme framework. *Expert Systems: International Journal of Knowledge Engineering and Neural Networks*, *42*(1), e13807. Advance online publication. DOI: 10.1111/exsy.13807

Budrionis, A., Miara, M., Miara, P., Wilk, S., & Bellika, J. G. (2021). Benchmarking PySyft federated learning framework on MIMIC-III dataset. *IEEE Access : Practical Innovations, Open Solutions*, *9*, 116869–116878. DOI: 10.1109/ACCESS.2021.3105929

Chelani, N., Tripathy, S., Kumhar, M., Bhatia, J., Saxena, V., Tanwar, S., & Nayyar, A. (2024). Federated Learning for Internet of medical healthcare: Issues and challenges. *Scalable Computing Practice and Experience*, *25*(5), 4442–4455. DOI: 10.12694/scpe.v25i5.2905

Crabtree, J. S., & Miele, L. (2022). Precision diagnostics in cancer: Predict, prevent, and personalize. In Progress in Molecular Biology and Translational Science (pp. 39–56). Elsevier. DOI: 10.1016/bs.pmbts.2022.03.005

Erel-Özçevik, M., Özçift, A., Özçevik, Y., & Yücalar, F. (2024). A genetic optimized federated learning approach for joint consideration of end-to-end delay and data privacy in vehicular networks. *Electronics (Basel)*, *13*(21), 4261. DOI: 10.3390/electronics13214261

Gao, W., Wang, D., & Huang, Y. (2023). Designing a Deep Learning-Driven Resource-Efficient Diagnostic System for Metastatic Breast Cancer: Reducing Long Delays of Clinical Diagnosis and Improving Patient Survival in Developing Countries. *Cancer Informatics*, *22*, 11769351231214446. DOI: 10.1177/11769351231214446 PMID: 38033362

Goel, N. (2023). Leveraging analytics and Big Data for informed decision-making: A comprehensive review. *INTERANTIONAL JOURNAL OF SCIENTIFIC RESEARCH IN ENGINEERING AND MANAGEMENT*, *07*(10), 1–11. DOI: 10.55041/IJSREM25934

Hirsch, D. (2019). From individual control to social protection: New paradigms for privacy law in the age of predictive analytics. SSRN Electronic Journal. DOI: 10.2139/ssrn.3449112

Kairouz, P., McMahan, H. B., Avent, B., Bellet, A., Bennis, M., Nitin Bhagoji, A., Bonawitz, K., Charles, Z., Cormode, G., Cummings, R., D'Oliveira, R. G. L., Eichner, H., El Rouayheb, S., Evans, D., Gardner, J., Garrett, Z., Gascón, A., Ghazi, B., Gibbons, P. B., … Zhao, S. (2021). Advances and open problems in federated learning. Foundations and Trends® in Machine Learning, 14(1–2), 1–210. DOI: 10.1561/2200000083

Kami, M., Pourshahbaz, A., Rezaei, O., Keshavarz Akhlaghi, A. A., Banihashem, S., Dehghanizadeh, Z., Olamie Koopaie, M., & Nosratabadi, M. (2024). Clinical utility and diagnostic validity of the hierarchical taxonomy of psychopathology for borderline personality disorder. *Iranian Journal of Psychiatry and Behavioral Sciences, 18*(4). Advance online publication. DOI: 10.5812/ijpbs-143833

Le Quoc, D., Beck, M., Bhatotia, P., Chen, R., Fetzer, C., & Strufe, T. (2019). Privacy-Preserving Data Analytics. In Encyclopedia of Big Data Technologies (pp. 1292–1300). Springer International Publishing. DOI: 10.1007/978-3-319-77525-8_152

Li, L. (2024). Application of artificial intelligence-driven federated learning based on machine learning and deep learning in medicine. In *Artificial Intelligence*. IntechOpen., DOI: 10.5772/intechopen.1008185

Li, W., Milletarì, F., Xu, D., Rieke, N., Hancox, J., Zhu, W., Baust, M., Cheng, Y., Ourselin, S., Cardoso, M. J., & Feng, A. (2019). Privacy-preserving federated brain tumour segmentation. In *Lecture Notes in Computer Science* (pp. 133–141). Springer International Publishing., DOI: 10.1007/978-3-030-32692-0_16

Liu, W., Zhang, Y.-H., Li, Y.-F., & Zheng, D. (2023). A fine-grained medical data sharing scheme based on federated learning. *Concurrency and Computation, 35*(20), e6847. Advance online publication. DOI: 10.1002/cpe.6847

Loftus, T. J., Ruppert, M. M., Shickel, B., Ozrazgat-Baslanti, T., Balch, J. A., Efron, P. A., Upchurch, G. R.Jr, Rashidi, P., Tignanelli, C., Bian, J., & Bihorac, A. (2022). Federated learning for preserving data privacy in collaborative healthcare research. *Digital Health, 8*, 20552076221134456. DOI: 10.1177/20552076221134455 PMID: 36325438

Nazir, S., & Kaleem, M. (2023). Federated learning for medical image analysis with deep neural networks. *Diagnostics (Basel), 13*(9), 1532. Advance online publication. DOI: 10.3390/diagnostics13091532 PMID: 37174925

Nguyen, D. C., Pham, Q.-V., Pathirana, P. N., Ding, M., Seneviratne, A., Lin, Z., Dobre, O., & Hwang, W.-J. (2023a). Federated Learning for smart healthcare: A survey. *ACM Computing Surveys, 55*(3), 1–37. DOI: 10.1145/3501296

Nguyen, D. C., Pham, Q.-V., Pathirana, P. N., Ding, M., Seneviratne, A., Lin, Z., Dobre, O., & Hwang, W.-J. (2023b). Federated Learning for smart healthcare: A survey. *ACM Computing Surveys*, *55*(3), 1–37. DOI: 10.1145/3501296

Nguyen, T. X., Ran, A. R., Hu, X., Yang, D., Jiang, M., Dou, Q., & Cheung, C. Y. (2022). Federated learning in ocular imaging: Current progress and future direction. *Diagnostics (Basel)*, *12*(11), 2835. DOI: 10.3390/diagnostics12112835 PMID: 36428895

Pfitzner, B., Steckhan, N., & Arnrich, B. (2021). Federated learning in a medical context: A systematic literature review. *ACM Transactions on Internet Technology*, *21*(2), 1–31. DOI: 10.1145/3412357

Predictive Analytics: The privacy pickle. (2019). Institute for Operations Research and the Management Sciences (INFORMS). DOI: 10.1287/LYTX.2013.06.02

Rajasegar, R. S., Gouthaman, P., Ponnusamy, V., Arivazhagan, N., & Nallarasan, V. (2024). Data privacy and ethics in data analytics. In *Studies in Big Data* (pp. 195–213). Springer Nature Singapore., DOI: 10.1007/978-981-97-0448-4_10

Rehman, M. H. U., Hugo Lopez Pinaya, W., Nachev, P., Teo, J. T., Ourselin, S., & Cardoso, M. J. (2023). Federated learning for medical imaging radiology. *The British Journal of Radiology*, *96*(1150), 20220890. DOI: 10.1259/bjr.20220890 PMID: 38011227

Roy, P. D., Gupta Chowdhory, U., Dey, A., & Husain Sagor, D. (2025). AI and Machine Learning in Healthcare: Advancing Diagnostics, Personalized Treatment, and Predictive Modeling. *Preprints*. DOI: 10.20944/preprints202504.0007.v1

Sadilek, A., Liu, L., Nguyen, D., Kamruzzaman, M., Serghiou, S., Rader, B., Ingerman, A., Mellem, S., Kairouz, P., Nsoesie, E. O., MacFarlane, J., Vullikanti, A., Marathe, M., Eastham, P., Brownstein, J. S., Arcas, B. A. Y., Howell, M. D., & Hernandez, J. (2021a). Privacy-first health research with federated learning. *NPJ Digital Medicine*, *4*(1), 132. DOI: 10.1038/s41746-021-00489-2 PMID: 34493770

Sadilek, A., Liu, L., Nguyen, D., Kamruzzaman, M., Serghiou, S., Rader, B., Ingerman, A., Mellem, S., Kairouz, P., Nsoesie, E. O., MacFarlane, J., Vullikanti, A., Marathe, M., Eastham, P., Brownstein, J. S., Arcas, B. A. Y., Howell, M. D., & Hernandez, J. (2021b). Privacy-first health research with federated learning. *NPJ Digital Medicine*, *4*(1), 132. DOI: 10.1038/s41746-021-00489-2 PMID: 34493770

Sandhu, S. S., Gorji, H. T., Tavakolian, P., Tavakolian, K., & Akhbardeh, A. (2023). Medical imaging applications of Federated Learning. *Diagnostics (Basel), 13*(19), 3140. Advance online publication. DOI: 10.3390/diagnostics13193140 PMID: 37835883

Silva, S., Altmann, A., Gutman, B., & Lorenzi, M. (2020). Fed-BioMed: A general open-source frontend framework for federated learning in healthcare. In Domain Adaptation and Representation Transfer, and Distributed and Collaborative Learning (pp. 201–210). Springer International Publishing. DOI: 10.1007/978-3-030-60548-3_20

Sohan, M. F., & Basalamah, A. (2023). A systematic review on federated learning in medical image analysis. *IEEE Access : Practical Innovations, Open Solutions, 11*, 28628–28644. DOI: 10.1109/ACCESS.2023.3260027

Wibawa, F., Catak, F. O., Sarp, S., & Kuzlu, M. (2022). BFV-based homomorphic encryption for privacy-preserving CNN models. *Cryptography, 6*(3), 34. DOI: 10.3390/cryptography6030034

Xia, Y., Yang, D., Li, W., Myronenko, A., Xu, D., Obinata, H., Mori, H., An, P., & Harmon, S. Turkbey Evrim and Turkbey, B., Wood, B., Patella Francesca and Stellato, E., Carrafiello, G., Ierardi, A., Yuille, A., & Roth, H. (2021). Auto-FedAvg: Learnable federated averaging for multi-institutional medical image segmentation. https://doi.org//arXiv.2104.10195DOI: 10.48550

Xu, J., Glicksberg, B. S., Su, C., Walker, P., Bian, J., & Wang, F. (2021a). Federated learning for healthcare informatics. *Journal of Healthcare Informatics Research, 5*(1), 1–19. DOI: 10.1007/s41666-020-00082-4 PMID: 33204939

Xu, J., Glicksberg, B. S., Su, C., Walker, P., Bian, J., & Wang, F. (2021b). Federated learning for healthcare informatics. *Journal of Healthcare Informatics Research, 5*(1), 1–19. DOI: 10.1007/s41666-020-00082-4 PMID: 33204939

Yang, X., & Xing, C. (2024). Federated medical learning framework based on blockchain and homomorphic encryption. *Wireless Communications and Mobile Computing, 2024*, 1–15. DOI: 10.1155/2024/8138644

Yaqoob, M. M., Alsulami, M., Khan, M. A., Alsadie, D., Saudagar, A. K. J., AlKhathami, M., & Khattak, U. F. (2023). Symmetry in privacy-based healthcare: A review of skin cancer detection and classification using federated learning. *Symmetry, 15*(7), 1369. DOI: 10.3390/sym15071369

Zhang, T., Zhang, S., Chen, Z., & Liu, D. (2021). PMFL: Partial Meta-Federated Learning for heterogeneous tasks and its applications on real-world medical records.

KEY TERMS AND DEFINITIONS

Federated Learning (FL): A decentralized machine learning approach where models are trained across multiple devices or institutions without sharing raw data, preserving privacy.

Data Sovereignty: The principle that data is subject to the laws and governance of the country or region in which it is collected and stored.

HIPAA: The Health Insurance Portability and Accountability Act, a U.S. law ensuring the protection and confidential handling of health information.

GDPR: The General Data Protection Regulation, an EU law that governs data protection and privacy for individuals in the European Union.

Differential Privacy (DP): A technique that introduces statistical noise to data or outputs, ensuring individual data points cannot be re-identified.

Secure Multiparty Computation (SMPC): A cryptographic method enabling multiple parties to jointly compute a function without revealing their individual inputs.

FedAvg: A model aggregation algorithm in FL that averages model weights from participating clients based on their data size.

FedProx: An extension of FedAvg that introduces a proximal term to better handle heterogeneous data across clients.

Non-IID Data: Data that is not independently and identically distributed across clients, often causing challenges in model training.

Trusted Execution Environment (TEE): A secure hardware-based area for executing sensitive computations, protecting them from external interference.

Chapter 14
The Next Decade of Healthcare:
Federated Learning as the Cornerstone of Medical AI Evolution

Urvashi Sugandh
Bennett University, India

Krishna Kant Agrawal
Galgotias University, India

Parvesh Tanwar
Galgotias University, India

Arvind Panwar
https://orcid.org/0000-0001-9957-6365
Galgotias University, India

Sarita Yadav
Bharati Vidyapeeth's College of Engineering, India

Achin Jain
https://orcid.org/0000-0002-3968-4169
Bharati Vidyapeeth's College of Engineering, India

ABSTRACT

The progress of artificial intelligence (AI) in healthcare is significantly hindered by data privacy concerns, regulatory constraints, and fragmented data silos, which challenge traditional centralized training models. This chapter presents Federated Learning (FL) as a cornerstone technology for the next era of medical AI. FL is a decentralized paradigm that allows multiple institutions to collaboratively train robust models without sharing raw patient data, thereby preserving privacy by design. The chapter examines FL's core principles and architectures, contrasting them with the limitations of centralized AI. It showcases real-world applications in diagnostics, drug discovery, and genomics, while also addressing the technical

DOI: 10.4018/979-8-3373-3306-9.ch014

and operational hurdles, such as data heterogeneity and security. Looking forward, we explore the future trajectory of FL, including its synergy with other privacy-enhancing technologies, the rise of personalized models (pFL).

1. INTRODUCTION: THE DAWN OF A COLLABORATIVE AI ERA IN MEDICINE

1.1. The Unfulfilled Promise of AI in Healthcare

Artificial intelligence (AI) has been touted for some time as a game-changer for healthcare, offering the potential for breakthroughs in diagnostics, clinical decision support, personalized medicine, and population health management(Jain, Dubey, Khan, et al., 2025). However, with unprecedented strides in deep learning, natural language processing, and algorithmic innovation over the last decade, the field finds itself in a state of limbo: if technology has evolved to what we have today, why isn't AI achieving its potential in transforming healthcare delivery across the globe?

Several factors underpin this paradox. AI tools for diagnosis have, in controlled research studies on curated datasets, shown extremely high sensitivity and specificity(Solanki et al., 2025). These achievements have ignited an exciting investment boom, with global healthcare AI spending forecasted to top $120 billion by 2032. However, the translation from laboratory to the clinic has been "sluggish and haphazard," said Runowicz. According to one recent study, fewer than 20% of hospitals internationally use AI in their regular medical routines. Pilot projects in the early stages of innovation are no exception; they remain local and change the world in never-disruptive pockets(Jain, Dubey, Pan, et al., 2025).

Yet this disparity is not due to lack of technology or its application in health care; it is based upon the nature of health care. Challenges of AI adoption Diversity of patients, variability of clinical protocols and sensitive medical data make the adoption of AI difficult(Jain, Dubey, Gupta, et al., 2025). The industry faces not only technical and operational challenges, but also intractably entrenched questions about trust, equity and governance.

1.2. The Data Privacy and Silo Conundrum

At the heart of the slow pace of emergence are conflicting demands to exploit gargantuan stores of health care data and provide for the protection of patient privacy. The vast majority of high-performance AI algorithms, especially deep learning-based algorithms, are heavily dependent on large amounts of annotated medical data(L. Zhou et al., 2025). However, real-world health data continues to exist in silo at different institutions, in proprietary formats such as those in electronic health record (EHR) systems, radiology archives, and clinical research databases.

This fragmentation is further reinforced by strict privacy regulations such as HIPAA in the US and the GDPR in Europe that appropriately protect consumer rights but at the same time choke off cooperative innovation(Verma & Khari, 2024). Hospitals and other research facilities are skittish about sharing patient data with outside parties — even when it's been anonymized — for fear of potential legal consequences and damage to their reputations(Mehrotra et al., 2024). The outcome is rampant "data silos" that are constraining the volume and variety of information available to build AI model(Agarwal et al., 2024).

Further, current centralized AI methods rely on pooling data in one place which raises significant issue with respect to privacy rights, unauthorized access and ethical misuse. The value citizens place in digital health solutions rests on strong privacy safeguards- something further bolstered in the wake of major events in cybersecurity in recent years. The tension is how to harmonize the ai-driven promise of improvement with the bedrock need for patient privacy and human-data stewardship(Jain et al., 2023).

1.3. Federated Learning as the Foundational Solution

Amid this landscape, federated learning (FL) has gained momentum as a powerful paradigm by which to realize the "full promise of medical AI" in a privacy-respecting, institution-silo-counteracting way(Azrour et al., 2024). Unlike conventional methods, FL lets numerous healthcare entities collectively train AI models on disparate datasets — ensuring that sensitive patient data never leaves the system where it's kept(Jian et al., 2024).

Different from centralized learning systems, federated learning is about orchestrating a symphony of decentralized data exchanges, ensuring robust learning while protecting local autonomy and regulation(Agbley et al., 2024). FL not only alleviates the privacy issue by sharing the training process to many nodes, but also enhances generalizability, fairness and robustness against some specific attacks. It is transformative of the underlying philosophy of AI development: away from a centralised, extractive model towards a mode of participation, carried out in the spirit of privacy preservation(Sharma et al., 2025). Figure 1 shows how Federated learning transform healthcare.

Figure 1. Federated learning transform healthcare

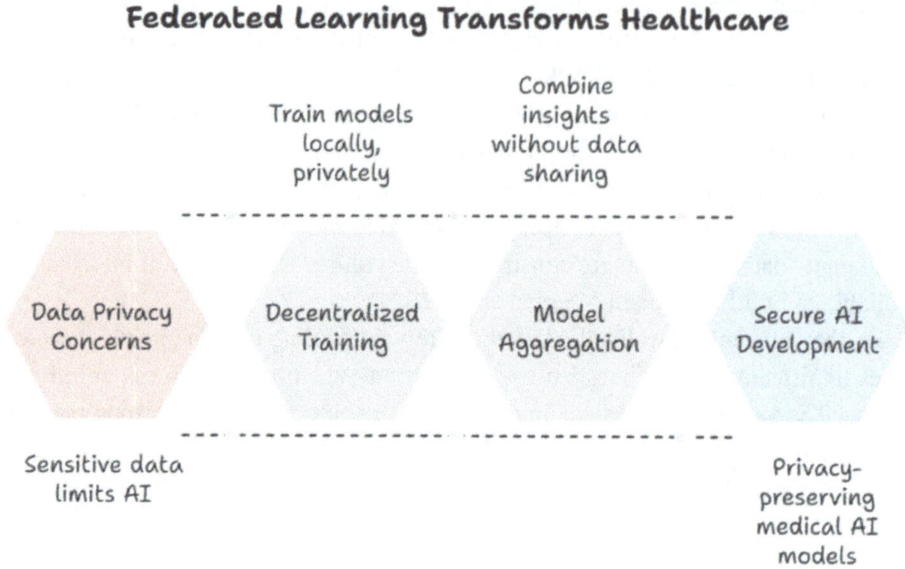

This chapter illustrates how federated learning will change the next decade of healthcare AI. In this context, we are all the more convinced that FL will play a central role to shape the development of medical AI in a time where collaboration, data security, and ethical rigour are central.

1.4. Chapter Roadmap and Objectives

To provide a clear picture of this novel paradigm, the chapter is organized in a considerate way. Section 2 discusses the drawbacks of centralized AI for healthcare, focusing on privacy issues, data silo, bias, and security problems. Section 3 then presents the core concepts behind federated learning, including its architectures, algorithms, and how this learning paradigm has introduced new solutions to tackle traditional problems. On top of this, in Section 4 we illustrate real-life scenarios, applications and case studies of federated learning in the main healthcare domains, proving the potential of the practice from diagnostics to population health. Section 5 details technical and deployment challenges with insights into active research trends and lessons learned to effectively realize federated learning. Finally, Section 6 also discusses the future of federated learning in healthcare and, in particular, opportunities for synergy with other privacy-enhancing technologies, and the roadmap for global adoption over the next decade. Lastly, Section 7 ties up the conclusions with a discussion of the results and reinforces the place of federated learning as the foundation of the progression of medical AI. At the end of each section a short summary leads into the next one, to maintain continuity and a logical progression, allowing for an unequivocal continuity through the chapter.

1.5. Summary: Setting the Stage for Paradigm Shift

This introductory section has framed the promise and limitations of AI in healthcare, emphasizing the critical impasse created by data privacy and institutional silos(Panwar et al., 2025). Federated learning emerges as a paradigm poised to resolve these challenges, setting the foundation for collaborative, secure, and effective medical AI. The next section will explore, in detail, why centralized AI approaches falter in healthcare—a necessary context for appreciating the revolutionary potential of FL(Haripriya et al., 2025).

2. THE IMPERATIVE FOR A PARADIGM SHIFT: LIMITATIONS OF CENTRALIZED AI IN HEALTHCARE

2.1. The Successes and Scaling Walls of Current Medical AI

The narrative of artificial intelligence in medicine is punctuated by significant, headline-grabbing successes. In radiology, deep learning models have demonstrated the ability to detect malignancies in mammograms, pathologies in retinal scans, and abnormalities in chest X-rays with accuracy that rivals, and sometimes exceeds, that of human experts(K et al., 2025). In pathology, AI algorithms can analyse gigapixel whole-slide images to identify cancerous tissues with remarkable precision, accelerating a traditionally labour-intensive process. These achievements, born from the centralized model of AI development, have been pivotal in proving the *potential* of machine intelligence in clinical contexts. They are the result of focused research efforts where large, well-annotated datasets were painstakingly collected and used to train sophisticated models in a controlled, centralized environment(Zhang et al., 2025).

However, such milestone victories often mask a more difficult truth: the wall of scale. The journey from a proof-of-concept model that works well on polished, controlled data to a real-world tool that works consistently across heterogeneous clinical environments is a strong impedance. A model trained on data from a single academic medical centre will likely have a severe performance drop when it is applied to a community hospital with diverse patient demographics, imaging devices, or clinical protocols(Nazir et al., 2025). This "lab-to-clinic" chasm illustrates an intrinsic limitation of the centralized model. It is great at solving tightly-formulated problems with great data, data for specific contexts, but is unable to produce generalisable, fair or scalable solutions unless for system-wide solutions in health system. The very model that brought these successes about -- the model of aggregating data into a single place -- is its biggest limitation.

2.2. The "Data-Hungry" Nature of Deep Learning vs. the Reality of Healthcare Data

Modern AI, particularly deep learning, is notoriously "data-hungry." The performance and robustness of these complex neural networks are directly proportional to the volume, variety, and quality of the data they are trained on(Y. Zhou et al., 2025). To develop an AI model capable of accurately diagnosing a rare disease, for instance, it requires exposure to a vast number of examples of that disease, along with a multitude of "normal" and other-pathology cases to learn from. This need for massive datasets is in direct conflict with the fragmented and protected nature of medical information.

The reality of healthcare data is one of scarcity and fragmentation. While the global volume of healthcare data is immense—estimated to be growing at a compound annual rate of 36%—it is not readily accessible. It is distributed across thousands of independent hospital networks, private clinics, research institutions, and national health systems, each with its own data infrastructure, standards, and governance policies(Kalpana et al., 2025). A single institution, even a large one, can rarely provide enough diverse data to train a model that is robust enough for widespread use. For example, training a model to detect a specific type of paediatric cancer may require data from dozens of specialized children's hospitals worldwide, as no single centre has a sufficient number of cases. The centralized model, which requires bringing all this data to one place, becomes logistically and legally untenable in such scenarios.

2.3. Core Challenges of the Centralized Model

The limitations of the centralized AI model in healthcare can be distilled into four interconnected challenges that form a systemic barrier to progress.

2.3.1. Data Governance, Privacy, and Regulatory Barriers (HIPAA, GDPR)

At the heart of these difficulties are a complex set of legal and ethical guidelines, among them patient's right to privacy. Laws like HIPAA (Health Insurance Portability and Accountability Act) in the US and the GDPR (General Data Protection Regulation) in EU have placed stringent restrictions on the utilization and transfer of Personal Health Information (PHI). While crucial for patient safety, those regulations translate into formidable barriers to the data pooling needed for the centralized model(Bhardwaj & Sumangali, 2025).

Obtaining the necessary clearances and patient consents to move data across institutional or international boundaries is a complex, time-consuming, and expensive process. Techniques like data de-identification or anonymization, while useful, are not foolproof. There remains a risk of re-identification, especially when linking datasets, which makes healthcare institutions highly risk-averse. GDPR, with its principle of "data minimization" and a data subject's "right to be forgotten," further complicates the creation of large, permanent data repositories for AI training(Ma et al., 2025). Consequently, the regulatory landscape, designed to protect individuals, inadvertently reinforces the very data silos that hinder the development of beneficial AI for the collective. Figure 2 shows the Core Challenges of the Centralized Model

Figure 2. Core Challenges of the Centralized Model

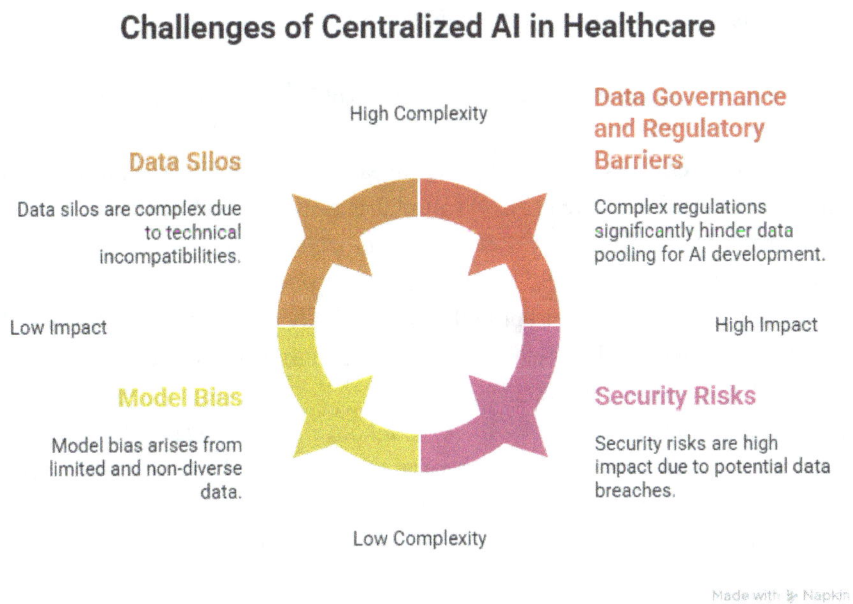

2.3.2. The Pervasiveness of Data Silos in Clinical Institutions

Beyond regulatory constraints, data silos are a natural and deeply entrenched feature of the healthcare ecosystem. They arise from a combination of factors:

- Competitive Interests: Healthcare institutions often view their clinical data as a strategic asset, providing a competitive advantage in research, clinical trials, and patient care. Sharing this asset can be perceived as diminishing its value(Alshareet & Awasthi, 2025).
- Technical Incompatibility: Hospitals use a wide array of Electronic Health Record (EHR) systems, Picture Archiving and Communication Systems (PACS), and other health IT infrastructure from different vendors. These systems often lack interoperability, using different data formats and standards, making data aggregation a technically daunting task(Li et al., 2025).
- Lack of Incentives: There is often no clear business or clinical incentive for a hospital to undertake the costly and risky process of sharing its data. The benefits of contributing to a larger data pool are often perceived as diffuse and long-term, while the costs and risks are immediate and concrete.

These silos lead to the development of AI models on small, institution-specific datasets, creating a landscape of fragmented, non-interoperable AI solutions that cannot be easily validated or adopted elsewhere.

2.3.3. Inherent Bias and Lack of Generalizability in Models

A direct consequence of training AI on siloed data is the creation of biased and non-generalizable models. An AI model is only as good as the data it learns from. If a model for detecting skin cancer is trained predominantly on images from light-skinned individuals, it will inevitably perform poorly and potentially produce harmful results when applied to individuals with darker skin tones. This is a well-documented failure that can perpetuate and even amplify existing health disparities(Choudhury et al., 2025).

Data silos exacerbate this problem. A model developed using data from one urban hospital may not be generalizable to a rural population, which may have different comorbidities, environmental exposure, and genetic background. Likewise, a model trained with images from an MRI machine of one manufacturer may not generalize when tested with images of another manufacturer's MRI machine. The centralized approach is inherently challenged when it comes to accessing a truly diverse range of data (across demographics, geographies, and devices) that is necessary to create AI that is not only robust but also equitable at scale. But the inability to generalize is not just a technical issue, it is also an ethical failing that undermines the applicability and reliability of medical AI(Yu et al., 2025).

2.3.4. Security Risks of Centralized Data Repositories

Finally, the centralized approach is a major cybersecurity weakness. We collect enormous quantities of sensitive patient data from various institutions and aggregate that data into large databases, granting attackers high-value targets, or "honey pots." Any compromise of such a repository would be catastrophic, with the prospect of millions of people's private medical details being put at risk(Shukla et al., 2025). The risks in terms of reputation, law, and currency of it all are too real for any institution who would like to contribute their datasets in a common pool. The risk, however, can never be eradicated even with the best security measures in place, and the risk of a single point of failure continues to be a bottleneck of the centralized architecture.

3. FEDERATED LEARNING: PRINCIPLES, ARCHITECTURES, AND A NEW COLLABORATIVE FRAMEWORK

3.1. Conceptual Framework: Training AI Models Without Moving Data

Having established the systemic limitations of centralized AI, the need for a fundamentally different approach becomes clear. Federated Learning (FL) provides this alternative by inverting the traditional data-aggregation model. Instead of moving vast and sensitive datasets to a central server for model training, FL brings the model training process to the data's source. This simple yet profound shift marks a new paradigm in collaborative machine learning, one that is particularly well-suited to the privacy-conscious and siloed environment of healthcare(Xing et al., 2025).

The conceptual framework of FL can be understood through an analogy. Imagine a consortium of expert radiologists from different hospitals aiming to develop a more accurate diagnostic protocol for a rare type of tumor. In the traditional, centralized approach, this would require collecting and sharing all patient scans at a central location a logistical and regulatory nightmare. In the federated approach, a general, initial protocol (the "global model") is sent to each radiologist. They each apply this protocol to their own local patient cases (training on "local data"), refine it based on their unique observations, and then send only their refinements not the patient scans themselves back to a coordinating body. This coordinator aggregates the insights from all participating radiologists to create an improved, more robust master protocol (the "updated global model"), which is then redistributed for the next round of refinement(Manocha et al., 2025).

This iterative cycle of local training and centralized aggregation of anonymized model updates (such as gradients or weights) allows the collective intelligence of the group to grow without any single radiologist ever having to share their confidential patient data. The core principle is “bringing the code to the data,” not the other way around. This enables knowledge to be extracted and shared in a secure, privacy-preserving manner, transforming isolated data silos into nodes in a collaborative learning network(Amin et al., 2025).

3.2. Core Architectural Models of Federated Learning

While the core principle remains consistent, FL can be implemented through several architectural models. The choice of architecture depends on the specific use case, the number of participants, and the level of trust between them. The two primary models are the client-server (or centralized) architecture and the peer-to-peer (or decentralized) architecture(Punitha & Preetha, 2025).

3.2.1. Client-Server Architecture (Centralized FL)

The client-server model is the most common and foundational architecture for federated learning, often referred to as centralized FL . It involves two main components: a central server (the coordinator) and multiple clients (e.g., hospitals, clinics, or research labs). The training process unfolds in a series of communication rounds, typically orchestrated as follows:

1. Initialization: The central server initializes a global AI model with a set of starting parameters and distributes it to a selection of participating clients.
2. Local Training: Each client trains the received model on its own private, local dataset. This training is performed for a set number of iterations, allowing the model to learn from the specific patterns present in that client's data.
3. Model Update Transmission: Upon completing the local training, each client sends its updated model parameters (e.g., the learned weights of the neural network) back to the central server. Critically, the raw data never leaves the client's secure environment.
4. Secure Aggregation: The central server aggregates the updates from all clients. It combines these individual updates, typically using a weighted averaging algorithm, to produce a single, improved global model that benefits from the collective knowledge of all participants.
5. Iteration: The server distributes this newly refined global model back to the clients, and the process repeats for multiple rounds until the model's performance converges or reaches a desired level of accuracy.

This architecture is powerful because it allows for the coordination of a large number of participants. However, it relies on a trusted central server to orchestrate the process and aggregate the model updates honestly. The central server represents a potential single point of failure and bottleneck, although it does not store the raw data itself. Figure 3 shows the Client-Server Architecture for Centralized FL

Figure 3. Shows the Client-Server Architecture for Centralized FL

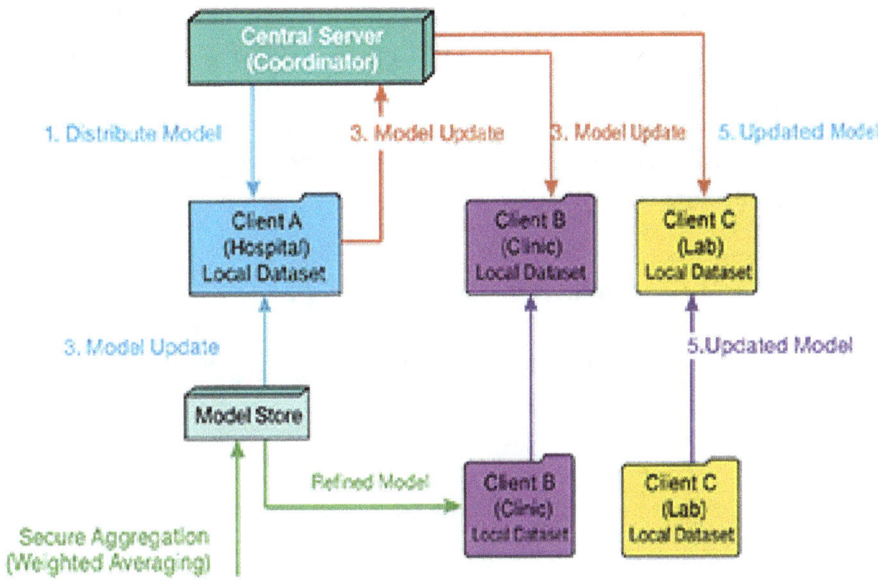

3.2.2. Peer-to-Peer Architecture (Decentralized FL)

In contrast to the client-server model, the peer-to-peer (P2P), or decentralized, architecture eliminates the need for a central coordinator. In this model, the clients (or "peers") communicate and share model updates directly with one another. The network topology can vary, but each client collaborates with a subset of other clients (its "neighbors").

The process in a decentralized FL system is more asynchronous:

1. Each client trains its model locally, similar to the centralized approach.
2. Instead of sending updates to a server, a client shares its updated model parameters directly with its neighbors in the network.

3. Each client is then responsible for aggregating the models received from its peers with its own local model to create an updated version.
4. This process of local training, sharing, and local aggregation propagates through the network, allowing a global consensus model to emerge organically over time without any central orchestration .

The primary advantage of the P2P architecture is its robustness. There is no single point of failure, making the system more resilient to server outages or attacks. It is particularly well-suited for scenarios where a natural trust hierarchy does not exist, such as collaborations between competing pharmaceutical companies. However, decentralized systems can be more complex to implement, may converge more slowly, and require more sophisticated communication and consensus protocols to ensure all clients eventually align on a consistent model. Figure 4 shows the Peer-to-Peer Architecture (Decentralized FL).

Figure 4. Peer-to-Peer Architecture (Decentralized FL)

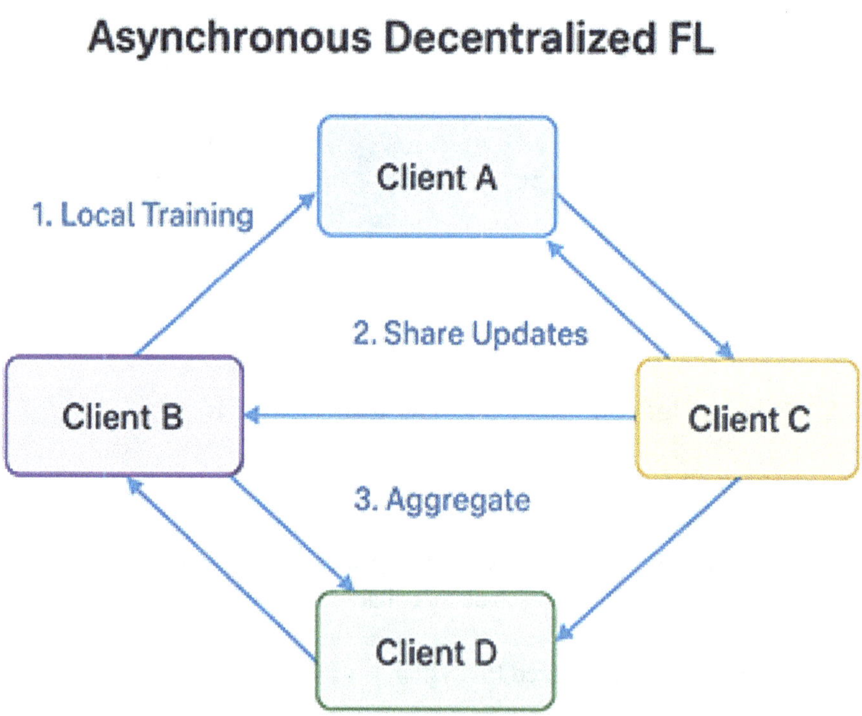

3.3. How FL Directly Addresses the Challenges of Centralized AI

The principles and architecture of federated learning provide direct and elegant solutions to the core challenges of the centralized model that were detailed in Section 2.

- Privacy and Regulation: FL's foundational promise is privacy-by-design. By ensuring raw data remains within the secure perimeter of the originating institution, it inherently complies with the spirit and letter of regulations like HIPAA and GDPR. Data transfer risks are minimized because only abstract model parameters, which are not considered protected health information, are exchanged(Wen et al., 2025).
- Data Silos: Rather than fighting to dismantle data silos, federated learning leverages them. It provides a robust technical and legal framework that allows institutions to collaborate and derive mutual benefit from their collective data without having to cede ownership, control, or competitive advantage. It turns a barrier into an asset.
- Bias and Generalizability: By enabling training across a wide consortium of institutions, FL allows models to learn from a far more diverse and representative patient population. The resulting global model is less susceptible to the biases inherent in a single-site dataset and is therefore more likely to generalize well across different demographics, geographies, and clinical settings, leading to more equitable and robust performance .
- Security: The federated model eliminates the high-stakes security risk of a centralized "honeypot" of patient data. While FL introduces new security considerations (which will be discussed in Section 5), it fundamentally decentralizes the risk. A breach at one client institution would not compromise the data of the entire network, making the overall system far more secure against catastrophic data loss .

3.4. Section Summary and Transition

This section has detailed the core tenets of federated learning, moving from its conceptual framework to its primary architectural models and foundational algorithms. We have established FL as a paradigm that trains AI by bringing the model to the data, thereby preserving privacy and working with, rather than against, the siloed nature of healthcare. The client-server and peer-to-peer architectures provide flexible frameworks for collaboration, while algorithms like FedAvg and FedProx provide the mathematical machinery to make this collaboration effective, even in the face of heterogeneous data. Most importantly, we have shown how this approach directly counters the primary limitations privacy, silos, bias, and security that have stalled the progress of centralized AI.

With this theoretical and architectural foundation laid, the discussion can now shift from the abstract to the concrete. Having understood *how* federated learning works, the next section will explore *where* it is working. We will examine real-world applications and case studies across key healthcare verticals, demonstrating the tangible impact that FL is already beginning to make in diagnostics, drug discovery, and beyond.

4. REAL-WORLD APPLICATIONS: FEDERATED LEARNING TRANSFORMING HEALTHCARE VERTICALS

The theoretical elegance of Federated Learning (FL) finds its ultimate validation in its practical application. Moving beyond conceptual frameworks, FL is actively being deployed across a spectrum of healthcare domains to solve tangible, high-stakes problems. By enabling collaboration among institutions that were previously isolated by privacy concerns, competitive interests, and regulatory barriers, federated learning is beginning to deliver on the long-standing promise of AI in medicine. This section showcases real-world examples and landmark case studies where FL is serving as the enabling technology for a new generation of medical intelligence(Ghadi et al., 2025).

4.1. Medical Imaging and Radiology: Enhancing Diagnostics Across Hospitals

Medical imaging is arguably the most mature domain for AI in healthcare, and it has become a fertile ground for federated learning. The reasons are twofold: imaging datasets are massive in size, making them difficult and costly to centralize, and they contain highly sensitive patient information. FL provides a natural solution to train robust diagnostic models across multiple hospitals without moving a single pixel of data(Shi et al., 2025).

A prominent example is the development of AI models for brain tumor segmentation. The task requires delineating the boundaries of a tumor from MRI scans, a critical step for surgical planning and radiation therapy. To train a highly accurate model, a vast and diverse set of scans from different patients, scanners, and hospitals is required. In a landmark study, a federated learning network spanning 20 institutions across the globe was used to train a brain tumor segmentation model. The resulting federated model significantly outperformed models trained on data from any single institution, demonstrating the power of collaboration in achieving state-of-the-art performance(Almogadwy & Alqarafi, 2025). The model learned to generalize across variations in imaging protocols and patient populations, a feat unattainable within a single data silo.

- *Case Study: NVIDIA FLARE (Federated Learning Application Runtime Environment)*

NVIDIA, a leader in AI computing, has heavily invested in enabling federated learning for healthcare through its open-source platform, NVIDIA FLARE . FLARE is not just a research tool but a production-ready system designed to make FL accessible and deployable for clinical institutions. It provides the underlying infrastructure for secure, multi-party collaboration, handling everything from secure communication to model aggregation and workflow orchestration. A notable application powered by FLARE is the EXAM (EMR CXR AI Model) project, a collaboration with Mass General Brigham. This initiative used FL to train a model on chest X-rays and electronic health record data to predict the future oxygen requirements of patients presenting with COVID-19 symptoms. By training the model across multiple hospitals, it achieved a high level of accuracy and robustness, providing clinicians with a valuable tool for patient triage and resource management during the pandemic, all while ensuring patient data remained securely within each hospital's firewall .

4.2. Genomics and Precision Medicine: Collaborative Research on Sensitive Genetic Data

Genomic data represents the blueprint of an individual's health and is perhaps the most sensitive form of personal information. The potential for AI to mine this data for insights into disease predisposition, drug response, and personalized therapies is immense. However, the risk of re-identification from genetic data is extremely high, making data sharing for research almost impossible under regulations like GDPR and HIPAA(Agbley et al., 2024).

Federated learning is breaking this deadlock. Researchers are now using FL to conduct Genome-Wide Association Studies (GWAS) across distributed datasets. In a traditional GWAS, the genomes of thousands of individuals are analyzed to find genetic variations associated with a particular disease. Using FL, multiple research centers can collaboratively perform these analyses without sharing any raw genetic sequences. Each site calculates summary statistics locally, and only these anonymized statistics are aggregated to identify significant genetic markers(Chen et al., 2024). This federated approach has been shown to produce results nearly identical to those from a centralized analysis, but without the immense privacy risks, opening the door for large-scale, international collaborations on a previously unimaginable scale .

4.3. Drug Discovery and Development: Accelerating Pharmaceutical R&D

The pharmaceutical industry is intensely competitive, with each company's chemical compound libraries and associated experimental data representing billions of dollars in research investment. This competitive landscape has historically prevented the kind of large-scale data sharing that could accelerate the discovery of new medicines. Federated learning offers a pre-competitive framework for collaboration, allowing companies to pool their collective knowledge without revealing their proprietary assets.

- *Case Study: The MELLODDY Drug Discovery Consortium*

The MELLODDY (Machine Learning Ledger Orchestration for Drug Discovery) project stands as one of the most ambitious demonstrations of federated learning to date. This three-year, €18 million public-private partnership involved 10 major pharmaceutical companies (including Amgen, Novartis, and Johnson & Johnson), several academic institutions, and tech startups . The goal was to train a multi-task predictive model on the combined chemical libraries of all participating pharma partners to better predict a compound's properties. Using a sophisticated FL platform, the partners collaboratively trained a model on a dataset of over 1.4 billion data points associated with millions of chemical compounds, one of the largest federated learning undertakings ever . The final "MELLODDY model" was proven to be more accurate than any model the companies could have trained on their own. This groundbreaking project demonstrated that even fierce competitors can collaborate to create a shared asset that benefits all, without any company having to expose its valuable proprietary compounds to others .

4.4. Smart Hospitals and IoT: Real-time Insights from Connected Devices

Modern hospitals are becoming increasingly instrumented, with a vast Internet of Things (IoT) ecosystem of bedside monitors, infusion pumps, ventilators, and wearable sensors generating a continuous stream of physiological data. This data holds the key to real-time predictive analytics, such as early warning systems for patient deterioration, sepsis onset, or cardiac events(Muhammed et al., 2024).

Centralizing this high-velocity, high-volume data stream for model training is often impractical due to bandwidth limitations and the need for low-latency predictions. Federated learning, particularly when combined with edge computing, offers an elegant solution. Models can be trained directly on hospital servers or even on the devices themselves. For example, a federated network could connect the ICUs of several hospitals to train a sepsis prediction model. Each hospital's model would learn from its local patient data streams, and the aggregated global model would benefit from the diverse clinical scenarios across the network, leading to a more robust and accurate early warning system. This approach allows for continuous model improvement in real-time without overwhelming network infrastructure or compromising patient data privacy(Barnawi et al., 2024).

5. NAVIGATING THE LABYRINTH: TECHNICAL AND IMPLEMENTATION HURDLES FOR FL IN HEALTHCARE

While the previous section highlighted the transformative potential of Federated Learning, the journey from a promising concept to a robust, scalable, and trustworthy healthcare infrastructure is fraught with challenges. The successful deployment of FL is not merely a matter of adopting a new algorithm; it requires overcoming significant technical hurdles inherent to distributed systems and navigating a complex landscape of operational, economic, and ethical considerations. This section delves into this labyrinth, systematically examining the key challenges and the emerging strategies being developed to mitigate them.

5.1. Technical Challenges and Mitigation Strategies

The core technical difficulties in federated learning stem from the inherent unpredictability and variability of real-world, decentralized environments. The data is not clean and uniform, the computing resources are not identical, and the communication channels are not perfect.

5.1.1. Addressing Statistical Heterogeneity (Non-IID Data)

Perhaps the most studied technical challenge in FL is statistical heterogeneity, which arises when the data distributions across clients are Not Independent and Identically Distributed (Non-IID) . In healthcare, this is the norm, not the exception. A model trained on data from one hospital's MRI scanner may not perform well on images from another manufacturer's machine. A community hospital's patient demographics (age, ethnicity, comorbidities) can differ vastly from those of a specialized urban cancer center. This heterogeneity can cause the local models trained at each client to diverge significantly, leading to slow, unstable, or even non-convergent training of the global model .

Mitigation Strategies:

- Advanced Aggregation Algorithms: Moving beyond the simple FedAvg, algorithms like FedProx introduce a proximal term that regularizes local updates, preventing them from straying too far from the global model and thereby ensuring more stable convergence . Other methods focus on robust aggregation, where the central server identifies and down-weights outlier updates that could destabilize the global model.
- Personalized Federated Learning (pFL): A growing consensus suggests that a single global model may not be optimal for every participating institution. pFL is an emerging branch of federated learning that aims to create customized models for each client . While still benefiting from the collective knowledge of the network, each hospital ends up with a model that is fine-tuned to its specific data distribution and patient population. This is achieved through techniques like model interpolation (mixing the global model with the local model) or meta-learning approaches.

5.1.2. Managing Systems Heterogeneity and Resource Constraints

Systems heterogeneity refers to the wide variability in the hardware (CPU, GPU, memory), network connectivity (bandwidth, latency), and power availability of the participating clients . In a healthcare federation, a large, well-funded research hospital may have dedicated servers with powerful GPUs, while a smaller, rural clinic might only have modest computational resources. This disparity means that some clients will be much slower at training their local models ("stragglers"), which can significantly slow down the entire synchronous training process, as the central server must wait for the slowest client in each round. Figure 5 shows the Technical Challenges and Mitigation Strategies

Mitigation Strategies:

- Asynchronous FL Protocols: Instead of waiting for all clients to report back in a given round, asynchronous protocols allow the server to update the global model as soon as it receives a certain number of client updates. This prevents stragglers from becoming a bottleneck for the entire network.
- Client Selection and Resource-Aware FL: The central server can be designed to be more intelligent about which clients it includes in each training round. It can prioritize clients with sufficient computational resources or adapt the complexity of the training task (e.g., number of local epochs) based on each client's reported capabilities, ensuring a more efficient and balanced training process.

Figure 5. Technical Challenges and Mitigation Strategies

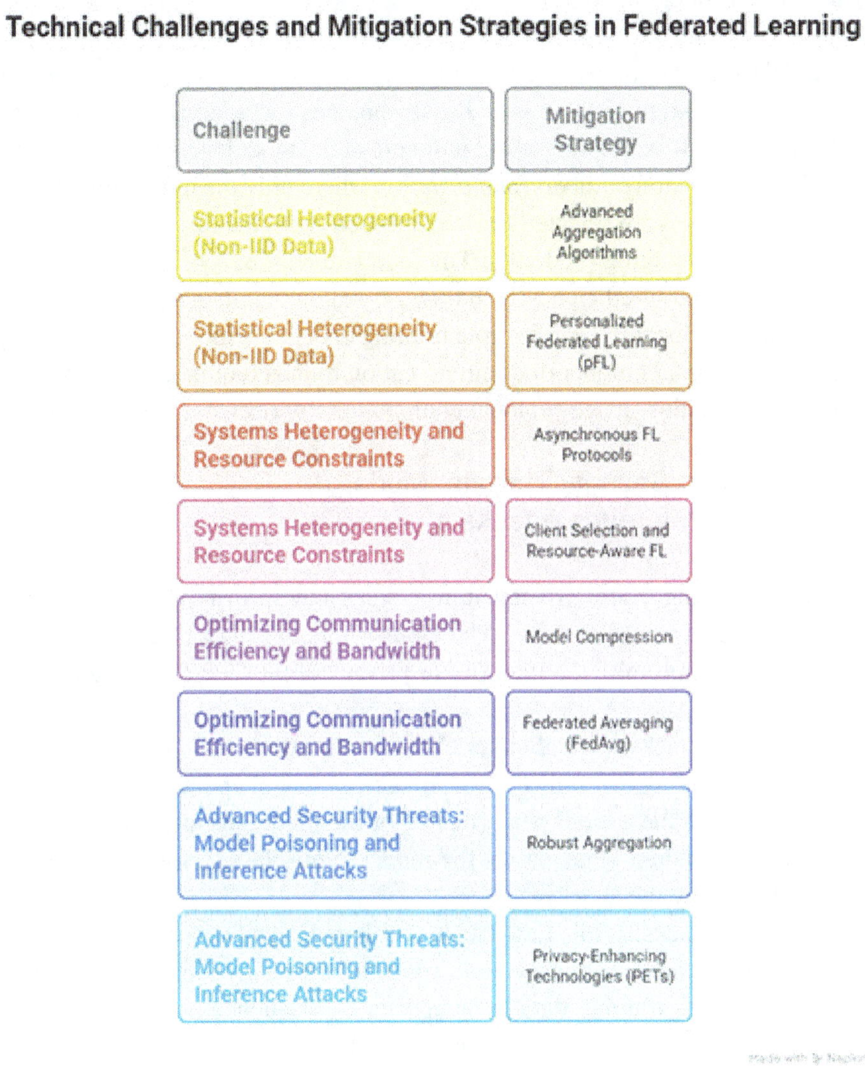

5.1.3. Optimizing Communication Efficiency and Bandwidth

In large-scale federated networks, especially those involving complex deep learning models with millions of parameters, communication can become the primary bottleneck. Transmitting these large model updates from hundreds or thousands of clients to a central server in every round can be prohibitively slow and expensive, particularly over limited or unreliable network connections(Li et al., 2024).

Mitigation Strategies:

- Model Compression: Before transmitting the model updates, clients can compress them to reduce their size. Key techniques include *quantization*, where the high-precision floating-point numbers of the model weights are converted to lower-precision numbers, and *pruning*, where only the most significant parameter updates are selected for transmission, with the rest being set to zero.
- Federated Averaging (FedAvg): The foundational FedAvg algorithm itself is a communication-efficiency technique. By allowing clients to perform more computation locally (i.e., multiple training epochs) before communicating, it reduces the total number of communication rounds required for the model to converge, trading increased local computation for decreased communication.

5.1.4. Advanced Security Threats: Model Poisoning and Inference Attacks

While FL is designed for privacy, it introduces new security vulnerabilities that do not exist in centralized systems. Malicious actors, posing as legitimate clients, can attempt to compromise the integrity or privacy of the federated system.

- Poisoning Attacks: A malicious client could attempt to poison the global model by sending carefully crafted, malicious model updates. The goal could be to degrade the overall performance of the model or, more insidiously, to create a "backdoor" that causes the model to misclassify specific inputs in a way desired by the attacker.
- Inference Attacks: While raw data is not shared, an adversary (either the central server or another client) could try to infer sensitive information about a client's private training data by analysing the sequence of model updates it sends. For example, they might be able to deduce whether a specific individual's data was used in the training process (a membership inference attack).

Mitigation Strategies:

- Robust Aggregation: The server can use aggregation rules that are robust to a certain percentage of malicious clients. For example, instead of a simple average, it could use algorithms that compute a geometric median of the updates, which is less sensitive to outliers.

- Privacy-Enhancing Technologies (PETs): To defend against inference attacks, FL can be combined with other PETs. *Differential Privacy* involves adding carefully calibrated statistical noise to the model updates before they are shared, providing mathematical guarantees that the presence of any single individual in the dataset cannot be determined. *Secure Multi-Party Computation (SMPC)* and *Homomorphic Encryption* are cryptographic techniques that allow the server to perform the aggregation computation on encrypted model updates, meaning the server never sees the individual client updates in plaintext.

5.2. Implementation and Operational Challenges

Beyond the purely technical aspects, building a successful federated learning ecosystem requires surmounting significant operational, economic, and governance hurdles.

5.2.1. Establishing Trust, Governance, and Consortium Models

Before a single line of code is written, a foundation of trust and a clear governance structure must be established among the participating institutions. Who owns the final, collaboratively trained model? Who is liable if the model produces an erroneous diagnostic and causes patient harm? How are new members admitted to the consortium, and under what conditions? These questions require the development of comprehensive legal frameworks and consortium agreements that clearly define data usage rights, intellectual property ownership, and liability. The MELLODDY project, for example, required extensive legal work to create a trusted framework that protected the proprietary interests of all 10 competing pharmaceutical partners.

5.2.2. The Economics of Federated Learning: Costs and Incentives

Participation in a federated network is not free. It requires computational resources, network bandwidth, and the time of skilled IT staff and data scientists at each client institution. A critical challenge is designing an economic model that provides clear incentives for organizations to join and contribute their data and resources. Incentives can be direct, such as payments for participation, or indirect, such as gaining access to a superior, collaboratively trained AI model that an institution could not develop on its own. For FL to be sustainable, the perceived benefits of participation must outweigh the costs.

5.2.3. Interoperability and Standardization Across Health Systems

Federated learning works best when the data across clients, while heterogeneous, adheres to a common structure and vocabulary. However, healthcare data is notoriously non-standardized. Different hospitals use different EHR vendors, coding systems (e.g., ICD-9 vs. ICD-10), and local terminologies. Before FL can even begin, a significant data harmonization effort is often required. This involves mapping local data representations to a Common Data Model (CDM), such as the Observational Medical Outcomes Partnership (OMOP) CDM. This preprocessing step is labour-intensive and requires deep domain expertise, representing a major upfront investment for any institution wishing to join a federated network.

5.2.4. The Evolving Regulatory and Ethical Landscape

While FL is a powerful tool for privacy, it does not provide a "get out of jail free" card for regulatory compliance. The legal landscape is still catching up with this technology. Under GDPR, for instance, there can be ambiguity about who is the "data controller" and who is the "data processor" in a federated network, with implications for legal responsibility. Furthermore, ethical questions remain. How do we ensure that the benefits of federated learning are distributed equitably? How do we handle a patient's "right to be forgotten" in a system where their data has influenced a global model that is now deployed across dozens of hospitals? Navigating this evolving regulatory and ethical terrain requires ongoing dialogue between technologists, ethicists, legal experts, and policymakers.

6. THE NEXT DECADE: THE FUTURE TRAJECTORY OF FEDERATED LEARNING IN MEDICINE

Having navigated the complexities and challenges of implementing Federated Learning (FL), the focus now shifts to the horizon. The ongoing research and innovation aimed at overcoming FL's current limitations are not merely incremental; they are paving the way for a more powerful, secure, and intelligent iteration of collaborative AI. Over the next decade, FL is poised to evolve from a specialized technique for privacy-preserving machine learning into a foundational component of a global, interconnected digital health ecosystem. This evolution will be driven by powerful synergies with other technologies, a shift towards personalization, and a deeper integration with the principles of responsible AI.

6.1. Synergies with Other Privacy-Enhancing Technologies (PETs)

Federated learning, while a powerful tool for privacy, is not a silver bullet. Its privacy protections primarily guard against the direct leakage of raw data. As discussed in the previous section, sophisticated inference attacks can still potentially extract sensitive information from the shared model updates. The future of secure medical AI, therefore, lies not in FL alone, but in its strategic combination with a suite of other Privacy-Enhancing Technologies (PETs), creating a multi-layered "defense-in-depth" strategy for data protection.

6.1.1. FL with Differential Privacy

Differential Privacy (DP) offers a mathematically rigorous definition of privacy. It ensures that the output of a computation (e.g., an aggregated model update) is statistically indistinguishable whether any single individual's data is included in the input dataset or not . When integrated with FL, DP is typically applied at the client level. Before a hospital sends its model update to the central server, it injects a carefully calibrated amount of statistical noise. This noise is just large enough to mask the contribution of any single patient, thus providing a strong, provable guarantee against membership inference attacks. The future will see the development of more sophisticated DP mechanisms that optimize the trade-off between privacy protection and model accuracy, allowing for strong guarantees with minimal impact on performance.

6.1.2. FL with Homomorphic Encryption

Homomorphic Encryption (HE) is a revolutionary form of cryptography that allows computations to be performed directly on encrypted data without ever decrypting it . In the context of FL, clients can encrypt their model updates before sending them to the central server. The server can then aggregate these encrypted updates into an encrypted global model. This is a paradigm shift for trust: it makes the central server's role purely computational, eliminating the need for it to be a trusted entity, as it never has access to the model updates in their plaintext form. While currently very computationally expensive, rapid advances in HE algorithms and hardware acceleration over the next decade are expected to make it a practical and powerful tool for securing federated networks, especially in high-stakes commercial or competitive collaborations.

6.1.3. FL with Secure Multi-Party Computation (SMPC)

Secure Multi-Party Computation (SMPC) is another cryptographic protocol that allows multiple parties to jointly compute a function over their inputs while keeping those inputs private. In the context of FL, SMPC can be used as an alternative to a central server for the aggregation step . The clients themselves can engage in a cryptographic protocol to collectively compute the average of their model updates, with no single client learning anything about another client's update beyond what is revealed by the final result. This is a key enabler for the fully decentralized, peer-to-peer FL architectures discussed in Section 3, fostering collaboration in environments where no central coordinator can be trusted or is desired.

6.2. The Rise of Personalized Federated Learning (pFL)

A significant evolution in the next decade will be the shift from a "one-size-fits-all" global model to Personalized Federated Learning (pFL). The core insight of pFL is that the ultimate goal for a participating hospital is not just to contribute to a strong global model, but to obtain a model that performs best for *its own* specific patient population and clinical environment. The statistical heterogeneity (Non-IID data) that is often seen as a problem to be solved is reframed by pFL as an opportunity for customization.

Future pFL frameworks will allow each client to learn a personalized model that is a sophisticated blend of the generalized knowledge from the global model and the specialized insights from its local data. This will involve advanced techniques like meta-learning, where the FL process learns an initial model that can be rapidly adapted with only a few local data samples, or multi-task learning, where the network simultaneously learns a shared representation of knowledge alongside personalized "heads" for each client. This move towards personalization will dramatically increase the clinical utility and adoption of FL, as institutions will receive a direct, tangible, and customized benefit from their participation.

6.3. The Role of FL in Building Unbiased, Fair, and Explainable AI (XAI)

As AI models become more integrated into clinical decision-making, ensuring they are fair, equitable, and transparent is a non-negotiable ethical imperative. Federated learning is uniquely positioned to be a cornerstone of this responsible AI movement in healthcare.

- Fairness and Bias Mitigation: By training on data from diverse global populations, FL naturally provides a mechanism to detect and mitigate biases that would be invisible in a single-site study. Future FL frameworks will incorporate fairness-aware algorithms that explicitly monitor model performance across different demographic subgroups (defined by race, sex, age, etc.) during the training process. If the model is found to be underperforming for a particular group at one site, the entire network can be leveraged to improve performance for that group, leading to more equitable models for all .
- Federated Explainable AI (XAI): A key barrier to AI adoption is the "black box" nature of many complex models. Clinicians are reluctant to trust a prediction without understanding *why* the model made it. Explainable AI (XAI) techniques aim to provide these explanations. In a federated setting, however, generating explanations is tricky as it cannot involve sharing the underlying data. The next decade will see the rise of Federated XAI, where new techniques will be developed to generate local explanations for a model's prediction at a given hospital, and even to create "global" explanations of the model's overall behaviour, all without violating the core privacy principles of the federated network.

6.4. Towards a Global Health Network: The Long-Term Vision

The culmination of these advancements points toward a truly transformative long-term vision: the creation of a global, federated health intelligence network. This would be a "learning health system" on a planetary scale, connecting hospitals, research centers, and public health agencies in a secure, collaborative ecosystem. Such a network could:

- Enable Real-Time Epidemiological Surveillance: New disease outbreaks or patterns of antibiotic resistance could be detected in near real-time by a federated model learning from data across a global network of hospitals, allowing for a much faster public health response than is currently possible.
- Revolutionize Clinical Trials: Recruitment for clinical trials for rare diseases could be dramatically accelerated by using a federated network to identify eligible patients across hundreds of hospitals without compromising their privacy. FL could even enable "in-silico" trials to be run on models trained on this vast, distributed data.
- Democratize Medical AI: Instead of AI expertise being concentrated in a few elite institutions, a global federated network would allow smaller or less-resourced hospitals to gain access to state-of-the-art AI models, helping to close the gap in healthcare quality between different regions.

6.5. Predictive Outlook: Key Milestones for the Next 10 Years

The path to this future can be charted through a series of expected milestones:

- Short-Term (1-3 Years): We will see the maturation and standardization of open-source FL platforms like NVIDIA FLARE and TensorFlow Federated, making it easier for institutions to participate. The first AI models trained using FL will likely receive regulatory clearance from bodies like the FDA and EMA for specific, non-critical diagnostic tasks.
- Mid-Term (3-6 Years): The emergence of "FL-as-a-Service" offerings from major cloud providers and specialized startups will lower the barrier to entry further. Clearer regulatory guidance on the legal and ethical aspects of FL will be established. We will see the first large-scale national FL networks for applications like population health management and cancer research.
- Long-Term (7-10 Years): Practical and efficient integration of FL with Homomorphic Encryption and other advanced PETs will become standard for high-security applications. Personalized FL will be a dominant paradigm, and FL will be deeply integrated into the workflows of smart hospitals for real-time predictive analytics. We may witness the formation of the first truly international, cross-continental federated health networks.

7. CONCLUSION

Throughout this chapter, we have embarked on a journey tracing the evolution of artificial intelligence in medicine, moving from a paradigm of centralized data aggregation to one of decentralized, collaborative intelligence. We began by confronting a critical paradox: despite spectacular algorithmic advances and proven successes in controlled settings, AI has yet to deliver on its promise of systemic, global transformation in healthcare. The reasons, as we explored, are not rooted in a failure of technology itself, but in the fundamental incompatibility of the centralized AI model with the realities of the healthcare ecosystem. The "data-hungry" nature of modern AI clashes with a landscape defined by stringent privacy regulations like HIPAA and GDPR, pervasive and fiercely guarded institutional data silos, the ethical imperative for unbiased and generalizable models, and the significant security risks of creating data "honeypots". These barriers have collectively formed a scaling wall, stalled progress and limiting the impact of medical AI to isolated pockets of innovation.

Looking to the next decade, the trajectory is clear. Federated Learning will become the cornerstone of medical AI's evolution, serving as the engine for a truly global, learning health system. Its synergy with technologies like differential privacy and homomorphic encryption, combined with a focus on fairness and explainability, will forge a new era of responsible and trustworthy AI. The future it promises is one where the collective medical knowledge of the world can be harnessed to accelerate research, improve diagnostics, and deliver better care for all, without compromising the fundamental right to privacy that lies at the heart of patient trust. The path forward requires continued multidisciplinary collaboration between technologists, clinicians, ethicists, and policymakers, but the foundation has been laid. The age of collaborative AI is dawning, and Federated Learning is its indispensable cornerstone.

REFERENCES

Agarwal, A., Verma, A., & Khari, M. (2024). Comparative assessment of machine learning methods for early prediction of diseases using health indicators. In *Approaches to Human-Centered AI in Healthcare* (pp. 160–186). IGI Global., DOI: 10.4018/979-8-3693-2238-3.ch007

Agbley, B. L. Y., Li, J. P., Haq, A. U., Bankas, E. K., Mawuli, C. B., Ahmad, S., Khan, S., & Khan, A. R. (2024). Federated Fusion of Magnified Histopathological Images for Breast Tumor Classification in the Internet of Medical Things. *IEEE Journal of Biomedical and Health Informatics, 28*(6), 3389–3400. DOI: 10.1109/JBHI.2023.3256974 PMID: 37028353

Almogadwy, B., & Alqarafi, A. (2025). Fused federated learning framework for secure and decentralized patient monitoring in healthcare 5.0 using IoMT. *Scientific Reports, 15*(1), 24263--. DOI: 10.1038/s41598-025-06574-w

Alshareet, O., & Awasthi, A. (2025). A Novel Framework for Integrating Blockchain-Driven Federated Learning with Neural Networks in E-Commerce. *Journal of Network and Systems Management, 33*(3), 56. Advance online publication. DOI: 10.1007/s10922-025-09928-x

Amin, M. S., Ahmad, S., & Loh, W. K. (2025). Federated learning for Healthcare 5.0: A comprehensive survey, taxonomy, challenges, and solutions. *Soft Computing, 29*(2), 673–700. DOI: 10.1007/s00500-025-10508-z

Azrour, M., Mabrouki, J., Guezzaz, A., Ahmad, S., Khan, S., & Benkirane, S. (2024). IoT, Machine Learning and Data Analytics for Smart Healthcare. In *IoT, Machine Learning and Data Analytics for Smart Healthcare* (pp. 1–94). CRC Press. DOI: 10.1201/9781003430735

Barnawi, A., Chhikara, P., Tekchandani, R., Kumar, N., & Alzahrani, B. (2024). A Differentially Privacy Assisted Federated Learning Scheme to Preserve Data Privacy for IoMT Applications. *IEEE Transactions on Network and Service Management, 21*(4), 4686–4700. DOI: 10.1109/TNSM.2024.3393969

Bhardwaj, T., & Sumangali, K. (2025). An explainable federated blockchain framework with privacy-preserving AI optimization for securing healthcare data. *Scientific Reports, 15*(1), 21799--. DOI: 10.1038/s41598-025-04083-4

Chen, J., Yi, C., Okegbile, S. D., Cai, J., & Shen, X. (2024). Networking Architecture and Key Supporting Technologies for Human Digital Twin in Personalized Healthcare: A Comprehensive Survey. *IEEE Communications Surveys and Tutorials, 26*(1), 706–746. DOI: 10.1109/COMST.2023.3308717

Choudhury, A., Sarma, K. K., Gulvanskii, V., Kaplun, D., & Dutta, L. (2025). Leveraging federated learning and edge computing for pandemic-resilient healthcare. *Scientific Reports, 15*(1), 20497--. DOI: 10.1038/s41598-025-00199-9

Ghadi, Y. Y., Shah, S. F. A., Waheed, W., Mazhar, T., Ahmad, W., Saeed, M. M., & Hamam, H. (2025). Integration of wearable technology and artificial intelligence in digital health for remote patient care. *Journal of Cloud Computing (Heidelberg, Germany), 14*(1), 39. Advance online publication. DOI: 10.1186/s13677-025-00759-4

Haripriya, R., Khare, N., & Pandey, M. (2025). Privacy-preserving federated learning for collaborative medical data mining in multi-institutional settings. *Scientific Reports, 15*(1), 12482--. DOI: 10.1038/s41598-025-97565-4

Jain, A., Bhatnagar, V., Rao, A. C. S., & Khari, M. (2023). Retina disease prediction using modified convolutional neural network based on Inception-ResNet model with support vector machine classifier. *Computational Intelligence, 39*(6), 1088–1111. DOI: 10.1111/coin.12601

Jain, A., Dubey, A. K., Gupta, M., Yadav, S., Panwar, A., Atanga, R., Lemos, B., & Mallik, S. (2025). Brain Stroke Prediction: A PSO Optimized Stacked Ensemble Machine Learning Approach with SMOTEEN Data Balancing. *BioRxiv*, 2025.06.05.657994. http://biorxiv.org/content/early/2025/06/08/2025.06.05.657994 .abstract

Jain, A., Dubey, A. K., Khan, S., Panwar, A., Alkhatib, M., & Alshahrani, A. M. (2025). A PSO weighted ensemble framework with SMOTE balancing for student dropout prediction in smart education systems. *Scientific Reports, 15*(1), 17463. DOI: 10.1038/s41598-025-97506-1 PMID: 40394143

Jain, A., Dubey, A. K., Pan, V. S. H., Mahfoudh, S., Althaqafi, T. A., Arya, V., Alhalabi, W., Singh, S. K., Jain, V., Panwar, A., Kumar, S., Hsu, C. H., & Gupta, B. B. (2025). Bayesian optimized CNN ensemble for efficient potato blight detection using fuzzy image enhancement. *Scientific Reports, 15*(1), 31259. DOI: 10.1038/s41598-025-15940-7 PMID: 40854933

Jian, W., Li, J. P., Akbar, M. A., Haq, A. U., Khan, S., Alotaibi, R. M., & Alajlan, S. A. (2024). SA-Bi-LSTM: Self Attention with Bi-Directional LSTM-Based Intelligent Model for Accurate Fake News Detection to Ensured Information Integrity on Social Media Platforms. *IEEE Access : Practical Innovations, Open Solutions, 12*, 48436–48452. DOI: 10.1109/ACCESS.2024.3382832

Kalpana, P., Tappari, S., Smitha, L., Madhavi, D., Naresh, K., & Vijayalakshmi, M. (2025). A novel end-to-end privacy preserving deep Aquila feed forward networks on healthcare 4.0 environment. *Discover Internet of Things*, *5*(1), 65. Advance online publication. DOI: 10.1007/s43926-025-00157-x

Li, X., Peng, L., Wang, Y. P., & Zhang, W. (2025). Open challenges and opportunities in federated foundation models towards biomedical healthcare. *BioData Mining, 18*(1), 2--. DOI: 10.1186/s13040-024-00414-9

Li, X., Zhang, L., Yang, J., & Teng, F. (2024). Role of Artificial Intelligence in Medical Image Analysis: A Review of Current Trends and Future Directions. *Journal of Medical and Biological Engineering*, *44*(2), 231–243. DOI: 10.1007/s40846-024-00863-x

Ma, Z., Ruhaiyem, N. I. R., Zhang, M., Musa, K. I., Hanis, T. M., Xiao, T., Hua, D., & Li, H. (2025). A review of federated learning technology and its research progress in healthcare applications. *Applied Intelligence*, *55*(10), 765. Advance online publication. DOI: 10.1007/s10489-025-06627-7

Manocha, A., Sood, S. K., & Bhatia, M. (2025). Federated learning-inspired smart ECG classification: An explainable artificial intelligence approach. *Multimedia Tools and Applications*, *84*(19), 21673–21696. DOI: 10.1007/s11042-024-20084-3

Mehrotra, M., Singh, K. P., & Singh, Y. B. (2024). Facial Emotion Recognition and Detection Using Convolutional Neural Networks with Low Computation Cost. *2024 2nd International Conference on Disruptive Technologies, ICDT 2024*, 1349–1354. DOI: 10.1109/ICDT61202.2024.10489678

Muhammed, D., Ahvar, E., Ahvar, S., Trocan, M., Montpetit, M. J., & Ehsani, R. (2024). Artificial Intelligence of Things (AIoT) for smart agriculture: A review of architectures, technologies and solutions. *Journal of Network and Computer Applications*, *228*, 103905. DOI: 10.1016/j.jnca.2024.103905

Nazir, A., Hussain, A., Singh, M., & Assad, A. (2025). Deep learning in medicine: Advancing healthcare with intelligent solutions and the future of holography imaging in early diagnosis. *Multimedia Tools and Applications*, *84*(17), 17677–17740. DOI: 10.1007/s11042-024-19694-8

Panwar, A., Gaba, P., Sugandh, U., & Bohra, N. (2025). Breaking the Centralization Barrier: Exploring Decentralized Federated Learning for Vehicle Number Plate Recognition in IoV. In *Federated Learning Based Intelligent Systems to Handle Issues and Challenges in IoVs (Part 2)* (pp. 102–139). Bentham Science Publishers. DOI: 10.2174/9789815322224125030006

Punitha, S., & Preetha, K. S. (2025). Enhancing reliability and security in cloud-based telesurgery systems leveraging swarm-evoked distributed federated learning framework to mitigate multiple attacks. *Scientific Reports, 15*(1), 27226--. DOI: 10.1038/s41598-025-12027-1

Sharma, N., Sugandh, U., Agarwal, J., Panwar, A., & Gaba, P. (2025). Federated Learning on Wheels: A Decentralized Approach to Privacy-Enhanced Data Collection in Internet of Vehicles. In *Federated Learning Based Intelligent Systems to Handle Issues and Challenges in IoVs (Part 2)* (pp. 1–33). Bentham Science Publishers. DOI: 10.2174/9789815322224125030003

Shi, Y., Zhang, J., Xue, M., Zeng, Y., Jia, G., Yu, Q., & Li, M. (2025). Vertical federated learning based on data subset representation for healthcare application. *Computer Methods and Programs in Biomedicine, 263*, 108623. DOI: 10.1016/j.cmpb.2025.108623 PMID: 39954511

Shukla, S., Rajkumar, S., Sinha, A., Esha, M., Elango, K., & Sampath, V. (2025). Federated learning with differential privacy for breast cancer diagnosis enabling secure data sharing and model integrity. *Scientific Reports, 15*(1), 13061--. DOI: 10.1038/s41598-025-95858-2

Solanki, S., Agarwal, J., Jain, A., Dubey, A. K., Panwar, A., & Priyadarshi, P. (2025). Evaluating Multi-Layer Perceptron and Recurrent Neural Networks for Speech Emotion Recognition. *2025 3rd International Conference on Communication, Security, and Artificial Intelligence, ICCSAI 2025, 3*, 349–354. DOI: 10.1109/ICCSAI64074.2025.11064042

Verma, A., & Khari, M. (2024). Vision-Based Accident Anticipation and Detection Using Deep Learning. *IEEE Instrumentation & Measurement Magazine, 27*(3), 22–29. DOI: 10.1109/MIM.2024.10505198

Wen, J., Li, X., Ye, X., Li, X., & Mao, H. (2025). A highly generalized federated learning algorithm for brain tumor segmentation. *Scientific Reports, 15*(1), 21053--. DOI: 10.1038/s41598-025-05297-2

Xing, H., Sun, R., Ren, J., Wei, J., Feng, C. M., Ding, X., Guo, Z., Wang, Y., Hu, Y., Wei, W., Ban, X., Xie, C., Tan, Y., Liu, X., Cui, S., Duan, X., & Li, Z. (2025). Achieving flexible fairness metrics in federated medical imaging. *Nature Communications, 16*(1), 3342--. DOI: 10.1038/s41467-025-58549-0

Yu, C., Shen, S., Wang, S., Zhang, K., & Zhao, H. (2025). Communication-Efficient Hybrid Federated Learning for E-Health with Horizontal and Vertical Data Partitioning. *IEEE Transactions on Neural Networks and Learning Systems, 36*(3), 5614–5628. DOI: 10.1109/TNNLS.2024.3383748 PMID: 38598400

Zhang, L., Fang, G., & Tan, Z. (2025). FedCCW: A privacy-preserving Byzantine-robust federated learning with local differential privacy for healthcare. *Cluster Computing*, *28*(3), 182. Advance online publication. DOI: 10.1007/s10586-024-04894-6

Zhou, L., Jain, A., Dubey, A. K., Singh, S. K., Gupta, N., Panwar, A., Kumar, S., Althaqafi, T. A., Arya, V., Alhalabi, W., & Gupta, B. B. (2025). FPA-based weighted average ensemble of deep learning models for classification of lung cancer using CT scan images. *Scientific Reports*, *15*(1), 19369. DOI: 10.1038/s41598-025-02015-w PMID: 40461493

Zhou, Y., Wu, Y., Su, Y., Li, J., Cai, J., You, Y., Zhou, J., Guo, D., & Qu, X. (2025). Cloud-magnetic resonance imaging system: In the era of 6G and artificial intelligence. *Magnetic Resonance Letters*, *5*(1), 200138. DOI: 10.1016/j.mrl.2024.200138 PMID: 40918039

Chapter 15

The Role of Federated Learning in AI-Powered Integrated Healthcare Solutions

Kahksha Ahmed
SAITM, India

Ankit Baranwal
SAITM, India

Neetu Sharma
Galgotias University, India

Puneet Garg
https://orcid.org/0000-0002-4635-546X
KIET Group of Institutions, India

Narinderjit Singh
INTI University, Malaysia

ABSTRACT

Federated Learning (FL) represents a revolutionary approach to artificial intelligence in the health care system, which addresses the important challenges of data lift, security and regulatory compliance, which enables severe ally insights. This paradigm allows health institutions to train the shared AI model without exchanging sensitive patient data, as the model travels where the data lives instead of centralizing the information. In an integrated health environment, FL provides facilitators for

DOI: 10.4018/979-8-3373-3306-9.ch015

spontaneous collaboration in quiet departments, specifications and organizations and at the same time maintain strict data above. Implementation of FL in the health care system enables a strong future analysis, individual remedies recommendations and enlarged clinical decision support systems that are attracted by diverse patient population without compromising privacy.

1. INTRODUCTION

Rapid progress in artificial intelligence (AI) has revolutionized the health care system, improved diagnosis, treatment plans and monitoring of the patient. AI-operated solutions have the ability to increase patient results, reduce medical errors and optimize hospital operations(Alowais et al., 2023). However, AI's complete capacity in the health care system is interrupted by challenges such as discontinuation of privacy considerations, security threats and inter -related problems between different health care. These issues occur because health data is extremely sensitive; the EU is subject to stringent restrictions such as the General Data Protection Regulation (GDPR), while the US is frequently subject to the Portability and Responsibility Act (HIPAA)(Malik et al., 2024).

Traditional AI models require large amounts of data, which are usually centralized in the same place for training. This centralization increases the concerns of the patient's privacy, data violations and unauthorized access. In addition, it is composed to collect different and representative data sets in many hospitals, research institutes and health professionals due to regulatory and operational obstacles. As a result, the (Khalid et al., 2023) AI models may suffer from prejudice, limited generality and incomplete information, affecting their credibility and efficiency.

Due to the increased incorporation of the technologies ML, NLP, and CV into healthcare, tasks such as diagnosis, treatment planning, patient monitoring and operational performance can be done with optimal efficiency. The scanning of massive amounts of medical data including X-rays, lab and genetic reports, and electronic health records becomes effortless with the use of AI. AI systems are able to detect patterns and make predictions with uncanny precision. The inclusion of these advanced technologies in medical workflows have proven to enhance clinical outcomes. Early disease detection, the customization of treatment plans, epidemic forecasting, and the automation of tedious tasks in hospitals can now be performed with the help of AI models. Therefore, AI can transform the delivery of healthcare services by improving accuracy and efficiency in services offered.

FL appears as a transformative paradigm that addresses these boundaries. Unlike traditional AI training methods, there are many health institutions to train raw patient data without collaborating. Instead, the AI model is locally trained in each participating institute, and only the collected model updates are shared. This decentralized approach not only improves privacy and security for data, but also provides the possibility of integrating different data sets from different geographical and demographic backgrounds, improves the AI model accuracy and justice (Yurdem et al., 2024).

Federated Learning (FL) Collaborate AI has emerged as an innovative approach to accommodate the model development and double the needs of strict data privacy. Instead of sending sensitive health data on a central server for training, FL AI models allow to be trained locally in hospitals or health institutions. Only model updates - for example, changes in weight or gradients - are shared with a central aggregator, not with raw data. This decentralized teaching technique ensures that the data remains within its original location, while they are still in accordance with privacy rules and contribute to the development of a global AI model. FL enables hospitals, laboratories and even portable equipment to work together to create a powerful machine learning model without the exchange of patient records. As a result, Federated learning is recognized as a basic technique for safe, morally and integrated AI-integrated health care. Federated Learning architecture showing in Fig 1 the iterative process of clients training locally and sending model weights to a central server for global aggregation

Figure 1. Federated Learning Approach (Upreti et al., 2024)

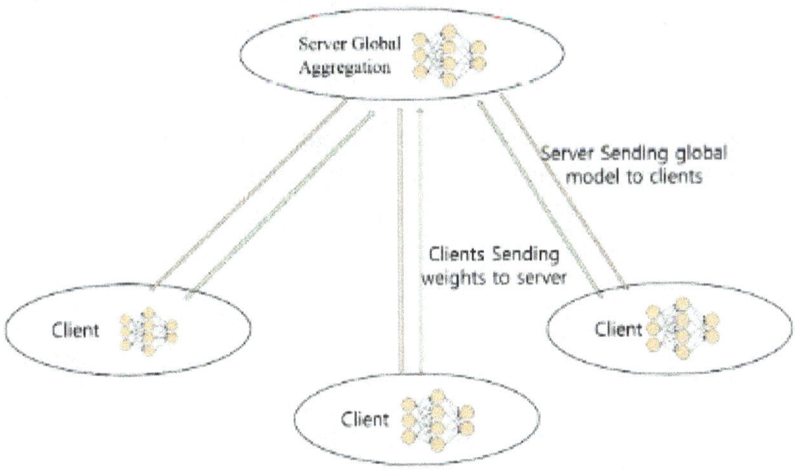

The importance of FL is out of privacy protection. By taking advantage of secure model aggregation, the FL transverse institutional collaboration enabled health professionals, pharmaceutical companies and research organizations to work together to collaborate. This collaborative structure accelerates medical research, facilitates initial disease detection and increases individual drug approach, and ensures compliance with data security rules (Yurdem et al., 2024)

In this chapter, we discover the role of Federal Learning in AI-controlled integrated health services, discussing the most important principles, applications, benefits, challenges and future instructions. When the health care system continues to embrace digital changes, FL stands as an important environment for scalable, safe and efficient AI-controlled health service infrastructure.

2. EVOLUTION OF MACHINE LEARNING STRUCTURE AND DEVELOPMENT OF FEDERATED LEARNING

Machine Learning (ML) has made significant development in recent decades, from simple algorithm trained on small datasets to a complex model that requires huge amounts of data and computational power. Originally, the ML model was often trained in a centralized way, where data collected from different sources were collected in a single depot or data center. This centralized structure made it easy to develop and adapt the model due to the availability of large, integrated data sets. However, as the amount of data increased and the fear of privacy and security increased, however, the limits of centralized ML became clear - especially in sensitive areas such as health care, finance and telecommunications.

The arrival of large data and spread of data-generating equipment, such as smartphones, portable sensors and IoT systems, led a distributed data landscape. Transfer of these massive and often sensitive data to a central server faces challenges related to bandwidth, delay, costs and most important privacy risk. Rules such as HIPAA in the health care system and GDPR in Europe implemented strict data sharing rules, and pushed researchers and industry leaders to reconsider traditional ML architecture.

Federated Learning (FL), a new paradigm that uses centralized data collection to convert the training process into decentralized, cooperative model creation, arose in response to these difficulties. The FL transmits the machine to the learning model, where the data stays, whether on the age unit, hospital server, or mobile unit, rather than transmitting the raw data to a central server. Only the model updates or parameters are sent to a coordinate server; each participant trains the model locally using their own personal data. This approach permits compliance with regulatory requirements, protects data privacy, and lessens the need for large data transit.

The Association Learning Data represents a significant development in the ML structure by enabling collaborative intelligence without compromising sovereignty. It benefits from progress in safe aggregation, difference in privacy and communication -efficient algorithms to solve the challenges of distributed data and asymmetrical environments. Today, FL person protection is speed as an effective solution for AI, especially in areas such as health care, where patient protection is crucial, and data silos are wide.

3. UNDERSTAND FEDERAL LEARNING IN HEALTH CARE

Federated Learning (FL) is an advanced machine learning paradigm designed to enable many decentralized institutions or equipment to train the AI model without the exchange of raw data. This decentralized teaching approach ensures that sensitive patient data live within its original institution, while it still contributes to the development of very accurate and strong AI models. Data addresses several regulatory and moral concerns related to AI in the FL health services, by preserving privacy and security (Upreti et al., 2024).

In traditional machine learning method, all data from different sources are collected and stored in one place to train the AI model. In the health care system, however, it improves serious privacy, security and legal concerns, as patients are confidential and protected by laws such as HIPAA (in the United States) and similar rules globally.

Federal learning solves this problem by keeping the data decentralized. It works like this:

- Each hospital models locally trained its own data.
- Only model updates (not yourself are not data) are shared with a central server.
- These updates are combined to improve the global model, which in turn is sent back to all participants.

3.1 Centralized vs. Federated Learning

In traditional centralized teaching, data from many sources or institutions are collected and collected into a single, central server or data warehouse. The AI model is then trained on this pool data set, which often results in very accurate and stronger models due to the amount and diversity of data. However, this approach presents important challenges in the health care system. The patient data is very sensitive, protected by strict privacy rules such as HIPAA and GDPR, and cannot be moved independently to institutions or geographical boundaries. In addition, centralization of large versions of data security risk, including data violations and unauthorized access, can lead to serious moral and legal consequences. In addition, centralized systems require significant infrastructure to store and manage large data sets, and data transfer can be expensive and slow, especially for large medical imaging files or genomic data.

On the other hand, Federated Learning (FL) provides a decentralized alternative, where the AI model is cooperating in many institutions without transferring raw data outside its local environment. Instead of collecting patient data in the same location, FL sends a model to each institution where it is locally trained on its personal data. Locally trained model updates, such as shield changes or weight adjustments, are then collected safely by a central server to update the global model. This approach significantly increases privacy and data security because the information of a sensitive patient never leaves the original site(Khan, 2024). FL also reduces data transfer overhead and complies with the legal framework as limited data sharing. While FL can sometimes be more composed to use and can meet challenges such as data Display or communication delay, it is quickly recognized as an important solution for privacy protection AI in the health care system.

In short, centralized education depends on data passation and has limitations due to privacy, security and legal concerns, while prioritizing data privacy by keeping Federated Learning Data Local and Sharing Model Parameters, distributing distributed health data safe in health data, Silo, included AI model development. This makes FL well adapted to sensitive domains, especially as health services where the patient's privacy is crucial. Comparison of Centralized, Distributed, and Federated Machine Learning architectures (Fig 2) in terms of data flow and model training approach.

Figure 2. Comparison of Centralized, Distributed, and Federated Machine Learning (Abdulrahman et al., 2021)

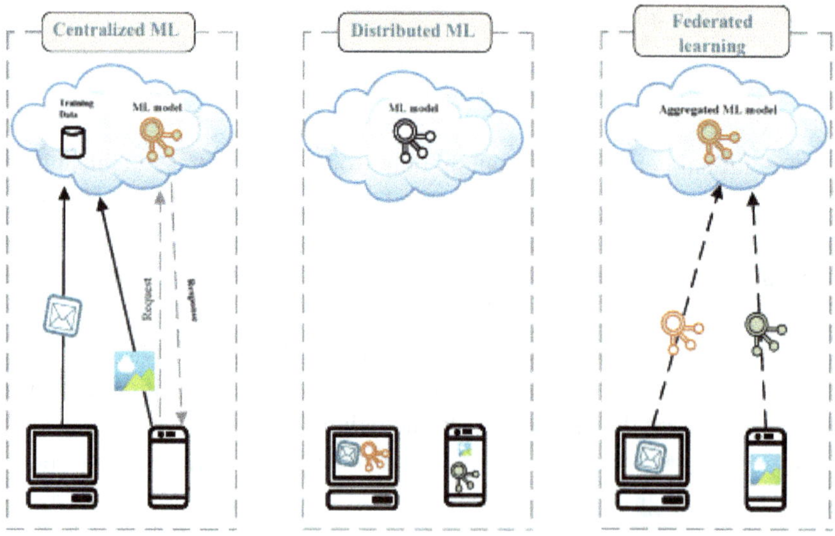

3.2 Types of Federal Learning

The three primary forms of data distribution in participating institutions that fall under the umbrella of Federal Learning (FL) are Federated transmission learning, vertical Federated learning, and horizontal Federated learning. Different data scenarios and use cases are addressed by each type, which is particularly pertinent in privacy-sensitive domains like the healthcare system. Fig. 3 depicts the approximate working principle. Federal Horizontal Learning (HFL). When different institutions have datasets about different people but with similar functions, horizontal Federated learning—also referred to as test-based Federated learning—applies. For instance, data such as age, penis, blood pressure, and diagnosis results can be gathered from two hospitals located in different cities. But every hospital treats a different set of patients. In this instance, even though the structure of the data is the same, patient records are not divided. In the health care system, HFL allows institutions to collaborate with the AI model, such as detecting heart disease, without highlighting personal health data. Each hospital trains locally the model and only shares the model updated with the central server. These updates are collected to improve over

3.2.2 Vertical Federated Learning (VFL)

Vertical Federal Learning, or function -based federal learning, is used when participating institutions have a variety of data (facilities) about the same set of individuals. This is often in collaboration between organizations such as hospitals and insurance companies. For example, a hospital may capture the patient's medical journal (eg test results, clinical notes), while an insurance provider maintains financial, behavior and lifestyle data on the same patient.

At VFL, both organizations work together to train a more comprehensive AI model without highlighting the dataset. Special techniques, such as safe unit adjustment, are used without revealing their identity to identify shared users. It enables more accurate and general predictions, such as exposed to long -term health risks or treatment ability. However, VFL is more complex to apply secure identity between different types of data due to the need for matching and coordination.

3.3.3 Federated Transfer Learning (FTL)

The union transfer learning is useful when both functions and computer tests vary in participants, and only a small overlap is present. This type of FL transfer combines the principles of learning and Federated learning to allow collaboration between institutions that have limited or different types of data. This rare disease is particularly relevant in scenarios such as research, where the data is rare and spread in global institutions.

For example, a research centre in Europe may have genomic data from cancer patients, while a hospital in Asia has environmental risk data and treatment reactions for different patients. By implementing the transfer of learning techniques, both institutions can still benefit from training each other with knowledge of each other.

Figure 3. Working principles of horizontal FL, vertical FL, and transfer FL (Hu et al., 2024)

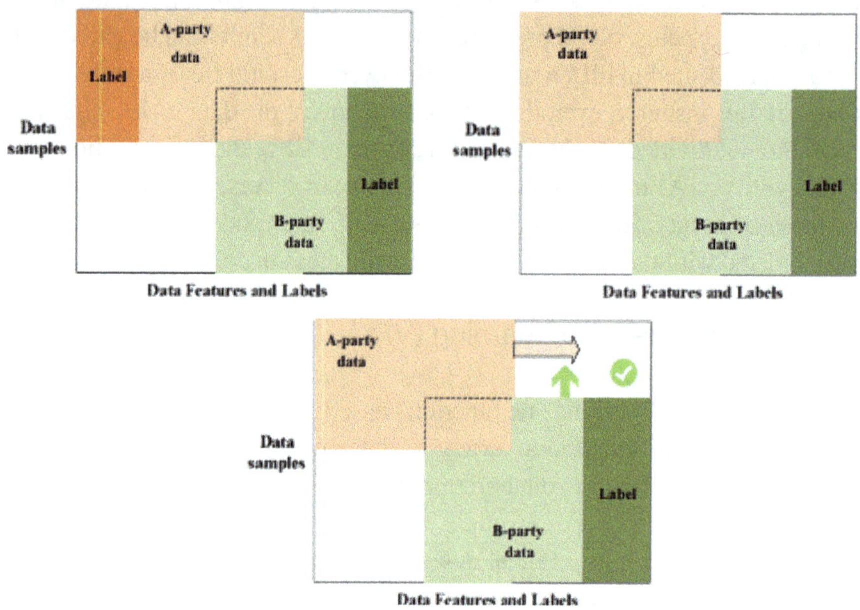

4. FEDERATED LEARNING ARCHITECTURE IN HEALTHCARE

4.1. System Component

- Customer (health services institutes and unit):
- These include hospitals, clinics, diagnostic laboratories, image centers and portable health equipment such as smartwatches or exercise tracks.
- Each client stores locally sensitive patient data and is responsible for training models on this data without moving externally.

- Customer varies in data size, quality and delivery, data inequality introduces challenges.
- They communicate model updates on the central server after the local training round.
- customers can also handle tasks before speeding up to prepare data for training.

4.2 Central Server (Coordinator)

As seen in Fig.4, this kind of FL architecture, in contrast to the centralized machine learning architecture, also needs a central server to collect each user's parameters; nevertheless, its primary goal was to safeguard user privacy.

- FL acts as an orchestrator for the system, and controls the training cycle of many customers.
- Incoming the global AI model and sends it to customers for local training.
- Agang Rieth collects the locally trained model updates from customers using algorithm as Federated Average (Fedavg).
- Communication planning, fault tolerance and client selection strategies to adapt performance and scalability.
- The O model ensures convergence and evaluates the overall global model performance.

4.3 Communication Network

- The O model provides secure, efficient and reliable transmission of model parameters (not raw data) between customers and servers.
- Communication protocols include encryption (eg TLS) to prevent frequent cutting or tampering.
- Bandwidth barriers and delay problems are addressed by optimizing update size and communication frequency (eg, sending updates only after several local ages).
- System can support the asynchronous or synchronous communication models based on design.

Figure 4. Client–server architecture (Hong et al., 2023)

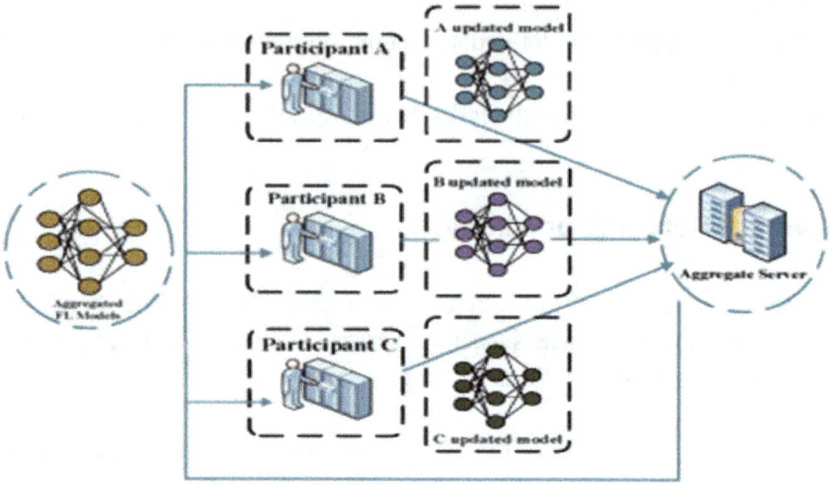

5. FEDERAL LEARNING APPROACH

By using a related machine learning methodology, Federated Learning (FL) enables numerous organizations or pieces of equipment to develop a common AI model without sharing or transferring raw data. In the healthcare system, where data privacy is of utmost importance, this approach is particularly helpful.

Step 1: Global Model Initiative

- A central authority (eg a research institute or supplier of cloud services) creates a base AI model.
- This model is often untrained or trained on publicly available medical data.
- It defines architecture (eg a nerve network for image classification).
- The model is then sent to many customers, such as hospitals, diagnostic laboratories or smart medical equipment.

Step 2: Local model training on customer equipment

- Each participating customer (eg a hospital) receives a global model and trains it locally by using its own patient data.
- This training includes many eras for learning based on local data characteristics (eg age group, type of disease, scanner solution).

- Training is on radius using local GPU or server.

Step 3: Send model updates to the server (not data

- After local training, the hospital does not share raw data.
- Instead, it sends model updates to the central server (such as weight change or difference in weight).
- These updates can be encrypted or preserved by using differences to prevent the reverse design of patient data.

Step 4: Local update collected on Central Server

- The central server receives updates from all hospitals.
- This uses an aggregation algorithm (for example, Federated average) to combine local updates and produce a better version of the model.
- Several hospitals participate, diversity and generalization of global models are better.

Step 5: Cooling of updated global models

- Better models are sent back to all participating hospitals and equipment.
- Each institution can now benefit from learning others without sharing private data.
- This cycle can be repeated in several rounds to continuously improve performance.

Step 6: Optional local fine adjustment (privatization)

- Some hospitals may choose to pursue global models for their local environment.
- It is useful when local data vary from global trends (eg rare conditions, regional diseases, specific demographics).

Step 7: Continuous monitoring and reaction

- Hospitals monitor how well the model performs in the real world scenarios.
- Feedback can be used to improve future model versions.
- Error or screen drops can be logged in to fix future FL cycles.

6. IMPORTANT PRINCIPLES OF FEDERAL EDUCATION

The Federated Learning cycle consists of decentralized processing, safe aggregation, adaptive training settings, and privacy-preserving strategies. In healthcare systems, each step guarantees the development of AI models that are secure, effective, and considerate of privacy shown Fig 5.

Figure 5. Principle of Federal Education

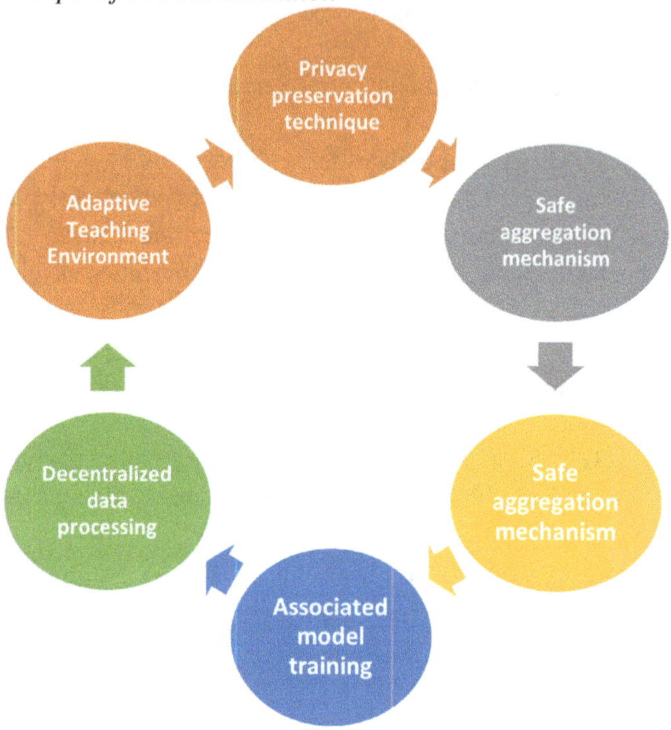

Decentralized data processing: Unlike traditional AI models, which require data centralization, FL ensures that all learning is local in health institutions. This eliminates the requirement for bulk data transfer and reduces contact with cyber security risk (Meurisch et al., 2020).

Associated model training: AI models are trained on the data sets of numerous hospitals, clinics, and medical research institutes; only encrypted model updates are sent to a central aggregator.

Safe aggregation mechanism: The central aggregator makes sure that the final AI model makes use of a variety of health data for health services by gathering model updates from various institutions without emphasizing specific data sets.

Privacy preservation method: To protect the patient, Federal Learning Models employs advanced cryptographic techniques like Secured Multi-Party Computation (SMPC), differential secrecy, and homomorine fish, as well as Advanced Multi-Party Computation (SMPC) (Mohammadi et al., 2024).

Adaptive Teaching Environment: FL Framework can dynamically adjust new data sources and ensure that the AI model remains updated with the latest medical progress and patient demographics

7. FEDERAL LEARNING APPLICATIONS IN HEALTHCARE

Medical imaging, EHR analysis, drug discovery, and remote patient monitoring are some of the major healthcare domains shown Fig 6 where AI and Federated Learning are revolutionizing the field. These apps make it possible to provide care in an effective, safe, and customized manner.

Figure 6. Federal Learning Applications in Healthcare

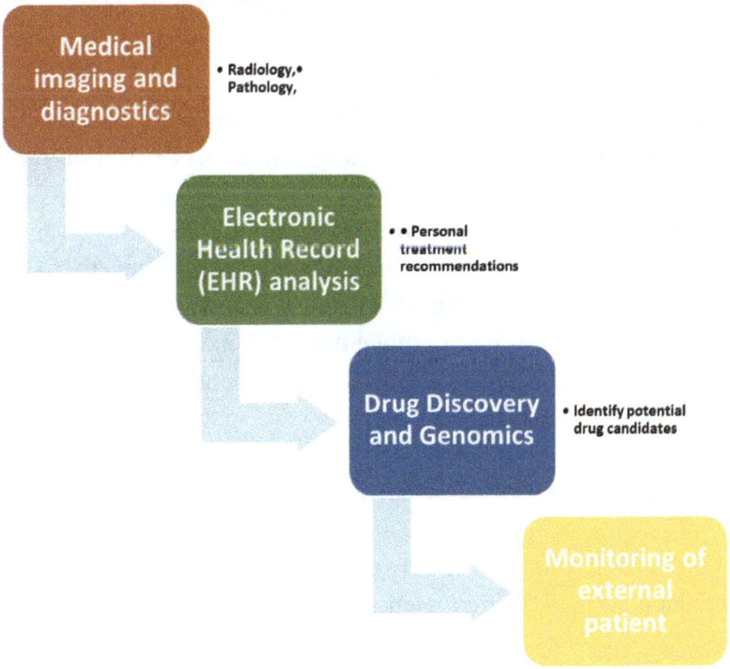

7.1. Medical imaging and diagnostics

FL enables collaboration between hospitals and research centers to train the AI model on a large, diverse medical imaging data set without violating the patient's privacy. This increases the accuracy of the disease detection in areas such as:

- **Radiology:** AI-Assisted FL models help detect deviations in MRI, CT scans and X-rays, which improve early diagnosis of diseases such as pneumonia, tumors and fractures (Beniwal et al., 2021).
- **Pathology:** FL-based model improves the identity of cancer cells in tissue samples and helps pathologists in quick and more accurate diagnosis.
- **Dermatology:** Trained AI models using FL can classify different skin diseases, identify conditions such as melanoma with high accuracy and help dermatologist in remote areas (Upadhyay et al., 2023)

7.2. Electronic Health Record (EHR) analysis

FL facilitates AI manual analysis of electronic health records in institutions without centralizing sensitive patient information. It supports:

- **Personal treatment recommendations:** By analyzing decentralized EHR data, AI models may suggest an analogue treatment based on the patient's history, genetics and lifestyle factors.

    Future analysis for the prevention of the disease: FL models help to identify risk patients by analyzing symptoms, genetic forecasts and lifestyle options, which enables preventive care measures.
- **Effective hospital resource management:** AI-operated FL models optimize the operation of the hospital, predicting the patient's influx, resource allocation and staffing requirements.

7.3. Drug Discovery and Genomics

By enabling safe AI collaboration between pharmaceutical companies, universities and research laboratories, floating intensifies drug discovery and genetic research:

- **Identify potential drug candidates:** AI models analyze giant datasets to predict promising compounds for drug development, reduce time and costs associated with traditional drug search methods.

- **Predicting drug responses in different populations:** By integrating genetic data from diverse population, the exact drug increases by sewing drug agents for specific genetic markers.
- **Understanding genetic factors that affect diseases:** FL data supports large -scale genetic analysis while maintaining confidentiality, promoting genetic disorders and personal medicine (Vora et al., 2023).

7.4. Monitoring of external patient

FL supports the AI model running on smart wearables and IoT Healthcare devices, which ensure personal health insight without compromising user data. Cases of use include:

- **Advance detection in real time:** AI-driven FL model-equipped devices detect irregularities in heart rate, oxygen level and blood pressure, and warn health professionals to potential health problems.
- **AI-driven notice of chronic disease management:** Patients with conditions such as diabetes or high blood pressure get reaction in real time and personal recommendations for their health management (Rahman et al., 2023).
- **Adaptive fitness and welfare program:** AI models analyze individual health matrix and propose adapted exercise and dietary plans, and promote active health management.

8. BENEFITS OF FEDERATED LEARNING IN INTEGRATED HEALTHCARE

Figure 7. Benefits Federal Learning in Healthcare (Upreti et al., 2024)

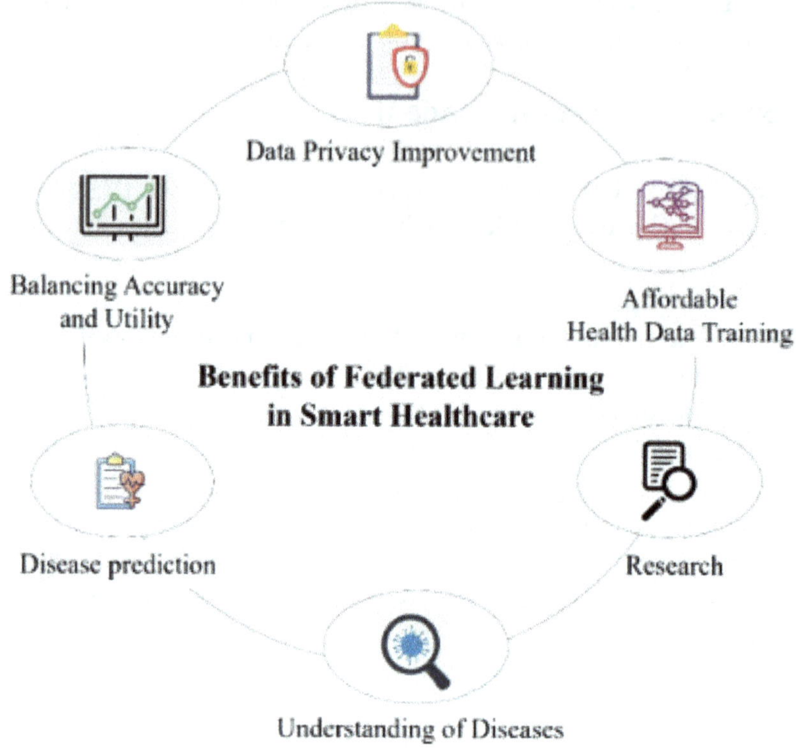

- **Enhanced Data Privacy and Security**: FL reduces the risk of data breaches and regulatory non-compliance because patient data stays with the original institution, complying with data protection regulations such as HIPAA and GDPR.
- **Improved AI Model Performance**: Training on diverse and decentralized datasets ensures AI models generalize better to real-world healthcare scenarios, enhancing diagnostic accuracy and treatment efficacy.
- **Regulatory Compliance**: FL enables healthcare institutions to adopt AI while maintaining compliance with stringent regulations, ensuring ethical and legal data usage.

- **Reduced Data Transfer Costs**: By eliminating the need to move large healthcare datasets, FL optimizes bandwidth and computational resources, making AI deployment more cost-effective.
- **Faster AI Deployment**: Institutions can benefit from improved AI models without waiting for data centralization and pre-processing, accelerating innovation in healthcare.
- **Understanding of Diseases**: Models trained on Federated (decentralized) healthcare data allow the discovery of diseases in diverse populations. This useful tool aids in understanding aspects like disease progression, risk factors and variations in demographics. This results in improved diagnosis, prognosis, and personalized treatment strategies.
- **Disease Prediction**: Health care predictive analytics: Health care predictive analytics uses massive datasets to predict the outbreak of diseases and risks to patient health. Federated Learning allows AI models to train on data distributed over numerous hospitals and clinics without requiring all the data to be centralized (Upreti et al., 2024).

9. IMPLEMENTATION OF FEDERATED LEARNING IN THE HEALTH CARE SYSTEM

The health care system involves many important components in practical implementation of FL:

- **Local AI training nodes**: Each participating hospital or health services run their own local AI training node, which processes data from electronic health records (EHR), medical imaging and portable equipment.
- **Federal Server for model aggregation**: A safe, centralized server collects model updates from local nodes and integrates them to limit the global AI model.
- **Privacy protection algorithm**: Technology such as differential privacy and the association average ensures that no individual patient data is compromised during model training.
- **Interoperability standards**: Healthcare institutions should use standardized data format and communication protocols to enable spontaneous integration of FL models into different systems and infrastructure.

By taking advantage of these components, Federated learning changes in A-driven health services, so that institutions can function safely through medical research, disease detection and protect personal treatment strategies (Zhang et al., 2024). The next section will detect specific applications of FL in various health services, including medical imaging, drug detection and monitoring of the patient at a distance.

10 THREAT MODELS OF FL

Even if the primary objective of Federated Learning (FL) is to maintain strict data privacy, security concerns are still present. With regards to safety, the unwanted attacks pose a greater risk and, in this case, model is a prime candidate for two concerns that arise during the initial design stage. Firstly, given the model's premise, the server typically observes every user's update and so if it is malicious, that model can certainly break the training procedure and control the global parameters, sweeping the value given of the model supplanting features update. Secondly, free joining and leaving users during FL work is permitted. Thus, with the presence of some active malevolent participants, these users can exploit this privilege to unmask global parameters, compromise personal data or vandalize global models. In both the passive and active attack modes, the attacker's main intention is to damage the unique attributes of the privacy preserving model. Such attributes are privacy, data integrity, and data accessibility (Lyu et al., 2020). In security matters, focus is often given to integrity and availability. Degradation of integrity and accessibility centres around the outcome of the machine learning models which is likely to disturb the normal operation of the model. The worrisome of integrity refers to motivating the model to act in a way that the model output is equal to the class label during prediction. There is some danger that mostly prevents the user from getting a correct output from the model or some models block the user from getting the features, for instance user-universe models become unreliable (Zhao et al., 2021).

When we discuss privacy, the emphasis is on privacy. Attacks based on privacy could unveil the information model and the model's inference data. Existing research suggests that privacy preserving algorithms still pose a risk to the user's privacy. Malicious customers frequently can guess precise data values included in the training sets, like where a person lives. Also, malicious customers can develop strategies on how they can infer and leak some sensitive identifying information of other customer data such as their participation in customer's metadata. They may also purport to hide the sensitive data for other parties to access, or even publicly make use of a fraction of the information which the user has covered concerning localization data. Hence, in this part, we analyse first the model for the FL's risk in detail (McMahan et al., 2017).

10.1 Internal against external

Being an autonomous branch, the most important feature of FL as a distributed teaching system is the link between the components, which is quite weak for attacks. External attacks can usually be classified into two categories: First, some attackers are external for models and focus on the communication lines between the model's subsystem (external attacks). Second, when the FL model occurs in broadcast server mode (internal attack), the user is attacked. An external attack will include predicting the purpose data or any model output information from Pri Mary(Sharma et al., 2025). On the other hand, internal attacks are less excusable, and the attackers apply to the attackers to be one or more users and servers in the learning system. Their intentions are to intervene in production from both models and distorting functionality by separating important data from other users. This fig 8 demonstrates that attackers have party-side knowledge (parameters, private datasets, partial outputs) in VFL systems and client-side knowledge (model access, local model details, client datasets) in HFL systems.

(1) **Single attack:** One of the goals might be to prevent the model from correctly classifying a specific high-confidence input structured set. One by one, the attacker who is part of the model for the selected attacks starts reallocating internal representation with their secret cache. As captured by the quote, "So the attack consists of blending in captured traffic with the transmitted traffic" so routing freely within the model and overcoming the hostile user's updates using increased traffic of corrupting users with their updates(Bhagoji et al., 2019).

(2) **Bijantin attacks:** The performance of the global model is impacted as the attacker uses your input to modify the production in order to modify the input into the correct model, making it harder to discover the system (Blanchard et al., 2017).

(3) **Sybil attacks:** -It is possible to copy anti-Dami participating accounts or choose participants who have already been compromised to launch more potent attacks on the FL system

Figure 8. Attacker capabilities in the HFL and VFL (Hu et al., 2024)

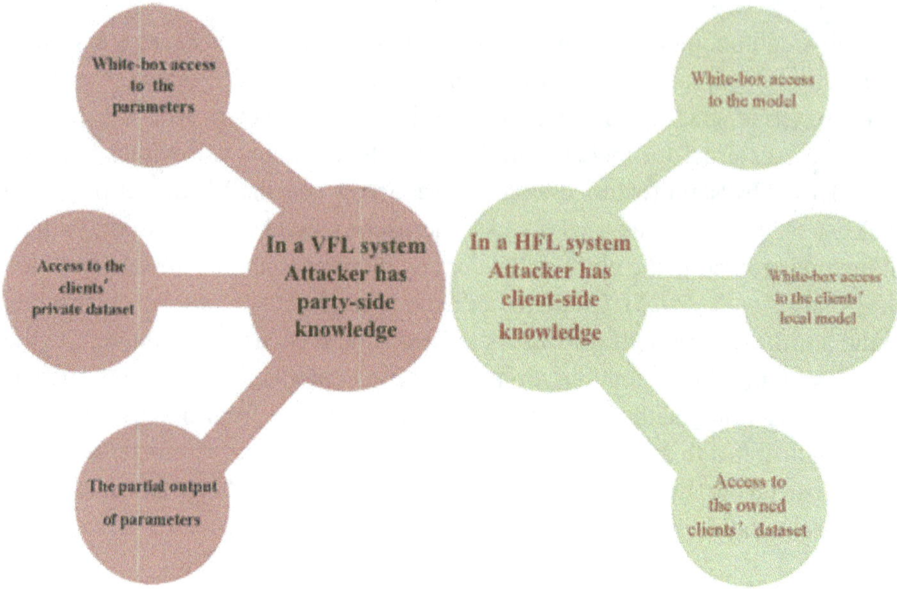

11. IMPLEMENTATION OF THE REAL WORLD OF FEDERAL LEARNING IN CASE STUDIES AND HEALTH SERVICES

Federated Learning (FL) is no longer a theoretical concept, but is adopted by major health organizations and technology companies around the world. It changes how the AI model is trained and distributed by activated to learn the partners while maintaining the patient's privacy and data security.

Below are some important case studies and the implementation of the real- world showing FL's power and versatility in the health care system

11.1 Google and Mayo Clinic – prophecy

Google Health participated to handle one of the most challenging health services with the Mayo Clinic: Exact and initial detection of breast cancer. Both organizations hold the huge and varied data sets with mammography images, which are important for training effective AI models. However, privacy rules and moral thoughts prohibit sharing raw patients at institutions. The union learning allowed these two veterans to train a deep learning model by placing data in their respective safe environment (Vasilev et al., 2025).

This collaboration produced a model with better generalization in different patient population and imaging units, which improves the model trained on the institute's data alone. The FL approach reduced false positivity and false negatively, which is important factor for the screening of breast cancer. Furthermore, the case highlighted how FL can accelerate medical AI innovation by following HIPAA and other privacy rules. It sets an example for equal cooperation in medical imaging and other domains of diagnostics.

11.2 Nvidia Clara - Federated Learning for Radiology

Nvidia Clara is a comprehensive AI platform designed for medical imaging and workflows in the health care system, which benefits from Federated Learning to strengthen cooperation model training on scale. Clara links many hospitals and radiology centers around the world, so they can train them locally sophisticated AI algorithms on high-dimensional depiction data such as CT scans, MRIs and PET scans.

Cutting privacy technologies are used in the platform, such as safe calculation of multiport, homomorphic encryption and differential secret to ensure that no sensitive patient data is leaked under the Federated procedure. Hospitals can jointly develop models for important tasks such as tumour department, lung knots detection and brain shooting that identify brain damage without compromising on the brain (Roth et al., 2022).

In addition to research, Nvidia Claras FL functions are distributed in clinical surroundings, increasing clinical accuracy and supporting radiologists in complex decision -making. The platform also complies with data protection laws in the courts, and shows federal learning scale and adaptability in global health care systems.

11.3 Find Covid-19 with Federated Learning Model

This demonstrated the ability to monitor infectious disease The COVID-19 epidemic created an immediate requirement for the exact clinical equipment worldwide, but sharing patient data on the limits was complicated by privacy and regulatory obstacles. Federated Learning offered an elegant solution by enabling hospitals and research institutes in many countries to develop the AI model that is the collaboration that analyzes the breast X -Strays and CT scans for signs of covid -19 infection (Garg et al., 2023).

Through the FL, the data within the infrastructure of each hospital remained, while the model updates were collected centrally. This collaborative approach accelerated the production of strong AI models responsible for different patient population and imaging variations. In addition, it increased the preparation of the epidemic by facilitating real -time updates and continuous model improvements such as new data.

In the case of this use, the role of Federated learning was emphasized to enable global health cooperation during crisis, while balanced the need for rapid innovation with strict privacy and moral standards in terms of use running beyond Covid-19.

11.4 Federated Learning in Mobile Health Apps

Mobile health and portable devices produce a huge amount of sensitive personal health data from heartbeat and oxygen levels in the blood to sleep quality and physical activity. Federated Learning has emerged as a playing technology that allows these apps to provide personal health insight by preserving the user's privacy. This local training method also enables fast model privatization and adaptation for individual users. Many M health applications have implemented FL for important health monitoring tasks such as detecting arrhythmias, predicting stress levels and assessing mental health conditions. For example, some smart watches use FLS that uses FL to continuously improve Alind -fibration detection algorithm based on decentralized user data (Maggo & Garg, 2022).

The use of FL in MHETT expands access to AI-controlled health services from the clinical environment to daily life, and strengthens patients with privacy conscious, real-time health monitoring and personal recommendations.

12. CHALLENGES AND LIMITATIONS

Implementing Federated Learning presents several difficulties, such as data inequity, communication lags, and processing overhead shown Fig 9. In healthcare settings, maintaining safety and navigating the complexities of integrating many systems continue to be top priorities (Rajput et al., 2024).

Figure 9. Federal Learning Challenges in Healthcare

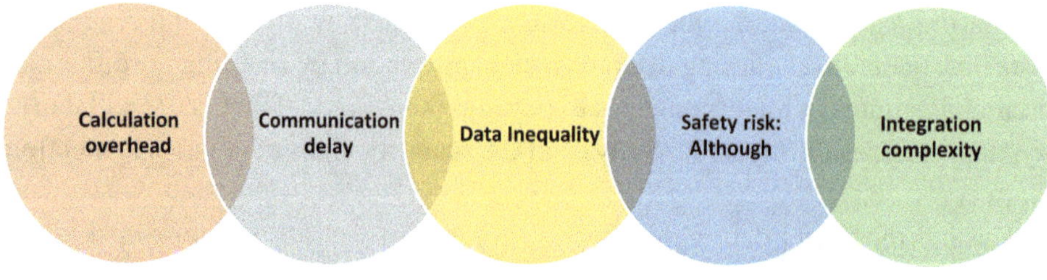

Calculation overhead: AI model on decentralized equipment requires important local calculation power to exercise, and requires advanced hardware infrastructure.

Communication delay: Model updates require secure and effective communication channels, which can introduce delays, especially in remote or underdeveloped areas.

Data Inequality: Differences in data formats, collection function and quality model in institutions can affect stability, and require strong standardization protocols.

Safety risk: Although FL data reduces exposure, harmful attacks and model - facing techniques persist, which requires continuous progress in cyber security.

Integration complexity: Applying to existing health care infrastructure requires differences between different systems and match frameworks, faced technical and logical challenges (Kalkatawi, 2025).

13. FUTURE INSTRUCTIONS AND INNOVATIONS

Federal Learning with Blockchain: By mixing off with blockchain technology, it can increase safety, traceability and transparency in the AI-operated health care system by ensuring tamper-proof data exchange (Kasralikar et al., 2025).

Individual Federal Learning Model: The AI model can be adapted to individual patients while maintaining collective intelligence from multiple sources, increasing the exact drug.

Edge AI in health services: Integration of FL with Edge AI can enable Ultra-fast medical insight to directly on devices such as mobile phones and smart watches, which reduces the dependence on cloud calculation (van Genderen et al., 2024).

Federal Transfer Learning: AI model for rare diseases can improve adaptability of rare diseases and reduce patient demographics by expanding medical research opportunities for rare diseases.

Supervisory authorities and ethical infrastructure: The ongoing development of global standards and guidelines will provide FL -adoption in mainstream health systems, which ensures moral AI distribution and patient confidence.

CONCLUSION

Federal Learning revolutionizes AI in the way of integrating into the health care system, providing a strong framework for privacy preservation that improves cooperation between medical institutions, research organizations and technology suppliers. By enabling decentralized training of the AI model, FL not only ensures compliance with strict data security law, but also accelerates the development of more accurate and general health services. The adoption of FL in the health care system has the ability to make significant advances in individual medical, initial disease detection and significant progress in monitoring a skilled patient. With its ability to collect insights from different data sets in many health institutions, FL AI helps to reduce bias in models, which improves the accuracy and treatment efficiency of the diagnosis.

Notwithstanding its many advantages, FL implementation continues to face obstacles such as computational overhead, communication impairments, and institutional standards for standardized protocols. In order to address these issues, governments, regulatory agencies, and health care system stakeholders must collaborate, invest in safe AI frameworks, and conduct ongoing research.

The future of federal learning in the health care system appears bright when we take a closer look. FL will play a significant role in encouraging the innovation of the global health care system since technological advancements increase privacy preservation AI techniques. The impact will be further strengthened by integrating FL with cutting-edge technologies like Blockchain, Edge Computing, and Safe Multi-Party computations, which opens the door to a health care system that is more effective, secure, and connected. Patients in the healthcare system can fully utilize AIS while preserving the integrity of their data by adopting Federated learning.

REFERENCES

Abdulrahman, S., Tout, H., Ould-Slimane, H., Mourad, A., Talhi, C., & Guizani, M. (2021). A survey on Federated learning: The journey from centralized to distributed on-site learning and beyond. *IEEE Internet of Things Journal, 8*(7), 5476–5497. DOI: 10.1109/JIOT.2020.3030072

Alowais, S. A., Alghamdi, S. S., Alsuhebany, N., Alqahtani, T., Alshaya, A. I., Almohareb, S. N., Aldairem, A., Alrashed, M., Bin Saleh, K., Badreldin, H. A., Al Yami, M. S., Al Harbi, S., & Albekairy, A. M. (2023). Revolutionizing healthcare: The role of artificial intelligence in clinical practice. *BMC Medical Education, 23*(1), 689. DOI: 10.1186/s12909-023-04698-z PMID: 37740191

Beniwal, S., Saini, U., Garg, P., & Joon, R. K. (2021). Improving performance during camera surveillance by integration of edge detection in IoT system. [IJEHMC]. *International Journal of E-Health and Medical Communications, 12*(5), 84–96. DOI: 10.4018/IJEHMC.20210901.oa6

Bhagoji, A. N., Chakraborty, S., Mittal, P., & Calo, S. (2019). Analyzing Federated learning through an adversarial lens. *International Conference on Machine Learning*, 634–643.

Blanchard, P., El Mhamdi, E. M., Guerraoui, R., & Stainer, J. (2017). Machine learning with adversaries: Byzantine tolerant gradient descent. *Advances in Neural Information Processing Systems*, 30.

Garg, P., Sharma, N., & Shukla, B. (2023). Predicting the Risk of Cardiovascular Diseases using Machine Learning Techniques. *International Journal of Intelligent Systems and Applications in Engineering, 11*(2s), 165–173.

Hong, Q., Jun, M., Bo, W., Sichao, T., Jiayi, Z., Biao, L., Tong, L., & Ruifeng, T. (2023). Application of Data-Driven technology in nuclear Engineering: Prediction, classification and design optimization. *Annals of Nuclear Energy, 194*, 110089. DOI: 10.1016/j.anucene.2023.110089

Hu, K., Gong, S., Zhang, Q., Seng, C., Xia, M., & Jiang, S. (2024). An overview of implementing security and privacy in Federated learning. *Artificial Intelligence Review, 57*(8), 204. DOI: 10.1007/s10462-024-10846-8

Kalkatawi, M. (2025). Beyond the upgrade: Unraveling the complexities of health information system migration. *Discover Health Systems, 4*(1), 7. DOI: 10.1007/s44250-025-00186-x

Kasralikar, P., Polu, O. R., Chamarthi, B., Rupavath, R. V. S. S. B., Patel, S., & Tumati, R. (2025). Blockchain for securing AI-driven healthcare systems: A systematic review and future research perspectives. *Cureus, 17*(4). Advance online publication. DOI: 10.7759/cureus.83136 PMID: 40438823

Khalid, N., Qayyum, A., Bilal, M., Al-Fuqaha, A., & Qadir, J. (2023). Privacy-preserving artificial intelligence in healthcare: Techniques and applications. *Computers in Biology and Medicine, 158*, 106848. DOI: 10.1016/j.compbiomed.2023.106848 PMID: 37044052

Khan, A. (2024). Optimisation methods based on soft computing for improving power system stability. *J. Electrical Systems, 20*(6s), 1051–1058. DOI: 10.52783/jes.2837

Lyu, L., Yu, H., & Yang, Q. (2020). Threats to Federated learning: A survey. *ArXiv Preprint ArXiv:2003.02133.*

Maggo, C., & Garg, P. (2022). From linguistic features to their extractions: Understanding the semantics of a concept. *2022 Fifth International Conference on Computational Intelligence and Communication Technologies (CCICT)*, 427–431. DOI: 10.1109/CCiCT56684.2022.00082

Malik, M., Garg, P., & Malik, C. (2024). Artificial intelligence-based prediction of health risks among women during menopause. *Artificial Intelligence and Machine Learning for Women's Health Issues*, 137–150.

McMahan, B., Moore, E., Ramage, D., Hampson, S., & y Arcas, B. A. (2017). Communication-efficient learning of deep networks from decentralized data. *Artificial Intelligence and Statistics*, 1273–1282.

Meurisch, C., Bayrak, B., & Mühlhäuser, M. (2020). Privacy-preserving AI services through data decentralization. *Proceedings of The Web Conference 2020*, 190–200. DOI: 10.1145/3366423.3380106

Mohammadi, S., Balador, A., Sinaei, S., & Flammini, F. (2024). Balancing privacy and performance in Federated learning: A systematic literature review on methods and metrics. *Journal of Parallel and Distributed Computing, 192*, 104918. DOI: 10.1016/j.jpdc.2024.104918

Rahman, A., Hossain, M. S., Muhammad, G., Kundu, D., Debnath, T., Rahman, M., Khan, M. S. I., Tiwari, P., & Band, S. S. (2023). Federated learning-based AI approaches in smart healthcare: Concepts, taxonomies, challenges and open issues. *Cluster Computing, 26*(4), 2271–2311. DOI: 10.1007/s10586-022-03658-4 PMID: 35996680

Rajput, R., Sukumar, V., Patnaik, P., Garg, P., & Ranjan, M. (2024). The Cognitive Analysis for an Approach to Neuroscience. *2024 International Conference on Automation and Computation (AUTOCOM)*, 524–528. DOI: 10.1109/AUTOCOM60220.2024.10486081

Roth, H. R., Cheng, Y., Wen, Y., Yang, I., Xu, Z., Hsieh, Y.-T., Kersten, K., Harouni, A., Zhao, C., Lu, K., & Associates. (2022). Nvidia flare: Federated learning from simulation to real-world. *ArXiv Preprint ArXiv:2210.13291.*

Sharma, S., Mittal, S., Tevatia, R., Tyagi, V. K., Garg, P., & Kapoor, S. (2025). Unlocking Workforce Potential. *AI-Powered Predictive Models for Employee Performance Evaluation.*, (May), 143–149. DOI: 10.63169/GCARED2025.p21

Upadhyay, D., Garg, P., Aldossary, S. M., Shafi, J., & Kumar, S. (2023). A linear quadratic regression-based synchronised health monitoring system (SHMS) for IoT applications. *Electronics (Basel)*, *12*(2), 309. DOI: 10.3390/electronics12020309

Upreti, D., Yang, E., Kim, H., & Seo, C. (2024). A Comprehensive Survey on Federated Learning in the Healthcare Area: Concept and Applications. *CMES-Computer Modeling in Engineering \& Sciences, 140*(3).

van Genderen, M. E., Cecconi, M., & Jung, C. (2024). Federated data access and Federated learning: Improved data sharing, AI model development, and learning in intensive care. *Intensive Care Medicine*, *50*(6), 974–977. DOI: 10.1007/s00134-024-07408-5 PMID: 38635044

Vasilev, Y., Rumyantsev, D., Vladzymyrskyy, A., Omelyanskaya, O., Pestrenin, L., Shulkin, I., Nikitin, E., Kapninskiy, A., & Arzamasov, K. (2025). Evolution of an Artificial Intelligence-Powered Application for Mammography. *Diagnostics (Basel)*, *15*(7), 822. DOI: 10.3390/diagnostics15070822 PMID: 40218172

Vora, L. K., Gholap, A. D., Jetha, K., Thakur, R. R. S., Solanki, H. K., & Chavda, V. P. (2023). Artificial intelligence in pharmaceutical technology and drug delivery design. *Pharmaceutics*, *15*(7), 1916. DOI: 10.3390/pharmaceutics15071916 PMID: 37514102

Yurdem, B., Kuzlu, M., Gullu, M. K., Catak, F. O., & Tabassum, M. (2024). Federated learning: Overview, strategies, applications, tools and future directions. *Heliyon*, *10*(19), e38137. DOI: 10.1016/j.heliyon.2024.e38137 PMID: 39391509

Zhang, F., Kreuter, D., Chen, Y., Dittmer, S., Tull, S., Shadbahr, T., Schut, M., Asselbergs, F., Kar, S., Sivapalaratnam, S., Williams, S., Koh, M., Henskens, Y., de Wit, B., D'Alessandro, U., Bah, B., Secka, O., Nachev, P., Gupta, R., & Roberts, M. (2024). Recent methodological advances in Federated learning for healthcare. *Patterns (New York, N.Y.)*, *5*(6), 101006. DOI: 10.1016/j.patter.2024.101006 PMID: 39005485

Zhao, Y., Chen, J., Zhang, J., Yang, Z., Tu, H., Han, H., Zhu, K., & Chen, B. (2021). User-Level Membership Inference for Federated Learning in Wireless Network Environment. *Wireless Communications and Mobile Computing*, *2021*(1), 5534270. DOI: 10.1155/2021/5534270

Compilation of References

Abadi, M., Chu, A., Goodfellow, I., McMahan, H. B., Mironov, I., Talwar, K., & Zhang, L. (2016). Deep learning with differential privacy. In *Proceedings of the 2016 ACM SIGSAC Conference on Computer and Communications Security* (pp. 308–318). ACM. https://doi.org/DOI: 10.1145/2976749.2978318

Abbas, S. R., Abbas, Z., Zahir, A., & Lee, S. W. (2024). Federated Learning in Smart Healthcare: A Comprehensive Review on Privacy, Security, and Predictive Analytics with IoT Integration. *Health Care*, *12*(24), 2587. DOI: 10.3390/healthcare12242587 PMID: 39766014

Abdulrahman, S., Tout, H., Ould-Slimane, H., Mourad, A., Talhi, C., & Guizani, M. (2021). A survey on Federated learning: The journey from centralized to distributed on-site learning and beyond. *IEEE Internet of Things Journal*, *8*(7), 5476–5497. DOI: 10.1109/JIOT.2020.3030072

Abreha, H. G., Hayajneh, M., & Serhani, M. A. (2022). Federated learning in edge computing: A systematic survey. *Sensors (Basel)*, *22*(2), 450. DOI: 10.3390/s22020450 PMID: 35062410

Acar, A., Aksu, H., Uluagac, A. S., & Conti, M. (2018). A survey on homomorphic encryption schemes: Theory and implementation. *ACM Computing Surveys*, *51*(4), 1–35. DOI: 10.1145/3214303

Adewunmi, M. C. (2025). Parents as catalysts for structural transformation toward inclusive and sustainable development. *International Journal of Social and Educational Innovation (IJSEIro)*, 42–64.

Adnan, M., Syed, M. H., Anjum, A., & Rehman, S. (2025). *A Framework for privacy-preserving in IoV using Federated Learning with Differential Privacy*. IEEE., DOI: 10.1109/ACCESS.2025.3526934

Agarwal, A., Verma, A., & Khari, M. (2024). Comparative assessment of machine learning methods for early prediction of diseases using health indicators. In *Approaches to Human-Centered AI in Healthcare* (pp. 160–186). IGI Global., DOI: 10.4018/979-8-3693-2238-3.ch007

Agbley, B. L. Y., Li, J. P., Haq, A. U., Bankas, E. K., Mawuli, C. B., Ahmad, S., Khan, S., & Khan, A. R. (2024). Federated Fusion of Magnified Histopathological Images for Breast Tumor Classification in the Internet of Medical Things. *IEEE Journal of Biomedical and Health Informatics*, *28*(6), 3389–3400. DOI: 10.1109/JBHI.2023.3256974 PMID: 37028353

Akter, M., Moustafa, N., Lynar, T., & Razzak, I. (2022). Edge intelligence: Federated learning-based privacy protection framework for smart healthcare systems. *IEEE Journal of Biomedical and Health Informatics*, *26*(12), 5805–5816. DOI: 10.1109/JBHI.2022.3192648 PMID: 35857737

Alanazi, A. S., Benlaria, H., & Alanazi, S. A. (2025). Sustainable assistive technology and employment opportunities for graduates with disability: Mediating role of government support. *Education and Information Technologies*, *30*(1), 257–278. DOI: 10.1007/s10639-024-12863-0

Alghamdi, W., Salama, R., Sirija, M., Abbas, A. R., & Dilnoza, K. (2023). Secure multi-party computation for collaborative data analysis. E3S Web of Conferences, 399, 04034. https://doi.org/DOI: 10.1051/e3sconf/202339904034

Al-Huthaifi, R., Li, T., Huang, W., Gu, J., & Li, C. (2023). Federated learning in smart cities: Privacy and security survey. *Information Sciences*, *632*, 833–857. DOI: 10.1016/j.ins.2023.03.033

Alibudbud, R. C., Aruta, J. J. B. R., Sison, K. A., & Guinto, R. R. (2025). Artificial intelligence in the era of planetary health: Insights on its application for the climate change-mental health nexus in the Philippines. *International Review of Psychiatry (Abingdon, England)*, *37*(1), 21–32. DOI: 10.1080/09540261.2024.2363373 PMID: 40035376

Ali, M., Naeem, F., Tariq, M., & Kaddoum, G. (2023). Federated Learning for Privacy Preservation in Smart Healthcare Systems: A Comprehensive Survey. *IEEE Journal of Biomedical and Health Informatics*, *27*(2), 778–789. DOI: 10.1109/JBHI.2022.3181823 PMID: 35696470

Almalki, J., Alshahrani, S. M., & Khan, N. A. (2024). A comprehensive secure system enabling healthcare 5.0 using federated learning, intrusion detection and blockchain. *PeerJ. Computer Science*, *10*, e1778. Advance online publication. DOI: 10.7717/peerj-cs.1778 PMID: 38259900

Almeida, D., & Beleg, J. (2025). Ethical implications of predictive analytics in personalized healthcare. In Navigating Privacy, Innovation, and Patient Empowerment Through Ethical Healthcare Technology (pp. 57–82). IGI Global. DOI: 10.4018/979-8-3693-7630-0.ch003

Almogadwy, B., & Alqarafi, A. (2025). Fused federated learning framework for secure and decentralized patient monitoring in healthcare 5.0 using IoMT. *Scientific Reports, 15*(1), 24263--. DOI: 10.1038/s41598-025-06574-w

Almufareh, M. F., Tehsin, S., Humayun, M., & Kausar, S. (2023). Intellectual disability and technology: An artificial intelligence perspective and framework. *Journal of Disability Research*, *2*(4), 58–70. DOI: 10.57197/JDR-2023-0055

Alowais, S. A., Alghamdi, S. S., Alsuhebany, N., Alqahtani, T., Alshaya, A. I., Almohareb, S. N., Aldairem, A., Alrashed, M., Bin Saleh, K., Badreldin, H. A., Al Yami, M. S., Al Harbi, S., & Albekairy, A. M. (2023). Revolutionizing healthcare: The role of artificial intelligence in clinical practice. *BMC Medical Education*, *23*(1), 689. DOI: 10.1186/s12909-023-04698-z PMID: 37740191

Alruwaili, M., Siddiqi, M. H., Idris, M., Alruwaili, S., Alanazi, A. S., & Khan, F. (2025). Advancing disability healthcare solutions through privacy-preserving federated learning with Theme framework. *Expert Systems: International Journal of Knowledge Engineering and Neural Networks*, *42*(1), e13807. Advance online publication. DOI: 10.1111/exsy.13807

Alshareet, O., & Awasthi, A. (2025). A Novel Framework for Integrating Blockchain-Driven Federated Learning with Neural Networks in E-Commerce. *Journal of Network and Systems Management*, *33*(3), 56. Advance online publication. DOI: 10.1007/s10922-025-09928-x

Amin, M. S., Ahmad, S., & Loh, W. K. (2025). Federated learning for Healthcare 5.0: A comprehensive survey, taxonomy, challenges, and solutions. *Soft Computing*, *29*(2), 673–700. DOI: 10.1007/s00500-025-10508-z

Andersen, H. U., Hangaard, S., Hommel, E., & Ridderstråle, M. (2018). Six-year follow-up after insulin pump initiation: HbA1c is significantly reduced without weight gain. *Journal of Diabetes Science and Technology*, *12*(2), 535–536. DOI: 10.1177/1932296817731424 PMID: 28927286

Antunes, R. S., André da Costa, C., Küderle, A., Yari, I. A., & Eskofier, B. (2022). Federated learning for healthcare: Systematic review and architecture proposal. [TIST]. *ACM Transactions on Intelligent Systems and Technology*, *13*(4), 1–23. DOI: 10.1145/3501813

Aouedi, O., Sacco, A., Piamrat, K., & Marchetto, G. (2023). Handling privacy-sensitive medical data with federated learning: Challenges and future directions. *IEEE Journal of Biomedical and Health Informatics*, *27*(2), 790–803. DOI: 10.1109/JBHI.2022.3185673 PMID: 35737624

Arefin, S. (2024). Strengthening Healthcare Data Security with Ai-Powered Threat Detection. [IJSRM]. *International Journal of Scientific Research and Management*, *12*(10), 1477–1483. DOI: 10.18535/ijsrm/v12i10.ec02

Arya, V., Bellamy, R. K., Chen, P. Y., Dhurandhar, A., Hind, M., Hoffman, S. C., & Zhang, Y. (2019). One explanation does not fit all: A toolkit and taxonomy of AI explainability techniques. arXiv. https://arxiv.org/abs/1909.03012

Asiimwe, R., Lam, S., Leung, S., Wang, S., Wan, R., Tinker, A., McAlpine, J. N., Woo, M. M. M., Huntsman, D. G., & Talhouk, A. (2021). From biobank and data silos into a data common: Convergence to support translational medicine. *Journal of Translational Medicine*, *19*(1), 493. DOI: 10.1186/s12967-021-03147-z PMID: 34863191

Ayaz, M., Pasha, M. F., Alzahrani, M. Y., Budiarto, R., & Stiawan, D. (2021). The Fast Health Interoperability Resources (FHIR) standard: Systematic literature review of implementations, applications, challenges and opportunities. *JMIR Medical Informatics*, *9*(7), e21929. DOI: 10.2196/21929 PMID: 34328424

Aziz, R., Banerjee, S., Bouzefrane, S., & Le Vinh, T. (2023). Exploring Homomorphic Encryption and Differential Privacy Techniques towards Secure Federated Learning Paradigm. *Future Internet*, *15*(9), 310. DOI: 10.3390/fi15090310

Azrour, M., Mabrouki, J., Guezzaz, A., Ahmad, S., Khan, S., & Benkirane, S. (2024). IoT, Machine Learning and Data Analytics for Smart Healthcare. In *IoT, Machine Learning and Data Analytics for Smart Healthcare* (pp. 1–94). CRC Press. DOI: 10.1201/9781003430735

Baalous, R., Poet, R., & Storer, T. (2018, April). Analyzing privacy policies of zero knowledge cloud storage applications on mobile devices. In 2018 Institute of Electrical and Electronics Engineers International Conference on Cloud Engineering (IC2E) 218-224. Institute of Electrical and Electronics Engineers. https://doi.org/DOI: 10.1109/IC2E.2018.00047

Babu, A. A., Jebamalar, G. B., Kumar, P., & Nalini, M. (2024, December). Blockchain Technology: Evolution and Future Prospects. In *2024 International Conference on Sustainable Communication Networks and Application (ICSCNA)* (pp. 381-387). IEEE. DOI: 10.1109/ICSCNA63714.2024.10864089

Bagdasaryan, E., Veit, A., Hua, Y., Estrin, D., & Shmatikov, V. (2020). How to backdoor federated learning. In Proceedings of the 23rd International Conference on Artificial Intelligence and Statistics (pp. 2938–2948). PMLR. http://proceedings.mlr.press/v108/bagdasaryan20a/bagdasaryan20a.pdf

Bagdasaryan, E., Veit, A., Hua, Y., Estrin, D., & Shmatikov, V. (2020, June). How to backdoor federated learning. In *International conference on artificial intelligence and statistics* (pp. 2938-2948). PMLR.

Balek, V., Sýkora, L., Sklenák, V., & Kliegr, T. (2024). LLM-based feature generation from text for interpretable machine learning. arXiv preprint arXiv:2409.07132. https://arxiv.org/pdf/2409.07132

Banabilah, S., Aloqaily, M., Alsayed, E., Malik, N., & Jararweh, Y. (2022). Federated learning review: Fundamentals, enabling technologies, and future applications. *Information Processing & Management*, *59*(6), 103061. DOI: 10.1016/j.ipm.2022.103061

Barnawi, A., Chhikara, P., Tekchandani, R., Kumar, N., & Alzahrani, B. (2024). A Differentially Privacy Assisted Federated Learning Scheme to Preserve Data Privacy for IoMT Applications. *IEEE Transactions on Network and Service Management*, *21*(4), 4686–4700. DOI: 10.1109/TNSM.2024.3393969

Barth, S. (2023, April 14). AI in healthcare. *ForeSee Medical*. https://www.foreseemed.com/artificial-intelligence-in-healthcare

Bashir, A. K., Victor, N., Bhattacharya, S., Huynh-The, T., Chengoden, R., Yenduri, G., Maddikunta, P. K. R., Pham, Q.-V., Gadekallu, T. R., & Liyanage, M. (2023). Federated learning for the healthcare metaverse: Concepts, applications, challenges, and future directions. *IEEE Internet of Things Journal*, *10*(24), 21873–21891. DOI: 10.1109/JIOT.2023.3304790

Baucas, M., Spachos, P., & Plataniotis, K. (2023). Federated learning and blockchain-enabled fog-IoT platform for wearables in predictive healthcare. *arXiv*. https://arxiv.org/abs/2301.04511

Bayerl, S. P., Frassetto, T., Jauernig, P., Riedhammer, K., Sadeghi, A. R., Schneider, T. & Weinert, C. (2020, March). Offline model guard: Secure and private ML on mobile devices. In 2020 Design, Automation & Test in Europe Conference & Exhibition, 460-465. Institute of Electrical and Electronics Engineers https://doi.org/.DOI: 10.23919/DATE48585.2020.9116560

Beam, A. L., Manrai, A. K., & Ghassemi, M. (2020). Challenges to the reproducibility of machine learning models in health care. *Journal of the American Medical Association*, *323*(4), 305–306. DOI: 10.1001/jama.2019.20866 PMID: 31904799

Beck, T., & Ward, H. (1961). An inventory for measuring depression. *Archives of General Psychiatry*, *4*(6), 561–571. DOI: 10.1001/archpsyc.1961.01710120031004 PMID: 13688369

Beniwal, S., Saini, U., Garg, P., & Joon, R. K. (2021). Improving performance during camera surveillance by integration of edge detection in IoT system. [IJEHMC]. *International Journal of E-Health and Medical Communications*, *12*(5), 84–96. DOI: 10.4018/IJEHMC.20210901.oa6

Benkhadra, K., Alahdab, F., Tamhane, S. U., McCoy, R. G., Prokop, L. J., & Murad, M. H. (2017). Continuous subcutaneous insulin infusion versus multiple daily injections in individuals with type 1 diabetes: A systematic review and meta-analysis. *Endocrine*, *55*(1), 77–84. DOI: 10.1007/s12020-016-1039-x PMID: 27477293

Berget, C., Lange, S., Messer, L., & Forlenza, G. P. (2020). A clinical review of the t:slim X2 insulin pump. *Expert Opinion on Drug Delivery*, *17*(12), 1675–1687. DOI: 10.1080/17425247.2020.1814734 PMID: 32842794

Berget, C., Messer, L. H., & Forlenza, G. P. (2019). A clinical overview of insulin pump therapy for the management of diabetes: Past, present, and future of intensive therapy. *Diabetes Spectrum*, *32*(3), 194–204. DOI: 10.2337/ds18-0091 PMID: 31462873

Bhagoji, A. N., Chakraborty, S., Mittal, P., & Calo, S. (2019). Analyzing Federated learning through an adversarial lens. *International Conference on Machine Learning*, 634–643.

Bhardwaj, T., & Sumangali, K. (2025). An explainable federated blockchain framework with privacy-preserving AI optimization for securing healthcare data. *Scientific Reports, 15*(1), 21799--. DOI: 10.1038/s41598-025-04083-4

Blanchard, S. (2025, May 13). Inside the cutting-edge NHS wards where robots assist surgeons – turning major ops into day cases. *The Scottish Sun*. https://www.thescottishsun.co.uk/health/14781345/million-pound-machine-keyhole-surgery-health-operations/

Blanchard, P., El Mhamdi, E. M., Guerraoui, R., & Stainer, J. (2017). Machine learning with adversaries: Byzantine tolerant gradient descent. *Advances in Neural Information Processing Systems*, 30.

Bogdanova, A., Attoh-Okine, N., & Sakurai, T. (2020). Risk and advantages of federated learning for health care data collaboration. *ASCE-ASME Journal of Risk and Uncertainty in Engineering Systems. Part A, Civil Engineering*, *6*(3), 04020027. Advance online publication. DOI: 10.1061/AJRUA6.0001078

Bonawitz, K.. (2023). Towards federated learning at scale: System design. *Proceedings of Machine Learning and Systems, 1*, 374–388. https://arxiv.org/abs/1902.01046

Bonawitz, K., Ivanov, V., Kreuter, B., Marcedone, A., McMahan, H. B., Patel, S., Ramage, D., Segal, A., & Seth, K. (2017). Practical secure aggregation for privacy-preserving machine learning. In *Proceedings of the 2017 ACM SIGSAC Conference on Computer and Communications Security* (pp. 1175-1191). DOI: 10.1145/3133956.3133982

Boopathi, S., & Khang, A. (2023). AI-integrated technology for a secure and ethical healthcare ecosystem. In *AI and IoT-Based Technologies for Precision Medicine* (pp. 36–59). IGI Global. DOI: 10.4018/979-8-3693-0876-9.ch003

Boughorbel, S., Jarray, F., Venugopal, N., Moosa, S., Elhadi, H., & Makhlouf, M. (2019). Federated uncertainty-aware learning for distributed hospital ehr data. *arXiv preprint arXiv:1910.12191.*

Brauneck, A., Schmalhorst, L., Kazemi Majdabadi, M. M., Bakhtiari, M., Völker, U., Baumbach, J., Baumbach, L., & Buchholtz, G. (2023). Federated machine learning, privacy-enhancing technologies, and data protection laws in medical research: Scoping review. *Journal of Medical Internet Research, 25*, e41588. DOI: 10.2196/41588 PMID: 36995759

Brien, M., Coutinho, F., Krishna, D., van der Haar, L., de Laat, J., Srinivasan, S. R., & Venkatachalapathy, N. (2023). Leveraging monitoring, evaluation, and learning to scale the Enabling Inclusion® program for children with disabilities in India and globally. *Frontiers in Public Health, 11*, 1165034. DOI: 10.3389/fpubh.2023.1165034 PMID: 38162603

Brisimi, T. S., Chen, R., Mela, T., Olshevsky, A., Paschalidis, I. C., & Shi, W. (2018). Federated learning of predictive models from federated electronic health records. *International Journal of Medical Informatics, 112*, 59–67. DOI: 10.1016/j.ijmedinf.2018.01.007 PMID: 29500022

Brown, T. B., Mann, B., Ryder, N., Subbiah, M., Kaplan, J., Dhariwal, P., & Amodei, D. (2020). *Language models are few-shot learners* (Vol. 33). Advances in Neural Information Processing Systems, https://arxiv.org/abs/2005.14165

Budrionis, A., Miara, M., Miara, P., Wilk, S., & Bellika, J. G. (2021). Benchmarking PySyft federated learning framework on MIMIC-III dataset. *IEEE Access : Practical Innovations, Open Solutions, 9*, 116869–116878. DOI: 10.1109/ACCESS.2021.3105929

Cardona-Acevedo, S., Agudelo-Ceballos, E., Cumpa Vásquez, J. T., Martínez Rojas, E., Valencia-Arias, A., Jimenez Garcia, J. A., & Benjumea-Arias, M. L. (2025, March). E-learning technologies at the secondary education level: Literature review. [). Frontiers Media SA.]. *Frontiers in Education, 10*, 1539763. DOI: 10.3389/feduc.2025.1539763

Cellamare, M., Van Gestel, A. J., Alradhi, H., Martin, F., & Moncada-Torres, A. (2022). A Federated Generalized Linear Model for Privacy-Preserving Analysis. *Algorithms, 15*(7), 243. DOI: 10.3390/a15070243

Chaddad, A., Wu, Y., & Desrosiers, C. (2023). Federated learning for healthcare applications. *IEEE Internet of Things Journal, 11*(5), 7339–7358. DOI: 10.1109/JIOT.2023.3325822

Chamikara, M. A. P., Bertok, P., Khalil, I., Liu, D., & Camtepe, S. (2021). Privacy preserving distributed machine learning with federated learning. *Computer Communications, 171*, 112–125. DOI: 10.1016/j.comcom.2021.02.014

Chandra, S., Fane, J., Azizi, N., McKenzie-Gray, M., Sager, M., & Dautenhahn, K. (2025). Integrating New Instructional Assistive Technology to Support Academic and Behavioural Instruction for Students with Learning Disabilities. *Journal of Special Education Technology* 01626434251314042. DOI: 10.1177/01626434251314042

Chattopadhyay, S., & Das, S. (2024). Safeguarding Privacy Through Federated Machine Learning Techniques. In *Emerging Technologies and Security in Cloud Computing* (pp. 295–318). IGI Global Scientific Publishing. DOI: 10.4018/979-8-3693-2081-5.ch013

Chelani, N., Tripathy, S., Kumhar, M., Bhatia, J., Saxena, V., Tanwar, S., & Nayyar, A. (2024). Federated Learning for Internet of medical healthcare: Issues and challenges. *Scalable Computing Practice and Experience, 25*(5), 4442–4455. DOI: 10.12694/scpe.v25i5.2905

Chen, Y., Yang, X., Qin, X., Yu, H., Chen, J., & Sun, J. (2021). FedHealth 2: Weighted federated transfer learning via batch normalization for personalized healthcare. In Machine Learning for Healthcare Conference (pp. 1-22).

Chen, J., Yi, C., Okegbile, S. D., Cai, J., & Shen, X. (2024). Networking Architecture and Key Supporting Technologies for Human Digital Twin in Personalized Healthcare: A Comprehensive Survey. *IEEE Communications Surveys and Tutorials, 26*(1), 706–746. DOI: 10.1109/COMST.2023.3308717

Chen, K., Chen, H., Conway, N., Hellerstein, J. M., & Parikh, T. S. (2011). Usher: Improving data quality with dynamic forms. *IEEE Transactions on Knowledge and Data Engineering, 23*(8), 1138–1153. DOI: 10.1109/TKDE.2011.31

Chen, M., Shlezinger, N., Poor, H. V., Eldar, Y. C., & Cui, S. (2021). Communication-efficient federated learning. *Proceedings of the National Academy of Sciences of the United States of America, 118*(17), e2024789118. DOI: 10.1073/pnas.2024789118 PMID: 33888586

Chen, Y., Lu, W., Qin, X., Wang, J., & Xie, X. (2024). MetaFed: Federated learning among federations with cyclic knowledge distillation for personalized healthcare. *IEEE Transactions on Neural Networks and Learning Systems, 35*(11), 16671–16682. DOI: 10.1109/TNNLS.2023.3297103 PMID: 37506019

Chen, Y., Qin, X., Wang, J., Yu, C., & Gao, W. (2020). FedHealth: A Federated Transfer Learning Framework for Wearable Healthcare. *IEEE Intelligent Systems, 35*(4), 83–93. DOI: 10.1109/MIS.2020.2988604

Chien, M. N., Chen, Y. J., Bai, C. H., & Huang, J. T. (2022). Continuous glucose monitoring system based on percutaneous microneedle array. *Micromachines, 13*(3), 478. DOI: 10.3390/mi13030478 PMID: 35334773

Choi, E., Schuetz, A., Stewart, W. F., & Sun, J. (2016). Using recurrent neural network models for early detection of heart failure onset. *Journal of the American Medical Informatics Association : JAMIA, 24*(2), 361–370. DOI: 10.1093/jamia/ocw112 PMID: 27521897

Choi, J., & Lee, S. (2017). *Efficient memory-mapped file I/O for in-memory file systems*. In *Proceedings of the 9th USENIX Workshop on Hot Topics in Storage and File Systems (HotStorage '17)*. USENIX Association.

Choi, R. Y., Coyner, A. S., Kalpathy-Cramer, J., Chiang, M. F., & Campbell, J. P. (2020). Introduction to machine learning, neural networks, and deep learning. *Translational Vision Science & Technology, 9*(2), 14. DOI: 10.1167/tvst.9.2.14 PMID: 32704420

Choudhury, A., Sarma, K. K., Gulvanskii, V., Kaplun, D., & Dutta, L. (2025). Leveraging federated learning and edge computing for pandemic-resilient healthcare. *Scientific Reports, 15*(1), 20497--. DOI: 10.1038/s41598-025-00199-9

Clements, M., Matuleviciene, V., Attvall, S., Ekelund, M., Pivodic, A., Dahlqvist, S., Fahlén, M., Haraldsson, B., & Lind, M. (2015). Predicting the effectiveness of insulin pump therapy on glycemic control in clinical practice: A retrospective study of patients with type 1 diabetes from 10 outpatient diabetes clinics in Sweden over 5 years. *Diabetes Technology & Therapeutics, 17*(1), 21–28. DOI: 10.1089/dia.2014.0139 PMID: 25470010

Cohen, B. M., & Mills, A. (2015). The Diagnostic Drawing Series (DDS) at thirty: Art therapy assessment and research. The Wiley handbook of art therapy, 558-568. https://doi.org/DOI: 10.1002/9781118306543.ch53

Cohen, I. G., & Mello, M. M. (2018). HIPAA and protecting health information in the 21st century. *Journal of the American Medical Association, 320*(3), 231–232. DOI: 10.1001/jama.2018.5630 PMID: 29800120

Crabtree, J. S., & Miele, L. (2022). Precision diagnostics in cancer: Predict, prevent, and personalize. In Progress in Molecular Biology and Translational Science (pp. 39–56). Elsevier. DOI: 10.1016/bs.pmbts.2022.03.005

Cubas, A. L. V., Provin, A. P., Dutra, A. R. D. A., Andrade Guerra, J. B. S. O. D., & Mussi, C. C. (2025). Forging a sustainable path: The QualEnv consortium's practices and strategies in promoting sustainable development in higher education institutions. *International Journal of Sustainability in Higher Education, 26*(1), 63–82. DOI: 10.1108/IJSHE-11-2023-0514

Cui, L., Qu, Y., Xie, G., Zeng, D., Li, R., Shen, S., & Yu, S. (2021). Security and privacy-enhanced federated learning for anomaly detection in IoT infrastructures. *IEEE Transactions on Industrial Informatics, 18*(5), 3492–3500. DOI: 10.1109/TII.2021.3107783

Dankar, F. K., & El Emam, K. (2013). Practicing differential privacy in health care: A review. *Transactions on Data Privacy*, 35–67. https://www.tdp.cat/issues11/tdp.a129a13.pdf

David, R., Duke, J., Jain, A., Janapa Reddi, V., & Jeffries, N., Li, Rhodes, R. (2021). Tensorflow lite micro: Embedded machine learning for tinyml systems. *Proceedings of Machine Learning and Systems, 3*, 800–811. https://proceedings.mlsys.org/paper_files/paper/2021/file/6c44dc73014d66ba49b28d483a8f8b0d-Paper.pdf

Dayan, I., Roth, H. R., Zhong, A., Harouni, A., Gentili, A., Abidin, A. Z., Lui, Y. W., Costa, A. B., Wood, B. J., Tsai, C. S., Li, K., Cheng, Y., McKenzie, S., Liu, A., Costa, A. F., Gidwani, M., Patel, V., Balachandar, N., Zhao, C., & Xu, D. (2021). Federated learning for predicting clinical outcomes in patients with COVID-19. *Nature Medicine, 27*(10), 1735–1743. DOI: 10.1038/s41591-021-01506-3 PMID: 34526699

Denny, J. C., Ritchie, M. D., Basford, M. A., Pulley, J. M., Bastarache, L., Brown-Gentry, K., Wang, D., Masys, D. R., Roden, D. M., & Crawford, D. C. (2010). PheWAS: Demonstrating the feasibility of a phenome-wide scan to discover gene–disease associations. *Bioinformatics (Oxford, England)*, *26*(9), 1205–1210. DOI: 10.1093/bioinformatics/btq126 PMID: 20335276

Dettmers, T., Pagnoni, A., Holtzman, A., & Smith, N. A. (2022). QLoRA: Efficient fine-tuning of quantized LLMs. *Proceedings of the 2023 International Conference on Machine Learning (ICML)*. https://arxiv.org/abs/2305.14314

Dhinakaran, D., Kumar, N. J., & Ponnuviji, N. P. (2025). Safeguarding confidentiality and privacy in cloud-enabled healthcare systems with spectrasafe encryption and dynamic k-anonymity algorithm. *Expert Systems with Applications*, *279*, 127584. DOI: 10.1016/j.eswa.2025.127584

Diaz-Rodríguez, N., Del Ser, J., Coeckelbergh, M., de Prado, M. L., Herrera-Viedma, E., & Herrera, F. (2023). Connecting the dots in trustworthy Artificial Intelligence: From AI principles, ethics, and key requirements to responsible AI systems and regulation. *Information Fusion*, *99*, 101896. DOI: 10.1016/j.inffus.2023.101896

Dobbelaere, T., Vereecken, P., & Detavernier, C. (2017). A USB-controlled potentiostat/galvanostat for thin-film battery characterization. *HardwareX*, *2*, 34–49. DOI: 10.1016/j.ohx.2017.08.001

Doshi-Velez, F., & Kim, B. (2017). Towards a rigorous science of interpretable machine learning. arXiv preprint arXiv:1702.08608.

Doshi-Velez, F., & Kim, B. (2017). Towards a rigorous science of interpretable machine learning. arXiv. https://arxiv.org/abs/1702.08608

Dubhir, T., Mishra, M., & Singhal, R. (2023, December). Benchmarking of quantization libraries in popular frameworks. In 2021 Institute of Electrical and Electronics Engineers International Conference on Big Data (Big Data) (pp. 3050-3055). https://Institute of Electrical and Electronics Engineersxplore.Institute of Electrical and Electronics Engineers.org/document/9671500

Dwork, C., McSherry, F., Nissim, K., & Smith, A. (2006). Calibrating noise to sensitivity in private data analysis. In *Lecture Notes in Computer Science* (pp. 265–284). Springer., DOI: 10.1007/11681878_14

Dwork, C., & Roth, A. (2014). The algorithmic foundations of differential privacy. *Foundations and Trends in Theoretical Computer Science*, *9*(3-4), 211–407. DOI: 10.1561/0400000042

Elayan, H., Aloqaily, M., & Guizani, M. (2022). Sustainability of Healthcare Data Analysis IoT-Based Systems Using Deep Federated Learning. *IEEE Internet of Things Journal*, *9*(10), 7338–7346. DOI: 10.1109/JIOT.2021.3103635

Erel-Özçevik, M., Özçift, A., Özçevik, Y., & Yücalar, F. (2024). A genetic optimized federated learning approach for joint consideration of end-to-end delay and data privacy in vehicular networks. *Electronics (Basel)*, *13*(21), 4261. DOI: 10.3390/electronics13214261

Esteva, A., Kuprel, B., Novoa, R. A., Ko, J., Swetter, S. M., Blau, H. M., & Thrun, S. (2017). Dermatologist-level classification of skin cancer with deep neural networks. *Nature*, *542*(7639), 115–118. DOI: 10.1038/nature21056 PMID: 28117445

European Commission. (2025, March 28). Artificial intelligence in healthcare. *Public Health*. https://health.ec.europa.eu/ehealth-digital-health-and-care/artificial-intelligence-healthcare_en

Fallah, A., Mokhtari, A., & Ozdaglar, A. E. (2020). Personalized federated learning with theoretical guarantees: A model-agnostic meta-learning approach. In Advances in Neural Information Processing Systems, 33 (pp. 3557–3568). https://proceedings.neurips.cc/paper/2020/file/24389bfe4fe2eba8bf9aa9203a44cdad-Paper.pdf

Fatima, E., Dhanda, N., & Zaidi, T. (2025, March). AI-Driven Detection of Stress, Anxiety, and Depression: Techniques, Challenges, and Future Perspectives. In 2025 3rd International Conference on Disruptive Technologies (ICDT) 118-123. Institute of Electrical and Electronics Engineers.

Fatourechi, M. M., Kudva, Y. C., Murad, M. H., Elamin, M. B., Tabini, C. C., & Montori, V. M. (2009). Clinical review: Hypoglycemia with intensive insulin therapy: A systematic review and meta-analyses of randomized trials of continuous subcutaneous insulin infusion versus multiple daily injections. *The Journal of Clinical Endocrinology and Metabolism*, *94*(3), 729–740. DOI: 10.1210/jc.2008-1415 PMID: 19088167

Fellows, E. K., & Batmunkh, D. (2025). Impact investing in childcare systems.

Fitzpatrick, K. K., Darcy, A., & Vierhile, M. (2017). Delivering Cognitive Behavior Therapy to Young Adults With Symptoms of Depression and Anxiety Using a Fully Automated Conversational Agent (Woebot): A Randomized Controlled Trial. *JMIR Mental Health*, *4*(2), e19. DOI: 10.2196/mental.7785 PMID: 28588005

Fredrikson, M., Jha, S., & Ristenpart, T. (2015). Model inversion attacks that exploit confidence information and basic countermeasures. In *Proceedings of the 22nd ACM SIGSAC Conference on Computer and Communications Security* (pp. 1322-1333). DOI: 10.1145/2810103.2813677

Galdón Sanz-Pastor, A., Justel Enríquez, A., Sánchez Bao, A., & Ampudia-Blasco, F. J. (2024). Current barriers to initiating insulin therapy in individuals with type 2 diabetes. *Frontiers in Endocrinology*, *15*, 1366368. DOI: 10.3389/fendo.2024.1366368 PMID: 38559691

Ganesan, I., Ponnuviji, N. P., Kumar, A. S., Nithya, M., Jambulingam, U., & Lalitha, S. D. (2024). Real-Time Event Detection and Predictive Analytics Using IoT and Deep Learning. In Industry Applications of Thrust Manufacturing: Convergence with Real-Time Data and AI (pp. 1-41). IGI Global Scientific Publishing. DOI: 10.4018/979-8-3693-4276-3.ch001

Gao, W., Wang, D., & Huang, Y. (2023). Designing a Deep Learning-Driven Resource-Efficient Diagnostic System for Metastatic Breast Cancer: Reducing Long Delays of Clinical Diagnosis and Improving Patient Survival in Developing Countries. *Cancer Informatics*, *22*, 11769351231214446. DOI: 10.1177/11769351231214446 PMID: 38033362

Garg, P., Sharma, N., & Shukla, B. (2023). Predicting the Risk of Cardiovascular Diseases using Machine Learning Techniques. *International Journal of Intelligent Systems and Applications in Engineering*, *11*(2s), 165–173.

Garza, M., Del Fiol, G., Tenenbaum, J., Walden, A., & Zozus, M. N. (2016). Evaluating common data models for use with a longitudinal community registry. *Journal of Biomedical Informatics*, *64*, 333–341. DOI: 10.1016/j.jbi.2016.10.016 PMID: 27989817

Ge, T., Hu, J., Wang, L., Wang, X., Chen, S. Q., & Wei, F. (2023). In-context autoencoder for context compression in a large language model. arXiv preprint arXiv:2307.06945. https://arxiv.org/pdf/2307.06945

Gerke, S., Minssen, T., & Cohen, G. (2020). Ethical and legal challenges of artificial intelligence-driven healthcare. In *Artificial Intelligence in Healthcare* (pp. 295–336). Academic Press. DOI: 10.1016/B978-0-12-818438-7.00012-5

Geyer, R. C., Klein, T., & Nabi, M. (2017). Differentially private federated learning: A client level perspective. arXiv. https://arxiv.org/abs/1712.07557

Ghadi, Y. Y., Shah, S. F. A., Waheed, W., Mazhar, T., Ahmad, W., Saeed, M. M., & Hamam, H. (2025). Integration of wearable technology and artificial intelligence in digital health for remote patient care. *Journal of Cloud Computing (Heidelberg, Germany)*, *14*(1), 39. Advance online publication. DOI: 10.1186/s13677-025-00759-4

Ghosh, S. S. (2025). ADAPTIVE LEARNING METHODS IN SPEECH-LANGUAGE PATHOLOGY. *The Routledge Handbook of the Sociopolitical Context of Language Learning*, 454.

Ghosh, M., & Bora, V. R. (2025). Evolution in blood glucose monitoring: A comprehensive review of invasive to non-invasive devices and sensors. *Discovery Medicine*, *2*(1), 74. DOI: 10.1007/s44337-025-00273-1

Ghosh, S., & Ghosh, S. K. (2023). FEEL: FEderated LEarning Framework for ELderly Healthcare Using Edge-IoMT. *IEEE Transactions on Computational Social Systems*, *10*(4), 1800–1809. DOI: 10.1109/TCSS.2022.3233300

Goel, N. (2023). Leveraging analytics and Big Data for informed decision-making: A comprehensive review. *INTERANTIONAL JOURNAL OF SCIENTIFIC RESEARCH IN ENGINEERING AND MANAGEMENT*, *07*(10), 1–11. DOI: 10.55041/IJSREM25934

Gong, Y., Fang, Y., & Guo, Y. (2016). Private Data Analytics on Biomedical Sensing Data via Distributed Computation. *IEEE/ACM Transactions on Computational Biology and Bioinformatics*, *13*(3), 431–444. DOI: 10.1109/TCBB.2016.2515610 PMID: 26761861

Gopi, B., Kokila, M. S., Bibin, C. V., Sasikala, D., Howard, E., & Boopathi, S. (2024). Distributed Technologies Using AI/ML Techniques for Healthcare Applications. In *Social Innovations in Education, Environment, and Healthcare* (pp. 375-396). IGI Global.

Gorini, A., Mazzocco, K., Triberti, S., Sebri, V., Savioni, L., & Riva, G. (2018). A P5 mHealth approach: Design rationale and technology components. *JMIR Mental Health*, *5*(3), e10232. DOI: 10.3389/fpsyg.2018.02066 PMID: 30429810

Gracious, L. A., Pajila, P. B., Johncy, G., Anish, T. P., & Prasanth, K. (2024, March). Towards Precision Oncology: A Study of Machine Learning Models for Breast Cancer Prediction. In *2024 10th International Conference on Advanced Computing and Communication Systems (ICACCS)* (Vol. 1, pp. 1938-1943). IEEE. DOI: 10.1109/ICACCS60874.2024.10717246

Gu, X., Li, M., & Xiong, L. (2021). PRECAD: Privacy-preserving and robust federated learning via crypto-aided differential privacy. *arXiv preprint arXiv:2110.11578*. https://arxiv.org/abs/2110.11578

Guan, Y., Li, Y., Zhang, T., & Liu, L. (2021). A federated learning framework for privacy-preserving prediction of mental health disorders. *Institute of Electrical and Electronics Engineers Journal of Biomedical and Health Informatics, 25*(8), 3088–3097. DOI: 10.3390/s25082374

Gulshan, V., Peng, L., Coram, M., Stumpe, M. C., Wu, D., Narayanaswamy, A., Venugopalan, S., Widner, K., Madams, T., Cuadros, J., Kim, R., Raman, R., Nelson, P. C., Mega, J. L., & Webster, D. R. (2016). Development and validation of a deep learning algorithm for detection of diabetic retinopathy in retinal fundus photographs. *Journal of the American Medical Association, 316*(22), 2402–2410. DOI: 10.1001/jama.2016.17216 PMID: 27898976

Guo, Z., Jin, R., Liu, C., Huang, Y., Shi, D., & Supryadi, Yu. L., Liu, Y., Li, J., Xiong, B., & Xiong, D. (2023). Evaluating large language models: A comprehensive survey. arXiv. https://arxiv.org/abs/2310.19736

Gupta, D., Kayode, O., Bhatt, S., Gupta, M., & Tosun, A. S. (2021). Hierarchical Federated Learning based Anomaly Detection using Digital Twins for Smart Healthcare. *Proceedings - 2021 IEEE 7th International Conference on Collaboration and Internet Computing, CIC 2021*, 16–25. DOI: 10.1109/CIC52973.2021.00013

Gupta, M., Singh, M., Sharma, A., Sukhija, N., Aggarwal, P. K., & Jain, P. (2023). Unification of machine learning and blockchain technology in healthcare industry. In *Innovations in Healthcare Informatics: From interoperability to data analysis* (pp. 185–206). Institution of Engineering and Technology. DOI: 10.1049/PBHE041E_ch6

Gupta, S., Huang, Y., Zhong, Z., Gao, T., Li, K., & Chen, D. (2022). Recovering private text in federated learning of language models. Advances in neural information processing systems, 35, 8130-8143. https://proceedings.neurips.cc/paper_files/paper/2022/file/35b5c175e139bff5f22a5361270fce87-Paper-Conference.pdf

Gupta, J., & Vegelin, C. (2016). Sustainable development goals and inclusive development. *International Environmental Agreement: Politics, Law and Economics, 16*(3), 433–448. DOI: 10.1007/s10784-016-9323-z

Gu, X., Sabrina, F., Fan, Z., & Sohail, S. (2023). A review of privacy enhancement methods for federated learning in healthcare systems. *International Journal of Environmental Research and Public Health, 20*(15), 6539. Advance online publication. DOI: 10.3390/ijerph20156539 PMID: 37569079

Hakak, S., Ray, S., Khan, W. Z., & Scheme, E. (2020). A Framework for Edge-Assisted Healthcare Data Analytics using Federated Learning. *Proceedings - 2020 IEEE International Conference on Big Data, Big Data 2020*, 3423–3427. DOI: 10.1109/BigData50022.2020.9377873

Hamilton, M. (1960). A rating scale for depression. *Journal of Neurology, Neurosurgery, and Psychiatry*, *23*(1), 56–62. DOI: 10.1136/jnnp.23.1.56 PMID: 14399272

Haripriya, R., Khare, N., & Pandey, M. (2025). Privacy-preserving federated learning for collaborative medical data mining in multi-institutional settings. *Scientific Reports, 15*(1), 12482--. DOI: 10.1038/s41598-025-97565-4

Hassan, A., Prasad, V. K., Bhattacharya, P., & Dutta, P. K. (Eds.). (2024). *Pioneering Smart Healthcare 5.0 with IoT, Federated Learning, and Cloud Security*. IGI Global.

Hassani, H., Huang, X., & Silva, E. S. (2024). Trustworthy federated learning: Privacy, security, and beyond. *arXiv*. https://arxiv.org/html/2411.01583

Hassani, H., Silva, E. S., & Al Kaabi, A. M. (2024). Federated learning, ethics, and the double black box problem in medical AI. *arXiv*. https://arxiv.org/html/2504.20656v1

Hassan, M. H., Vyas, C., Grieve, B., & Bartolo, P. (2021). Recent advances in enzymatic and non-enzymatic electrochemical glucose sensing. *Sensors (Basel), 21*(14), 4672. DOI: 10.3390/s21144672 PMID: 34300412

Heller, A., & Feldman, B. (2008). Electrochemical glucose sensors and their applications in diabetes management. *Chemical Reviews, 108*(7), 2482–2505. DOI: 10.1021/cr068069y PMID: 18465900

Hirsch, D. (2019). From individual control to social protection: New paradigms for privacy law in the age of predictive analytics. SSRN Electronic Journal. DOI: 10.2139/ssrn.3449112

Hong, Q., Jun, M., Bo, W., Sichao, T., Jiayi, Z., Biao, L., Tong, L., & Ruifeng, T. (2023). Application of Data-Driven technology in nuclear Engineering: Prediction, classification and design optimization. *Annals of Nuclear Energy, 194*, 110089. DOI: 10.1016/j.anucene.2023.110089

https://www.usenix.org/system/files/conference/hotstorage17/hotstorage17-paper-hoi.pdfUsenix

Huang, D., Ye, X., & Sakurai, T. (2024). Multi-party collaborative drug discovery via federated learning. *Computers in Biology and Medicine, 171*, 108181. DOI: 10.1016/j.compbiomed.2024.108181 PMID: 38428094

Huang, L., Yin, Y., Fu, Z., Zhang, S., Deng, H., & Liu, D. (2020). LoAdaBoost: Loss-based AdaBoost federated machine learning with reduced computational complexity on IID and non-IID intensive care data. *PLoS One*, *15*(4), e0230706. DOI: 10.1371/journal.pone.0230706 PMID: 32302316

Hu, K., Gong, S., Zhang, Q., Seng, C., Xia, M., & Jiang, S. (2024). An overview of implementing security and privacy in federated learning. *Artificial Intelligence Review*, *57*(8), 204. DOI: 10.1007/s10462-024-10846-8

Indu, V. T., Elumalai, M., & Gracious, L. A. (2026). Optimization Algorithms for Machine Learning Model Enhancement in Healthcare. In *AI Model Design and Data Management for Disease Prediction* (pp. 159–192). IGI Global Scientific Publishing.

Insilico Medicine. (n.d.). IPF – Phase 1. https://insilico.com/blog/ipf-phase1

Ishak, H., Matore, M. E. E. M., & Nor, H. A. M. (2025). Bibliometric analysis of adaptive behavior research: Advancing Sustainable Development Goals (SDGs) for children with disabilities. *Journal of Lifestyle and SDGs Review*, *5*(2), e03405. DOI: 10.47172/2965-730X.SDGsReview.v5.n02.pe03405

Jahan, N., Rashid, I. B., Al Numan, O., Hasan, A. T., & Begum, N. (2021, July). Collaborative AI in smart healthcare system. In *2021 International Conference on Automation, Control and Mechatronics for Industry 4.0 (ACMI)* (pp. 1-5). IEEE.

Jain, P., Sharma, S., Arora, S., Shokeen, V., Aggarwal, P. K., & Singh, M. (2024). Edge computing-based design for IoT security. In *Network Optimization in Intelligent Internet of Things Applications: Principles and Challenges* (pp. 298–309). CRC Press. DOI: 10.1201/9781003405535-22

Jain, A., Bhatnagar, V., Rao, A. C. S., & Khari, M. (2023). Retina disease prediction using modified convolutional neural network based on Inception-ResNet model with support vector machine classifier. *Computational Intelligence*, *39*(6), 1088–1111. DOI: 10.1111/coin.12601

Jain, A., Dubey, A. K., Gupta, M., Yadav, S., Panwar, A., Atanga, R., Lemos, B., & Mallik, S. (2025). Brain Stroke Prediction: A PSO Optimized Stacked Ensemble Machine Learning Approach with SMOTEEN Data Balancing. *BioRxiv*, 2025.06.05.657994. http://biorxiv.org/content/early/2025/06/08/2025.06.05.657994.abstract

Jain, A., Dubey, A. K., Khan, S., Panwar, A., Alkhatib, M., & Alshahrani, A. M. (2025). A PSO weighted ensemble framework with SMOTE balancing for student dropout prediction in smart education systems. *Scientific Reports*, *15*(1), 17463. DOI: 10.1038/s41598-025-97506-1 PMID: 40394143

Jain, A., Dubey, A. K., Pan, V. S. H., Mahfoudh, S., Althaqafi, T. A., Arya, V., Alhalabi, W., Singh, S. K., Jain, V., Panwar, A., Kumar, S., Hsu, C. H., & Gupta, B. B. (2025). Bayesian optimized CNN ensemble for efficient potato blight detection using fuzzy image enhancement. *Scientific Reports*, *15*(1), 31259. DOI: 10.1038/s41598-025-15940-7 PMID: 40854933

Jain, J., & Jaiswal, U. K. (2025). Revolutionizing medicine: The impact of artificial intelligence in healthcare. In Gupta, S., Gupta, U., Sharma, M., & Malik, K. (Eds.), *Generative intelligence in healthcare: Transforming patient care with AI creativity* (pp. 176–209). CRC Press., DOI: 10.1201/9781003539483-8

Jajal, P., Jiang, W., Tewari, A., Kocinare, E., Woo, J., Sarraf, A., & Davis, J. C. (2024). Interoperability in deep learning: A user survey and failure analysis of onnx model converters. In Proceedings of the 33rd Association for Computing Machinery SIGSOFT International Symposium on Software Testing and Analysis 1466-1478) https://dl.acm.org/doi/pdf/10.1145/3650212.3680374

Jebreel, N. M., Domingo-Ferrer, J., Blanco-Justicia, A., & Sánchez, D. (2022). Enhanced security and privacy via fragmented federated learning. *IEEE Transactions on Neural Networks and Learning Systems*, *35*(5), 6703–6717. DOI: 10.1109/TNNLS.2022.3212627 PMID: 36260588

Jiang, A. Q., Sablayrolles, A., Mensch, A., Bamford, C., Chaplot, D. S., de las Casas, D., Bressand, F., Lengyel, G., Lample, G., Saulnier, L., Lavaud, L. R., Lachaux, M.-A., Stock, P., Le Scao, T., Lavril, T., Wang, T., Lacroix, T., & El Sayed, W. (2023). *Mistral 7B*. arXiv. https://arxiv.org/abs/2310.06825

Jiang, F., Jiang, Y., Zhi, H., Dong, Y., Li, H., Ma, S., Wang, Y., Dong, Q., Shen, H., & Wang, Y. (2017). Artificial intelligence in healthcare: Past, present and future. *Stroke and Vascular Neurology*, *2*(4), 230–243. DOI: 10.1136/svn-2017-000101 PMID: 29507784

Jiang, Y., Konečný, J., Rush, K., & Kannan, S. (2019). Improving federated learning personalization via model agnostic meta learning. arXiv. https://arxiv.org/abs/1909.12488

Jian, W., Li, J. P., Akbar, M. A., Haq, A. U., Khan, S., Alotaibi, R. M., & Alajlan, S. A. (2024). SA-Bi-LSTM: Self Attention with Bi-Directional LSTM-Based Intelligent Model for Accurate Fake News Detection to Ensured Information Integrity on Social Media Platforms. *IEEE Access : Practical Innovations, Open Solutions*, *12*, 48436–48452. DOI: 10.1109/ACCESS.2024.3382832

Ji, S., Zhang, T., Ansari, L., Fu, J., Tiwari, P., & Cambria, E. (2022). MentalBERT. In *Proceedings of the Thirteenth Language Resources and Evaluation Conference*, pages 7184–7190, Marseille, France. European Language Resources Association.

Johnson, K. (2020, April 16). Health care organizations use NVIDIA's Clara federated learning to improve mammogram analysis AI. *VentureBeat*. https://venturebeat.com/ai/healthcare-organizations-use-nvidias-clara-federated-learning-to-improve-mammogram-analysis-ai/

Johnson, A. E., Pollard, T. J., Shen, L., Lehman, L. W. H., Feng, M., Ghassemi, M., Moody, B., Szolovits, P., Anthony Celi, L., & Mark, R. G. (2016). MIMIC-III, a freely accessible critical care database. *Scientific Data*, *3*(1), 1–9. DOI: 10.1038/sdata.2016.35 PMID: 27219127

Joshi, A. M., Jain, P., & Mohanty, S. P. (2020, July). Secure-iGLU: A secure device for noninvasive glucose measurement and automatic insulin delivery in IoMT framework. In 2020 IEEE Computer Society annual symposium on VLSI (ISVLSI) (pp. 440-445). IEEE. https://doi.org/DOI: 10.1109/ISVLSI49217.2020.00-17

Jun, M. (2025). Platform framework for blockchain-enhanced healthcare AIoT systems. *Frontiers in Communications and Networks*, *6*, 1538965. Advance online publication. DOI: 10.3389/frcmn.2025.1538965

Kairouz, P., McMahan, H. B., Avent, B., Bellet, A., Bennis, M., Bhagoji, A. N., ... & Zhao, S. (2021). Advances and open problems in federated learning. *Foundations and trends® in machine learning, 14*(1–2), 1-210.

Kairouz, P., McMahan, H. B., Avent, B., Bellet, A., Bennis, M., Nitin Bhagoji, A., Bonawitz, K., Charles, Z., Cormode, G., Cummings, R., D'Oliveira, R. G. L., Eichner, H., El Rouayheb, S., Evans, D., Gardner, J., Garrett, Z., Gascón, A., Ghazi, B., Gibbons, P. B., … Zhao, S. (2021). Advances and open problems in federated learning. Foundations and Trends® in Machine Learning, 14(1–2), 1–210. DOI: 10.1561/2200000083

Kaissis, G. A., Makowski, M. R., Rückert, D., & Braren, R. F. (2020). Secure, privacy-preserving and federated machine learning in medical imaging. *Nature Machine Intelligence*, *2*(6), 305–311. DOI: 10.1038/s42256-020-0186-1

Kaissis, G., Ziller, A., Passerat-Palmbach, J., Ryffel, T., Usynin, D., Trask, A., Lima, I.Jr, Mancuso, J., Jungmann, F., Steinborn, M.-M., Saleh, A., Makowski, M., Rueckert, D., & Braren, R. (2021). End-to-end privacy preserving deep learning on multi-institutional medical imaging. *Nature Machine Intelligence*, *3*(6), 473–484. DOI: 10.1038/s42256-021-00337-8

Kakao Healthcare. (n.d.). Kakao Healthcare to link data platform with 17 major hospitals. *Pulse*. https://pulse.mk.co.kr/news/english/11290677

Kalkatawi, M. (2025). Beyond the upgrade: Unraveling the complexities of health information system migration. *Discover Health Systems*, *4*(1), 7. DOI: 10.1007/s44250-025-00186-x

Kalluri, K. (2022). Federate machine learning: A secure paradigm for collaborative AI in privacy-sensitive domains. *International Journal on Science and Technology*, *13*(4), 1–13. DOI: 10.5281/zenodo.14551746

Kalpana, P., Tappari, S., Smitha, L., Madhavi, D., Naresh, K., & Vijayalakshmi, M. (2025). A novel end-to-end privacy preserving deep Aquila feed forward networks on healthcare 4.0 environment. *Discover Internet of Things*, *5*(1), 65. Advance online publication. DOI: 10.1007/s43926-025-00157-x

Kami, M., Pourshahbaz, A., Rezaei, O., Keshavarz Akhlaghi, A. A., Banihashem, S., Dehghanizadeh, Z., Olamie Koopaie, M., & Nosratabadi, M. (2024). Clinical utility and diagnostic validity of the hierarchical taxonomy of psychopathology for borderline personality disorder. *Iranian Journal of Psychiatry and Behavioral Sciences*, *18*(4). Advance online publication. DOI: 10.5812/ijpbs-143833

Karimireddy, S. P., Kale, S., Mohri, M., Reddi, S., Stich, S., & Suresh, A. T. (2020, November). Scaffold: Stochastic controlled averaging for federated learning. In *International conference on machine learning* (pp. 5132-5143). PMLR.

Karumbunathan, L.S. (2022). Nvidia jetson agx orin series. https://www.nvidia.com/content/dam/en-zz/Solutions/gtcf21/jetson-orin/nvidia-jetson-agx-orin-technical-brief.pdf

Kasralikar, P., Polu, O. R., Chamarthi, B., Rupavath, R. V. S. S. B., Patel, S., & Tumati, R. (2025). Blockchain for securing AI-driven healthcare systems: A systematic review and future research perspectives. *Cureus*, *17*(4). Advance online publication. DOI: 10.7759/cureus.83136 PMID: 40438823

Khalid, N., Qayyum, A., Bilal, M., Al-Fuqaha, A., & Qadir, J. (2023). Privacy-preserving artificial intelligence in healthcare: Techniques and applications. *Computers in Biology and Medicine*, *158*, 106848. DOI: 10.1016/j.compbiomed.2023.106848 PMID: 37044052

Khan, A. (2024). Optimisation methods based on soft computing for improving power system stability. *J. Electrical Systems*, *20*(6s), 1051–1058. DOI: 10.52783/jes.2837

Khang, A. (Ed.). (2023). *AI and IoT-based technologies for precision medicine*. IGI Global. DOI: 10.4018/979-8-3693-0876-9

Khang, A. (Ed.). (2024). *AI-Driven Innovations in Digital Healthcare: Emerging Trends, Challenges, and Applications: Emerging Trends*. Challenges, and Applications.

Khang, A., Jadhav, B., & Sayyed, M. (2024). Role of cutting-edge technologies and deep learning frameworks in the digital healthcare sector. In *AI-driven innovations in digital healthcare: emerging trends, challenges, and applications* (pp. 1–22). IGI Global Scientific Publishing. DOI: 10.4018/979-8-3693-3218-4.ch001

Klein Brinke, J., Van Der Linden, M., & Havinga, P. (2024). Using Federated Learning and Channel State Information-Based Sensing for Scalable and Realistic At-Home Healthcare. *ACM International Conference Proceeding Series*, 186–193. DOI: 10.1145/3655693.3660254

Kokila, M. S., Fenil, E., Ponnuviji, N. P., & Nirmala, G. (2024). Securing cloud-based medical data: An optimal dual kernal support vector approach for enhanced EHR management. *International Journal of System Assurance Engineering and Management, 15*(7), 3495–3507. DOI: 10.1007/s13198-024-02356-1

Krishna, K. (2022). Optimizing query performance in distributed NoSQL databases through adaptive indexing and data partitioning techniques. International Journal of Creative Research Thoughts (IJCRT). https://ijcrt.org/viewfulltext.php

Krishna, K., & Thakur, D. (2021). Automated Machine Learning (AutoML) for real-time data streams: Challenges and innovations in online learning algorithms. [JETIR]. *Journal of Emerging Technologies and Innovative Research, 8*(12).

Krishnan, S., Anand, A. J., Srinivasan, R., Kavitha, R., & Suresh, S. (2024). *Federated Learning*. CRC Press.

Kroenke, K., Spitzer, R. L., & Williams, J. B. (2021). The PHQ-9: Validity of a brief depression severity measure. *Journal of General Internal Medicine, 16*(9), 606–613. https://onlinelibrary.wiley.com/doi/pdf/10.1046/j.1525-1497.2001.016009606.x. DOI: 10.1046/j.1525-1497.2001.016009606.x PMID: 11556941

Kulkarni, V., Kulkarni, M., & Pant, A. (2020, July). Survey of personalization techniques for federated learning. In *2020 fourth world conference on smart trends in systems, security and sustainability (WorldS4)* (pp. 794-797). IEEE. DOI: 10.1109/WorldS450073.2020.9210355

Kumar, P., & Sharma, M. K. (2024). AI-Driven System for Early Detection and Diagnosis of Cataracts by Image Recognition and Machine Learning Algorithms. In *AI-Driven Innovations in Digital Healthcare: Emerging Trends, Challenges, and Applications* (pp. 168-184). IGI Global Scientific Publishing. DOI: 10.4018/979-8-3693-3218-4.ch008

Kumar, P., Jain, J., Jaiswal, U. K., Yadav, D., & Solanki, B. (2024). Childhood asthma disease prediction using classification algorithms of supervised machine learning. In 2024 1st International Conference on Advanced Computing and Emerging Technologies (ACET) (pp. 1–6). IEEE. DOI: 10.1109/ACET61898.2024.10730050

Kumar, S., Lakshminarayanan, A., Chang, K., Guretno, F., Mien, I. H., Kalpathy-Cramer, J., Krishnaswamy, P., & Singh, P. (2022). Towards More Efficient Data Valuation in Healthcare Federated Learning Using Ensembling. *Lecture Notes in Computer Science (Including Subseries Lecture Notes in Artificial Intelligence and Lecture Notes in Bioinformatics), 13573 LNCS*, 119–129. DOI: 10.1007/978-3-031-18523-6_12

Kumar, A., Vajpayee, A., & Sanghani, P. (2024). IoT-infused care: Disentanglement family dynamics and coping strategies in the realm of intellectually disabled children. In Gupta, S. K., Karras, D. A., & Natarajan, R. (Eds.), *Revolutionizing Healthcare: AI Integration with IoT for Enhanced Patient Outcomes* (Vol. 7). Springer., DOI: 10.1007/978-3-031-65022-2_14

Kumar, Y., & Singla, R. (2021). Federated learning systems for healthcare: Perspective and recent progress. In *Studies in computational intelligence* (pp. 141–156). Springer., DOI: 10.1007/978-3-030-70604-3_6

Lainidi, O., Jendeby, M. K., Montgomery, A., Mouratidis, C., Paitaridou, K., Cook, C., Johnson, J., & Karakasidou, E. (2023). An integrative systematic review of employee silence and voice in healthcare: What are we really measuring? *Frontiers in Psychiatry, 14*, 1111579. DOI: 10.3389/fpsyt.2023.1111579 PMID: 37304444

Lalar, S., Kumar, T., Kumar, R., & Kumar, S. (2025). Unlocking Potential: The Role of Artificial Intelligence in Revolutionizing Special Education for Inclusive Learning. In *Impacts of Generative AI on the Future of Research and Education* (pp. 201-232). IGI Global.

Le Quoc, D., Beck, M., Bhatotia, P., Chen, R., Fetzer, C., & Strufe, T. (2019). Privacy-Preserving Data Analytics. In Encyclopedia of Big Data Technologies (pp. 1292–1300). Springer International Publishing. DOI: 10.1007/978-3-319-77525-8_152

Lee, T., Shiau, J., Chen, C., Yun, W., Wuu, C., Huang, Y., Yeh, S., Chen, H., & Chao, P. (2025). A machine learning model for predicting breast cancer recurrence and supporting personalized treatment decisions through comprehensive feature selection and explainable ensemble learning. *Cancer Management and Research, 17*, 917–932. DOI: 10.2147/CMAR.S514693 PMID: 40357238

Lehne, M., Sass, J., Essenwanger, A., Schepers, J., & Thun, S. (2019). Why digital medicine depends on interoperability. *NPJ Digital Medicine*, *2*(1), 79. DOI: 10.1038/s41746-019-0158-1 PMID: 31453374

Lesiuk, T., Kauffman, M. A., Fleszar-Pavlovic, S. E., Esquives, B. N., Brito, A. E., Wang, T., & Penedo, F. J. (2025). A hybrid eHealth mindfulness-based music therapy intervention for adults receiving an allogeneic hematopoietic stem cell transplant. *Music Therapy Perspectives*, *43*(1), miaf004.

Li, T., Sahu, A. K., Zaheer, M., Sanjabi, M., Talwalkar, A., & Smith, V. (2020). Federated optimization in heterogeneous networks. *Proceedings ofMachine learning and systems, 2*, 429-450.

Li, X., Peng, L., Wang, Y. P., & Zhang, W. (2025). Open challenges and opportunities in federated foundation models towards biomedical healthcare. *BioData Mining, 18*(1), 2--. DOI: 10.1186/s13040-024-00414-9

Li, H., Cai, Z., Wang, J., Tang, J., Ding, W., Lin, C.-T., & Shi, Y. (2024). FedTP: Federated learning by transformer personalization. *IEEE Transactions on Neural Networks and Learning Systems*, *35*(10), 13426–13440. DOI: 10.1109/TNNLS.2023.3269062 PMID: 37220054

Li, K. (2025). A Blockchain-Integrated Federated Learning Approach for Secure Data Sharing and Privacy Protection in Multi-Device Communication. *Applied Artificial Intelligence*, *39*(1), 2442770. Advance online publication. DOI: 10.1080/08839514.2024.2442770

Li, L. (2024). Application of artificial intelligence-driven federated learning based on machine learning and deep learning in medicine. In *Artificial Intelligence*. IntechOpen., DOI: 10.5772/intechopen.1008185

Lilhore, U. K., Simaiya, S., Poongodi, M., & Dutt, V. (Eds.). (2024). *Federated Learning and Privacy-preserving in Healthcare AI*. IGI Global. DOI: 10.4018/979-8-3693-1874-4

Li, Q., Wen, Z., Wu, Z., Hu, S., Wang, N., Li, Y., Liu, X., & He, B. (2021). A survey on federated learning systems: Vision, hype and reality for data privacy and protection. *IEEE Transactions on Knowledge and Data Engineering, 35*(4), 3347–3366. DOI: 10.1109/TKDE.2021.3124599

Li, S., Liu, P., Nascimento, G. G., Wang, X., Leite, F. R. M., Chakraborty, B., Hong, C., Ning, Y., Xie, F., Teo, Z. L., Ting, D. S. W., Haddadi, H., Ong, M. E. H., Peres, M. A., & Liu, N. (2023). Federated and distributed learning applications for electronic health records and structured medical data: A scoping review. *Journal of the American Medical Informatics Association : JAMIA, 30*(12), 2041–2049. DOI: 10.1093/jamia/ocad170 PMID: 37639629

Li, T., Sahu, A. K., Talwalkar, A., & Smith, V. (2020). Federated learning: Challenges, methods, and future directions. *IEEE Signal Processing Magazine, 37*(3), 50–60. DOI: 10.1109/MSP.2020.2975749

Liu, Y., Ott, M., Goyal, N., Du, J., Joshi, M., Chen, D., & Stoyanov, V. (2020). RoBERTa: A robustly optimized BERT pretraining approach. arXiv preprint arXiv:1907.11692. https://arxiv.org/abs/1907.11692

Liu, W., Zhang, Y.-H., Li, Y.-F., & Zheng, D. (2023). A fine-grained medical data sharing scheme based on federated learning. *Concurrency and Computation, 35*(20), e6847. Advance online publication. DOI: 10.1002/cpe.6847

Liu, X., Li, H., Xu, G., Chen, Z., Huang, X., & Lu, R. (2021). Privacy-enhanced federated learning against poisoning adversaries. *IEEE Transactions on Information Forensics and Security, 16*, 4574–4588. DOI: 10.1109/TIFS.2021.3108434

Liu, Y., Kang, Y., Xing, C., Chen, T., & Yang, Q. (2020). A secure federated transfer learning framework. *IEEE Intelligent Systems, 35*(4), 70–82. DOI: 10.1109/MIS.2020.2988525

Liu, Y., Yu, Q., Luo, X., Yang, L., & Cui, Y. (2021). Continuous monitoring of diabetes with an integrated microneedle biosensing device through 3D printing. *Microsystems & Nanoengineering, 7*(1), 75. DOI: 10.1038/s41378-021-00302-w PMID: 34631143

Li, W., Milletarì, F., Xu, D., Rieke, N., Hancox, J., Zhu, W., Baust, M., Cheng, Y., Ourselin, S., Cardoso, M. J., & Feng, A. (2019). Privacy-preserving federated brain tumour segmentation. In *Medical Image Computing and Computer Assisted Intervention – MICCAI 2019* (pp. 133–141). Springer., DOI: 10.1007/978-3-030-32692-0_16

Li, X., Gu, Y., Dvornek, N., Staib, L. H., Ventola, P., & Duncan, J. S. (2020). Multi-site fMRI analysis using privacy-preserving federated learning and domain adaptation: ABIDE results. *Medical Image Analysis*, *65*, 101765. DOI: 10.1016/j.media.2020.101765 PMID: 32679533

Li, X., Huang, K., Yang, W., Wang, S., & Zhang, Z. (2019). On the convergence of FedAvg on non-IID data. In *International Conference on Learning Representations*.

Li, X., Zhang, L., Yang, J., & Teng, F. (2024). Role of Artificial Intelligence in Medical Image Analysis: A Review of Current Trends and Future Directions. *Journal of Medical and Biological Engineering*, *44*(2), 231–243. DOI: 10.1007/s40846-024-00863-x

Loftus, T. J., Ruppert, M. M., Shickel, B., Ozrazgat-Baslanti, T., Balch, J. A., Efron, P. A., Upchurch, G. R.Jr, Rashidi, P., Tignanelli, C., Bian, J., & Bihorac, A. (2022). Federated learning for preserving data privacy in collaborative healthcare research. *Digital Health*, *8*, 20552076221134455. DOI: 10.1177/20552076221134455 PMID: 36325438

Long, Y., Zhang, J., Wang, G., & Fu, J. (2023). Hierarchical federated learning with global differential privacy. *Electronic Research Archive*, *31*(7), 3741–3758. DOI: 10.3934/era.2023190

Lu, M. Y., Chen, R. J., Kong, D., Lipkova, J., Singh, R., Williamson, D. F., Chen, T. Y., & Mahmood, F. (2022). Federated learning for computational pathology on gigapixel whole slide images. *Medical Image Analysis*, *76*, 102298. DOI: 10.1016/j.media.2021.102298 PMID: 34911013

Lundberg, S. M., & Lee, S. I. (2017). A unified approach to interpreting model predictions. In Advances in Neural Information Processing Systems, 30. https://proceedings.neurips.cc/paper_files/paper/2017/file/8a20a8621978632d76c43dfd28b67767-Paper.pdf

Luo, J., Zhang, Y., Zhang, Z., Zhang, J., Mu, X., Wang, H., & Xu, Z. (2024, August). SecFormer: Fast and Accurate Privacy-Preserving Inference for Transformer Models via SMPC. In Findings of the Association for Computational Linguistics ACL 2024 13333-13348. https://aclanthology.org/2024.findings-acl.790.pdf

Luo, H., Sun, Q., Xu, C., Zhao, P., Lou, J., Tao, C., Geng, X., Lin, Q., Chen, S., Tang, Y., & Zhang, D. (2023). WizardMath: Empowering mathematical reasoning for large language models via reinforced Evol-Instruct. arXiv. https://arxiv.org/abs/2308.09583

Lyu, L., Yu, H., & Yang, Q. (2020). Threats to Federated learning: A survey. *ArXiv Preprint ArXiv:2003.02133.*

Madsen, K. P., Olsen, K. R., Rytter, K., Willaing, I., Pedersen-Bjergaard, U., Schmidt, S., Nørgaard, K., & Kjær, T. (2023). Effects of initiating insulin pump therapy in the real world: A nationwide, register-based study of adults with type 1 diabetes. *Diabetes Research and Clinical Practice*, *196*, 110225. DOI: 10.1016/j.diabres.2022.110225 PMID: 36535513

Maggo, C., & Garg, P. (2022). From linguistic features to their extractions: Understanding the semantics of a concept. *2022 Fifth International Conference on Computational Intelligence and Communication Technologies (CCICT)*, 427–431. DOI: 10.1109/CCiCT56684.2022.00082

Magoutas, B., Schmidt, K. U., Mentzas, G., & Stojanovic, L. (2010). An adaptive e-questionnaire for measuring user perceived portal quality. *International Journal of Human-Computer Studies*, *68*(10), 729–745. DOI: 10.1016/j.ijhcs.2010.06.003

Maheshwaran, T., Muthumarilakshmi, S., Suganya, K., Maheswari, B., & Girija, P. (2024). Securing E-Commerce Strategies With Cloud, Blockchain, AI, and ML. In *Strategies for E-Commerce Data Security: Cloud, Blockchain, AI, and Machine Learning* (pp. 470-500). IGI Global.

Malik, M., Garg, P., & Malik, C. (2024). Artificial intelligence-based prediction of health risks among women during menopause. *Artificial Intelligence and Machine Learning for Women's Health Issues*, 137–150.

Malviya, R., & Rajput, S. (2025). Advances and Insights into AI-Created Disability Supports.

Mammen, P. M. (2021). Federated learning: Opportunities and challenges. *arXiv preprint arXiv:2101.05428.*

Manea, L., Gilbody, S., & McMillan, D. (2015). A diagnostic meta-analysis of the Patient Health Questionnaire-9 (PHQ-9) algorithm scoring method as a screen for depression. *General Hospital Psychiatry*, *37*(1), 67–75. DOI: 10.1016/j.genhosppsych.2014.09.009 PMID: 25439733

Mangairkarasi, S., Ramana, T. V., Vaishnavi, R., Agalya, S., Sathya, V., & Subramanian, R. S. (2025). Advancing Healthcare Through Artificial Intelligence: Applications, Challenges, and Future Directions. In *Responsible AI for Digital Health and Medical Analytics* (pp. 113-134). IGI Global Scientific Publishing.

Manjunathan, N., Shanmugapriya, D., Girija, P., Vasudevan, M., & Murugesan, S. (2024, September). Ensemble Learning: Importance, Applications, Challenges, and Future Work. In *2024 International Conference on Integration of Emerging Technologies for the Digital World (ICIETDW)* (pp. 1-6). IEEE. Li, L., Fan, Y., Tse, M., & Lin, K. Y. (2020). A review of applications in federated learning. *Computers & Industrial Engineering*, *149*, 106854.

Manocha, A., Sood, S. K., & Bhatia, M. (2025). Federated learning-inspired smart ECG classification: An explainable artificial intelligence approach. *Multimedia Tools and Applications*, *84*(19), 21673–21696. DOI: 10.1007/s11042-024-20084-3

Manov, A. E., Chauhan, S., Dhillon, G., Dhaliwal, A., Antonio, S., Donepudi, A., Jalal, Y. N., Nazha, J., Banal, M., & House, J. (2023). The effectiveness of continuous glucose monitoring devices in managing uncontrolled diabetes mellitus: A retrospective study. *Cureus*, *15*(7), e42545. DOI: 10.7759/cureus.42545 PMID: 37637581

Mathew, U. O., Rodriguez, D. Z., Rosa, R. L., Ayub, M. S., & Adasme, P. (2024). Advancing Healthcare 5.0 through Federated Learning: Opportunity for Security Enforcement using Blockchain. *2024 32nd International Conference on Software, Telecommunications and Computer Networks, SoftCOM 2024*. DOI: 10.23919/SoftCOM62040.2024.10722012

Ma, Z., Ruhaiyem, N. I. R., Zhang, M., Musa, K. I., Hanis, T. M., Xiao, T., Hua, D., & Li, H. (2025). A review of federated learning technology and its research progress in healthcare applications. *Applied Intelligence*, *55*(10), 765. Advance online publication. DOI: 10.1007/s10489-025-06627-7

McMahan, B., Moore, E., Ramage, D., Hampson, S., & y Arcas, B. A. (2017). Communication-efficient learning of deep networks from decentralized data. *Artificial Intelligence and Statistics*, 1273–1282.

McMahan, H. B., Moore, E., Ramage, D., Hampson, S., & Arcas, B. A. (2017). Communication-efficient learning of deep networks from decentralized data. Proceedings of the 20th International Conference on Artificial Intelligence and Statistics (AISTATS), 54, 1273–1282. http://proceedings.mlr.press/v54/mcmahan17a.html

McMahan, H. B., Moore, E., Ramage, D., Hampson, S., & Arcas, B. A. Y. (2017). Communication-efficient learning of deep networks from decentralized data. In Proceedings of the 20th International Conference on Artificial Intelligence and Statistics (pp. 1273–1282). PMLR. http://proceedings.mlr.press/v54/mcmahan17a/mcmahan17a.pdf

McMahan, B., Moore, E., Ramage, D., Hampson, S., & Arcas, B. A. (2017, April). Communication-efficient learning of deep networks from decentralized data. In *Artificial intelligence and statistics* (pp. 1273–1282). PMLR.

McMahan, H. B., Moore, E., Ramage, D., Hampson, S., & Arcas, B. A. (2017). Communication-efficient learning of deep networks from decentralized data. *Proceedings of the 20th International Conference on Artificial Intelligence and Statistics (AISTATS)*, 54, 1273–1282. https://arxiv.org/abs/1602.05629

Mehrotra, M., Singh, K. P., & Singh, Y. B. (2024). Facial Emotion Recognition and Detection Using Convolutional Neural Networks with Low Computation Cost. *2024 2nd International Conference on Disruptive Technologies, ICDT 2024*, 1349–1354. DOI: 10.1109/ICDT61202.2024.10489678

Meloni, G. N. (2016). Building a microcontroller-based potentiostat: An inexpensive and versatile platform for teaching electrochemistry and instrumentation. *Journal of Chemical Education*, *93*(7), 1320–1322. DOI: 10.1021/acs.jchemed.5b00961

Mendieta, M., Yang, T., Wang, P., Lee, M., Ding, Z., & Chen, C. (2022). Local learning matters: Rethinking data heterogeneity in federated learning. In *Proceedings of the IEEE/CVF Conference on Computer Vision and Pattern Recognition* (pp. 8387–8396). CVPR., https://openaccess.thecvf.com/content/CVPR2022/html/Mendieta_Local_Learning_Matters_Rethinking_Data_Heterogeneity_in_Federated_Learning_CVPR_2022_paper.html DOI: 10.1109/CVPR52688.2022.00821

Meurisch, C., Bayrak, B., & Mühlhäuser, M. (2020). Privacy-preserving AI services through data decentralization. *Proceedings of The Web Conference 2020*, 190–200. DOI: 10.1145/3366423.3380106

Miner, A. S., Milstein, A., Schueller, S., Hegde, R., Mangurian, C., & Linos, E. (2016). Smartphone-Based Conversational Agents and Responses to Questions About Mental Health, Interpersonal Violence, and Physical Health. *JAMA Internal Medicine, 176*(5), 619–625. DOI: 10.1001/jamainternmed.2016.0400 PMID: 26974260

Mitra, A., ... "Orca 2: Teaching small language models how to reason." arXiv preprint arXiv:2311.11045 (2023). https://arxiv.org/abs/2311.11045

Mittelstadt, B. D., Allo, P., Taddeo, M., Wachter, S., & Floridi, L. (2016). The ethics of algorithms: Mapping the debate. *Big Data & Society*, *3*(2), 1–21. DOI: 10.1177/2053951716679679

Mo, F., & Haddadi, H. (2019, March). Efficient and private federated learning using tee. In *Proc. EuroSys Conf.,* Dresden, Germany (p. 1).

Mohammadi, S., Balador, A., Sinaei, S., & Flammini, F. (2024). Balancing privacy and performance in Federated learning: A systematic literature review on methods and metrics. *Journal of Parallel and Distributed Computing*, *192*, 104918. DOI: 10.1016/j.jpdc.2024.104918

Mohiddin, A. (2022). Insulin and diabetes mellitus [Review]. *International Journal of Science and Research (Raipur, India)*, *11*(12), 1299–1302. DOI: 10.21275/MR22125112434

Montagna, S., Aguzzi, G., Ferretti, S., Pengo, M. F., Klopfenstein, L. C., Ungolo, M., & Magnini, M. (2024, March). LLM-based solutions for healthcare Chatbots: a comparative analysis. In 2024 Institute of Electrical and Electronics Engineers International Conference on Pervasive Computing and Communications Workshops and other Affiliated Events, 346-351, Institute of Electrical and Electronics Engineers. DOI: 10.1109/PerComWorkshops59983.2024.10503257

Mothukuri, V., Parizi, R. M., Pouriyeh, S., Huang, Y., Dehghantanha, A., & Srivastava, G. (2021). A survey on security and privacy of federated learning. *Future Generation Computer Systems*, *115*, 619–640. DOI: 10.1016/j.future.2020.10.007

Muazu, T., Mao, Y., Muhammad, A. U., Ibrahim, M., Kumshe, U. M. M., & Samuel, O. (2024). A federated learning system with data fusion for healthcare using multi-party computation and additive secret sharing. *Computer Communications*, *216*, 168–182. DOI: 10.1016/j.comcom.2024.01.006

Muhammed, D., Ahvar, E., Ahvar, S., Trocan, M., Montpetit, M. J., & Ehsani, R. (2024). Artificial Intelligence of Things (AIoT) for smart agriculture: A review of architectures, technologies and solutions. *Journal of Network and Computer Applications*, *228*, 103905. DOI: 10.1016/j.jnca.2024.103905

Murthy, P., & Thakur, D. (2022). Cross-layer optimization techniques for enhancing consistency and performance in distributed NoSQL database. International Journal of Enhanced Research in Management & Computer Applications, 35.

Murthy, P., & Mehra, A. (2021). Exploring neuromorphic computing for ultra-low latency transaction processing in edge database architectures. *Journal of Emerging Technologies and Innovative Research*, *8*(1), 25–26.

Naranjo, D., Tanenbaum, M. L., Iturralde, E., & Hood, K. K. (2016). Diabetes technology: Uptake, outcomes, barriers, and the intersection with distress. *Journal of Diabetes Science and Technology*, *10*(4), 852–858. DOI: 10.1177/1932296816650900 PMID: 27234809

Narwaria, M., & Jaiswal, S. (2024). Multicriteria client selection model using class topper optimization based optimal federated learning for healthcare informatics. *Cluster Computing*, *27*(8), 10325–10342. DOI: 10.1007/s10586-024-04466-8

Natarajan, R., Krishna, S., & Ranjith, C. P. (2025). A Novel Federated Learning Framework for Healthcare Applications Using Wearable Devices. *2025 IEEE 4th International Conference on AI in Cybersecurity, ICAIC 2025*. https://doi.org/DOI: 10.1109/ICAIC63015.2025.10848974

Nayan, T., Guo, Q., Al Duniawi, M., Botacin, M., Uluagac, S., & Sun, R. (2024). {SoK}: All You Need to Know About {On-Device} {ML} Model Extraction-The Gap Between Research and Practice. In 33rd USENIX Security Symposium (USENIX Security 24) pp. 5233-5250. https://www.usenix.org/system/files/usenixsecurity24-nayan.pdf

Nazir, A., Hussain, A., Singh, M., & Assad, A. (2025). Deep learning in medicine: Advancing healthcare with intelligent solutions and the future of holography imaging in early diagnosis. *Multimedia Tools and Applications*, *84*(17), 17677–17740. DOI: 10.1007/s11042-024-19694-8

Nazir, S., & Kaleem, M. (2023). Federated learning for medical image analysis with deep neural networks. *Diagnostics (Basel)*, *13*(9), 1532. Advance online publication. DOI: 10.3390/diagnostics13091532 PMID: 37174925

Nederlof, M., Stoker, L. J., Egberts, T. C., & Heerdink, E. R. (2024). Instructions for clinical and biomarker monitoring in the Summary of Product Characteristics (SmPC) for psychotropic drugs: Overview and applicability in clinical practice. *Journal of Psychopharmacology (Oxford, England)*, *29*(12), 1248–1254. DOI: 10.1177/0269881115609016 PMID: 26464457

Nguyen, D. C., Ding, M., Pathirana, P. N., Seneviratne, A., Li, J., & Poor, H. V. (2021). Federated learning for internet of things: A comprehensive survey. *IEEE Communications Surveys and Tutorials*, *23*(3), 1622–1658. DOI: 10.1109/COMST.2021.3075439

Nguyen, D. C., Pham, Q. V., Pathirana, P. N., Ding, M., Seneviratne, A., Lin, Z., Dobre, O., & Hwang, W. J. (2022). Federated learning for smart healthcare: A survey. *ACM Computing Surveys*, *55*(3), 1–37. DOI: 10.1145/3501296

Nguyen, T. V., Dakka, M. A., Diakiw, S. M., Ver Milyea, M. D., Perugini, M., Hall, J. M. M., & Perugini, D. (2022). A novel decentralized federated learning approach to train on globally distributed, poor quality, and protected private medical data. *Scientific Reports*, *12*(1), 8888. DOI: 10.1038/s41598-022-12833-x PMID: 35614106

Nguyen, T. X., Ran, A. R., Hu, X., Yang, D., Jiang, M., Dou, Q., & Cheung, C. Y. (2022). Federated learning in ocular imaging: Current progress and future direction. *Diagnostics (Basel), 12*(11), 2835. DOI: 10.3390/diagnostics12112835 PMID: 36428895

Niu, Q., Li, H., Liu, Y., Qin, Z., Zhang, L. B., Chen, J., & Lyu, Z. (2024). Toward the internet of medical things: Architecture, trends and challenges. *Mathematical Biosciences and Engineering, 21*(1), 650–678. DOI: 10.3934/mbe.2024028 PMID: 38303438

Nkonge, K. M., Nkonge, D. K., & Nkonge, T. N. (2023). Insulin therapy for the management of diabetes mellitus: A narrative review of innovative treatment strategies. *Diabetes Therapy : Research, Treatment and Education of Diabetes and Related Disorders, 14*(11), 1801–1831. DOI: 10.1007/s13300-023-01468-4 PMID: 37736787

Novotney, S., Mukherjee, S., Ahmed, Z., & Stolcke, A. (2022). CUE vectors: Modular training of language models conditioned on diverse contextual signals. https://arxiv.org/pdf/2106.01978

NVIDIA. (2021, October 20). *Federated learning helps hospitals predict COVID patients' oxygen needs*. NVIDIA Blog. https://blogs.nvidia.com/blog/federated-learning-covid-oxygen-needs/

Oh, W., & Nadkarni, G. N. (2023). Federated learning in health care using structured medical data. *Advances in Kidney Disease and Health, 30*(1), 4–16. DOI: 10.1053/j.akdh.2022.11.007 PMID: 36723280

Orlando, L. A., Buchanan, A. H., Hahn, S. E., Christianson, C. A., Powell, K. P., Skinner, C. S., & Henrich, V. C. (2013). Development and validation of a primary care-based family health history and decision support program (MeTree). *North Carolina Medical Journal, 74*(4), 287–296. https://pmc.ncbi.nlm.nih.gov/articles/PMC5215064/pdf/nihms838194.pdf. DOI: 10.18043/ncm.74.4.287 PMID: 24044145

Oyedokun, T. T. (2025). Assistive Technology and Accessibility Tools in Enhancing Adaptive Education. In *Advancing Adaptive Education: Technological Innovations for Disability Support* (pp. 125-162). IGI Global Scientific Publishing.

Panda, S., Dubey, R., Jena, B., Pareek, V., Tsai, L., & Saxena, S. (2025). Federated learning frameworks in smart e-healthcare: A systematic literature review with bias evaluation. *Applied Soft Computing, 171*, 112747. Advance online publication. DOI: 10.1016/j.asoc.2025.112747

Panwar, A., Gaba, P., Sugandh, U., & Bohra, N. (2025). Breaking the Centralization Barrier: Exploring Decentralized Federated Learning for Vehicle Number Plate Recognition in IoV. In *Federated Learning Based Intelligent Systems to Handle Issues and Challenges in IoVs (Part 2)* (pp. 102–139). Bentham Science Publishers. DOI: 10.2174/97898153222241250300006

Papernot, N., Song, S., Mironov, I., Raghunathan, A., Talwar, K., & Erlingsson, Ú. (2018). Scalable private learning with pate. *arXiv preprint arXiv:1802.08908.*

Passerat-Palmbach, J., Farnan, T., Miller, R., Gross, M. S., Flannery, H. L., & Gleim, B. (2020). A blockchain-orchestrated federated learning architecture for healthcare consortia. *arXiv preprint arXiv:1910.12603.*

Patel, M., Dayan, I., Fishman, E. K., Flores, M., Gilbert, F. J., Guindy, M., Koay, E. J., Rosenthal, M., Roth, H. R., & Linguraru, M. G. (2023). Accelerating artificial intelligence: How federated learning can protect privacy, facilitate collaboration, and improve outcomes. *Health Informatics Journal, 29*(4), 14604582231207744. DOI: 10.1177/14604582231207744 PMID: 37864543

Patel, V., Saxena, S., Lund, C., Thornicroft, G., Baingana, F., Bolton, P., & Unützer, J. (2018). The Lancet Commission on global mental health and sustainable development. *Lancet, 392*(10157), 1553–1598. DOI: 10.1016/S0140-6736(18)31612-X PMID: 30314863

Pati, S., Baid, U., Edwards, B., Sheller, M., Wang, S., Reina, G. A., Foley, P., Gruzdev, A., Karkada, D., Davatzikos, C., Sako, C., Ghodasara, S., Bilello, M., Mohan, S., Vollmuth, P., Brugnara, G., Preetha, C. J., Sahm, F., Maier-Hein, K., & Bakas, S. (2022). Federated learning enables big data for rare cancer boundary detection. *Nature Communications, 13*(1), 7346. Advance online publication. DOI: 10.1038/s41467-022-33407-5 PMID: 36470898

Patwari, P., & Vajpayee, A. (2024). Exploring the Interplay of Educational Social Media Usage, Procrastination, and Subjective Well-being in the Context of Industry 5.0 Education. In Tripathi, S., & Rosak-Szyrocka, J. (Eds.). (2024*). Impact of Artificial Intelligence on Society* (1st ed.). Chapman and Hall/CRC. Pp:119-133.

Pfitzner, B., Steckhan, N., & Arnrich, B. (2021). Federated learning in a medical context: A systematic literature review. *ACM Transactions on Internet Technology, 21*(2), 1–31. DOI: 10.1145/3412357

Pinto-Coelho, L. (2023). How artificial intelligence is shaping medical imaging technology: A survey of innovations and applications. *Bioengineering (Basel, Switzerland), 10*(12), 1435. Advance online publication. DOI: 10.3390/bioengineering10121435 PMID: 38136026

Pistolesi, M., Frangioni, G., Fraboni, F., Fabbri, E., & Masci, F. (2025). How will technology change people's home care in the next 20 years? A strategic foresight study. *Ergonomics*, *68*(3), 406–424. DOI: 10.1080/00140139.2024.2334428 PMID: 38533589

Pitt, K. M., Mikuls, A., Ousley, C. L., Boster, J. B., Mahmoudi, M., McCarthy, J., & Burnison, J. (2025). Considering whether brain–computer interfaces have prospective potential to support children who have the physical abilities for touch-based AAC access: A forum manuscript. *Augmentative and Alternative Communication*, 1–9. DOI: 10.1080/07434618.2025.2495897 PMID: 40454682

Pitts, L. N., Armstrong, A., Fleming, L., Fazeli, P. L., Landier, W., & Ladores, S. (2025). The application and evolution of the social-ecological model for adolescent and young adult readiness for transition: A scoping review. *Journal of Pediatric Health Care*, *39*(3), 355–376. DOI: 10.1016/j.pedhc.2024.12.004 PMID: 39772328

Poirot, M. G., Vepakomma, P., Chang, K., Kalpathy-Cramer, J., Gupta, R., & Raskar, R. (2019). Split learning for collaborative deep learning in healthcare. arXiv preprint arXiv:1912.12115.

Ponnuviji, N. P., Nirmala, G., Kokila, M. S., & Priyadharshini, S. I. (2025). Optimizing Image Retrieval in Cloud Servers with TN-AGW: A Secure and Efficient Approach. *Journal of The Institution of Engineers (India): Series B*, *106*(2), 459-473.

Ponnuviji, N. P., Sumaiya Begum, A., Gnanasekaran, T., Rajendiran, M., & Shenbaga Ezhil, S. (2023, April). Leveraging Random Forest for Intelligent IoT Systems in Industrial Environments. In *International Conference on Internet of Things* (pp. 46-57). Cham: Springer Nature Switzerland.

Poria, S., Cambria, E., Hazarika, D., & Vij, P. (2019). A deeper look into conversational AI: A survey of open-domain dialogue systems. *Information Fusion*, *54*, 124–144. DOI: 10.1016/j.inffus.2019.07.001

Predictive Analytics: The privacy pickle. (2019). Institute for Operations Research and the Management Sciences (INFORMS). DOI: 10.1287/LYTX.2013.06.02

Price, W. N.II, & Cohen, I. G. (2019). Privacy in the age of medical big data. *Nature Medicine*, *25*(1), 37–43. DOI: 10.1038/s41591-018-0272-7 PMID: 30617331

Priyadharshini, S. I., Irene, D. S., Beulah, J. R., & Ponnuviji, N. P. (2025). Enhancing real-time health monitoring with hybrid recurrent long short-term tyrannosaurus search for menstrual cups. *Biomedical Signal Processing and Control*, *100*, 107065. DOI: 10.1016/j.bspc.2024.107065

Punitha, S., & Preetha, K. S. (2025). Enhancing reliability and security in cloud-based telesurgery systems leveraging swarm-evoked distributed federated learning framework to mitigate multiple attacks. *Scientific Reports, 15*(1), 27226--. DOI: 10.1038/s41598-025-12027-1

Punreddy, A. R. (2023). *Federated Learning for Protecting Medical Data Privacy* [Master of Science, San Jose State University]., DOI: 10.31979/etd.cfgv-t6wa

Purohit, R. M., Verma, J. P., Jain, R., & Kumar, A. (2025). FedBlocks: Federated learning and blockchainbased privacy-preserved pioneering framework for IoT healthcare using IPFS in web 3.0 era. *Cluster Computing, 28*(2), 139. DOI: 10.1007/s10586-024-04738-3

Qi, J., Zhou, Q., Lei, L., & Zheng, K. (2021). Federated reinforcement learning: techniques, applications, and open challenges. In *Intelligence and Robotics* (Vol. 1, pp. 18–57). OAE Publishing Inc., DOI: 10.20517/ir.2021.02

Qu, L., Zhou, Y., Liang, P. P., Xia, Y., Wang, F., & Adeli, E.. (2022). Rethinking architecture design for tackling data heterogeneity in federated learning. In *Proceedings of the IEEE/CVF Conference on Computer Vision and Pattern Recognition (CVPR 2022)* (pp. 10051–10061). IEEE. DOI: 10.1109/CVPR52688.2022.00982

Radford, A., Wu, J., Child, R., Luan, D., Amodei, D., & Sutskever, I. (2019). Language models are unsupervised multitask learners. OpenAI. https://cdn.openai.com/better-language-models/language_models_are_unsupervised_multitask_learners.pdf

Rahaman, M., Arya, V., Orozco, S. M., & Pappachan, P. (2024). Secure multi-party computation (SMPC) protocols and privacy. In Innovations in Modern Cryptography, pp. 190-214. IGI Global. https://doi.org/DOI: 10.4018/979-8-3693-5330-1.ch008

Rahman, A., Hossain, M. S., Muhammad, G., Kundu, D., Debnath, T., Rahman, M., Khan, M. S. I., Tiwari, P., & Band, S. S. (2023). Federated learning-based AI approaches in smart healthcare: Concepts, taxonomies, challenges and open issues. *Cluster Computing, 26*(4), 2271–2311. DOI: 10.1007/s10586-022-03658-4 PMID: 35996680

Rajasegar, R. S., Gouthaman, P., Ponnusamy, V., Arivazhagan, N., & Nallarasan, V. (2024). Data privacy and ethics in data analytics. In *Studies in Big Data* (pp. 195–213). Springer Nature Singapore., DOI: 10.1007/978-981-97-0448-4_10

Rajendran, S., Xu, Z., Pan, W., Ghosh, A., & Wang, F. (2023). Data heterogeneity in federated learning with electronic health records: Case studies of risk prediction for acute kidney injury and sepsis diseases in critical care. *PLOS Digital Health, 2*(3), e0000117. DOI: 10.1371/journal.pdig.0000117 PMID: 36920974

Rajkomar, A., Dean, J., & Kohane, I. (2019). Machine learning in medicine. *The New England Journal of Medicine, 380*(14), 1347–1358. DOI: 10.1056/NEJMra1814259 PMID: 30943338

Rajkomar, A., Hardt, M., Howell, M. D., Corrado, G., & Chin, M. H. (2018). Ensuring fairness in machine learning to advance health equity. *Annals of Internal Medicine, 169*(12), 866–872. DOI: 10.7326/M18-1990 PMID: 30508424

Rajkomar, A., Oren, E., Chen, K., Dai, A. M., Hajaj, N., Hardt, M., Liu, P. J., Liu, X., Marcus, J., Sun, M., Sundberg, P., Yee, H., Zhang, K., Zhang, Y., Flores, G., Duggan, G. E., Irvine, J., Le, Q., Litsch, K., & Dean, J. (2018). Scalable and accurate deep learning with electronic health records. *NPJ Digital Medicine, 1*(1), 18. DOI: 10.1038/s41746-018-0029-1 PMID: 31304302

Rajput, R., Sukumar, V., Patnaik, P., Garg, P., & Ranjan, M. (2024). The Cognitive Analysis for an Approach to Neuroscience. *2024 International Conference on Automation and Computation (AUTOCOM)*, 524–528. DOI: 10.1109/AUTOCOM60220.2024.10486081

Ramaiah, M. S., Nagarajan, S. K. S., Whig, P., & Dutta, P. K. (2025). AI-powered innovations transforming adaptive education for disability support. In *Advancing Adaptive Education: Technological Innovations for Disability Support* (pp. 73–100). IGI Global Scientific Publishing.

Ramesh, P., Bhargavi, V. S., Shiney, S. A., Dinesh, M. G., & Nalini, M. (2024, October). Exploring the Transformative Impact of Machine Learning in Healthcare: Applications, Challenges, and Future Directions. In *2024 2nd International Conference on Self Sustainable Artificial Intelligence Systems (ICSSAS)* (pp. 620-627). IEEE.

Regulatory Affairs Professionals Society. (n.d.). The global regulatory landscape for AI/ML-enabled medical devices. *RAPS*. https://www.raps.org/News-and-Articles/News-Articles/2024/9/The-global-regulatory-landscape-for-AI-ML-enabled

Rehman, M. H. U., Hugo Lopez Pinaya, W., Nachev, P., Teo, J. T., Ourselin, S., & Cardoso, M. J. (2023). Federated learning for medical imaging radiology. *The British Journal of Radiology, 96*(1150), 20220890. DOI: 10.1259/bjr.20220890 PMID: 38011227

Reilly, J. B., Kim, J. G., Cooney, R., DeWaters, A. L., Holmboe, E. S., Mazotti, L., & Gonzalo, J. D. (2023). Breaking down silos between medical education and health systems: Creating an integrated multilevel data model to advance the systems-based practice competency. *Academic Medicine, 99*(2), 146–152. DOI: 10.1097/ACM.0000000000005294 PMID: 37289829

Ribeiro, M. T., Singh, S., & Guestrin, C. (2016, August). "Why should I trust you?": Explaining the predictions of any classifier. In Proceedings of the 22nd ACM SIGKDD International Conference on Knowledge Discovery and Data Mining (pp. 1135–1144). ACM. https://doi.org/DOI: 10.1145/2939672.2939778

Ribet, F., Stemme, G., & Roxhed, N. (2018). Real-time intradermal continuous glucose monitoring using a minimally invasive microneedle-based system. *Biomedical Microdevices*, *20*(4), 101. DOI: 10.1007/s10544-018-0349-6 PMID: 30523421

Rideout, V., & Fox, S. (2018), Digital Health Practices, Social Media Use, and Mental Well-Being Among Teens and Young Adults in the U.S.1-96, https://digitalcommons.providence.org/publications/1093/

Ridley, E. L. (2021, September 16). Strength in numbers: Federated learning boosts AI for COVID-19. *AuntMinnie*. https://www.auntminnie.com/clinical-news/digital-x-ray/article/15629249/strength-in-numbers-federated-learning-boosts-ai-for-covid-19

Rieke, N., Hancox, J., Li, W., Milletari, F., Roth, H. R., Albarqouni, S., Bakas, S., Galtier, M. N., Landman, B. A., Maier-Hein, K., Ourselin, S., Sheller, M., Summers, R. M., Trask, A., Xu, D., Baust, M., & Cardoso, M. J. (2020). The future of digital health with federated learning. *NPJ Digital Medicine*, *3*(1), 119. Advance online publication. DOI: 10.1038/s41746-020-00323-1 PMID: 33015372

Rimon, M. T. I., Hasan, M. W., Hassan, M. F., & Cesmeci, S. (2024). Advancements in insulin pumps: A comprehensive exploration of insulin pump systems, technologies, and future directions. *Pharmaceutics*, *16*(7), 944. DOI: 10.3390/pharmaceutics16070944 PMID: 39065641

Rose, R. M., Varun, C. M., Sivasakthi, K., Kennady, R., & Lekha, D. (2025, May). Leveraging AI and IoT Data for Predictive Modelling and Preventive Healthcare. In *2025 Third International Conference on Augmented Intelligence and Sustainable Systems (ICAISS)* (pp. 628-633). IEEE. DOI: 10.1109/ICAISS61471.2025.11041733

Roth, H. R., Cheng, Y., Wen, Y., Yang, I., Xu, Z., Hsieh, Y.-T., Kersten, K., Harouni, A., Zhao, C., Lu, K., & Associates. (2022). Nvidia flare: Federated learning from simulation to real-world. *ArXiv Preprint ArXiv:2210.13291.*

Roth, H. R., Chang, K., Singh, P., Neumark, N., Li, W., Gupta, V., & Kalpathy-Cramer, J. (2020, September). Federated learning for breast density classification: A real-world implementation. In *MICCAI Workshop on Domain Adaptation and Representation Transfer* (pp. 181-191). Cham: Springer International Publishing. DOI: 10.1007/978-3-030-60548-3_18

Roussou, A. M., Argyrakou, C. C., & Milakis, E. D. (2025). Integrating STEAM and theatrical methods in early childhood environmental education: A framework for holistic learning. *International Journal of Geography. Geology and Environment, 7*(2), 19–42.

Roy, P. D., Gupta Chowdhory, U., Dey, A., & Husain Sagor, D. (2025). AI and Machine Learning in Healthcare: Advancing Diagnostics, Personalized Treatment, and Predictive Modeling. *Preprints*. DOI: 10.20944/preprints202504.0007.v1

Rydzewski, P. (2025). Digital inequality and sustainable development. *Problemy Ekorozwoju, 20*(1), 96–108. DOI: 10.35784/preko.6691

Sadilek, A., Liu, L., Nguyen, D., Kamruzzaman, M., Serghiou, S., Rader, B., Ingerman, A., Mellem, S., Kairouz, P., Nsoesie, E. O., MacFarlane, J., Vullikanti, A., Marathe, M., Eastham, P., Brownstein, J. S., Arcas, B. A. Y., Howell, M. D., & Hernandez, J. (2021). Privacy-first health research with federated learning. *NPJ Digital Medicine, 4*(1), 132. DOI: 10.1038/s41746-021-00489-2 PMID: 34493770

Sandhu, S. S., Gorji, H. T., Tavakolian, P., Tavakolian, K., & Akhbardeh, A. (2023). Medical imaging applications of Federated Learning. *Diagnostics (Basel), 13*(19), 3140. Advance online publication. DOI: 10.3390/diagnostics13193140 PMID: 37835883

Saraswat, D., Bhattacharya, P., Verma, A., Prasad, V. K., Tanwar, S., Sharma, G., Bokoro, P. N., & Sharma, R. (2022). Explainable AI for healthcare 5.0: Opportunities and challenges. *IEEE Access : Practical Innovations, Open Solutions, 10*, 84486–84517. DOI: 10.1109/ACCESS.2022.3197671

Sattler, F., Wiedemann, S., Müller, K., & Samek, W. (2019). Sparse binary compression: Towards distributed deep learning with minimal communication. In *Proceedings of the International Joint Conference on Neural Networks (IJCNN)* (pp. 1–8). IEEE. https://doi.org/DOI: 10.1109/IJCNN.2019.8852172

Scalcon, F. P., Tahal, R., Ahrabi, M., Huangfu, Y., Ahmed, R., Nahid-Mobarakeh, B., & Emadi, A. (2024, June). AI-Powered Video Monitoring: Assessing the NVIDIA Jetson Orin Devices for Edge Computing Applications. In 2024 Institute of Electrical and Electronics Engineers Transportation Electrification Conference and Expo (ITEC) pp. 1-6. Institute of Electrical and Electronics Engineers.

Schick, T., & Schütze, H. "It's not just size that matters: Small language models are also few-shot learners." arXiv preprint arXiv:2009.07118 (2020). https://arxiv.org/pdf/2009.07118

Selvaraju, R. R., Cogswell, M., Das, A., Vedantam, R., Parikh, D., & Batra, D. (2017). Grad-CAM: Visual explanations from deep networks via gradient-based localization. *International Journal of Computer Vision, 128*(2), 336–359. DOI: 10.1007/s11263-019-01228-7

Shahsavari, Y., Dambri, O. A., Baseri, Y., Hafid, A. S., & Makrakis, D. (2024). *Integration of Federated Learning and Blockchain in Healthcare: A Tutorial.*

Sharma, N., Sugandh, U., Agarwal, J., Panwar, A., & Gaba, P. (2025). Federated Learning on Wheels: A Decentralized Approach to Privacy-Enhanced Data Collection in Internet of Vehicles. In *Federated Learning Based Intelligent Systems to Handle Issues and Challenges in IoVs (Part 2)* (pp. 1–33). Bentham Science Publishers. DOI: 10.2174/9789815322224125030003

Sharma, S., Mittal, S., Tevatia, R., Tyagi, V. K., Garg, P., & Kapoor, S. (2025). Unlocking Workforce Potential. *AI-Powered Predictive Models for Employee Performance Evaluation.*, (May), 143–149. DOI: 10.63169/GCARED2025.p21

Sheller, M. J., Edwards, B., Reina, G. A., Martin, J., Pati, S., Kotrotsou, A., Milchenko, M., Xu, W., Marcus, D., Colen, R. R., Bakas, S., & Davatzikos, C. (2020). Federated learning in medicine: Facilitating multi-institutional collaborations without sharing patient data. *Scientific Reports, 10*(1), 12598. DOI: 10.1038/s41598-020-69250-1 PMID: 32724046

Shen, H., Chang, H., Dong, B., Luo, Y., & Meng, H. (2023). Efficient llm inference on cpus. arXiv preprint, https://arxiv.org/pdf/2311.00502

Shiny Irene, D., Ponnuviji, N. P., & Kalaivani, A. (2025). EHECA-HSWS: A Holistic Method for Improving Menstrual Health App User Experience. *Journal of the Institution of Electronics and Telecommunication Engineers*, 1–12. DOI: 10.1080/03772063.2025.2508330

Shi, Y., Zhang, J., Xue, M., Zeng, Y., Jia, G., Yu, Q., & Li, M. (2025). Vertical federated learning based on data subset representation for healthcare application. *Computer Methods and Programs in Biomedicine, 263*, 108623. DOI: 10.1016/j.cmpb.2025.108623 PMID: 39954511

Shokri, R., Stronati, M., Song, C., & Shmatikov, V. (2017, May). Membership inference attacks against machine learning models. In *2017 IEEE symposium on security and privacy (SP)* (pp. 3-18). IEEE. DOI: 10.1109/SP.2017.41

Shokri, R., & Shmatikov, V. (2015). Privacy-preserving deep learning. In **Proceedings of the 22nd ACM SIGSAC Conference on Computer and Communications Security (CCS '15)*. Association for Computing Machinery, New York, NY, USA, 1310–1321. https://doi.org/DOI: 10.1145/2810103.2813687

Shukla, S., Rajkumar, S., Sinha, A., Esha, M., Elango, K., & Sampath, V. (2025). Federated learning with differential privacy for breast cancer diagnosis enabling secure data sharing and model integrity. *Scientific Reports, 15*(1), 13061--. DOI: 10.1038/s41598-025-95858-2

Silva, S., Altmann, A., Gutman, B., & Lorenzi, M. (2020). Fed-BioMed: A general open-source frontend framework for federated learning in healthcare. In Domain Adaptation and Representation Transfer, and Distributed and Collaborative Learning (pp. 201–210). Springer International Publishing. DOI: 10.1007/978-3-030-60548-3_20

Silva, S., Gutman, B. A., Romero, E., Thompson, P. M., Altmann, A., & Lorenzi, M. (2019, April). Federated learning in distributed medical databases: Meta-analysis of large-scale subcortical brain data. In *2019 IEEE 16th international symposium on biomedical imaging (ISBI 2019)* (pp. 270-274). IEEE.

Singh, M., Gupta, M., Sharma, A., Jain. Parita, & Aggarwal, P. (2023). *Role of Deep Learning in Healthcare Industry: Limitations, Challenges and Future Scope* (Vol. 11). BENTHAM SCIENCE PUBLISHERS. DOI: 10.2174/97898150802301230201

Singh, M., Sukhija, N., Sharma, A., Gupta, M., & Aggarwal, P. K. (2021). Security and Privacy Requirements for IoMT-Based Smart Healthcare System: Challenges, Solutions, and Future Scope. In *Big Data Analysis for Green Computing*. Concepts and Applications., DOI: 10.1201/9781003032328-2

Smuha, N. A. (2019). The EU approach to ethics guidelines for trustworthy artificial intelligence. Computer Law Review International, 20(4), 97-106. https://www.europarl.europa.eu/cmsdata/196377/AI%20HLEG_Ethics%20Guidelines%20for%20Trustworthy%20AI.pdf

Sohan, M. F., & Basalamah, A. (2023). A systematic review on federated learning in medical image analysis. *IEEE Access : Practical Innovations, Open Solutions, 11*, 28628–28644. DOI: 10.1109/ACCESS.2023.3260027

Solanki, S., Agarwal, J., Jain, A., Dubey, A. K., Panwar, A., & Priyadarshi, P. (2025). Evaluating Multi-Layer Perceptron and Recurrent Neural Networks for Speech Emotion Recognition. *2025 3rd International Conference on Communication, Security, and Artificial Intelligence, ICCSAI 2025, 3*, 349–354. DOI: 10.1109/ICCSAI64074.2025.11064042

Sprenkamp, K., Fernández, J. D., Eckhardt, S., & Zavolokina, L. (2024). Overcoming intergovernmental data sharing challenges with federated learning. *Data & Policy*, *6*, e19. Advance online publication. DOI: 10.1017/dap.2024.19

Sundari, V. M., Rose, R. M., Sassirekha, S. M., Nalini, M., & Girija, P. (2024, November). Deep Learning: Techniques, Taxonomy, Applications, and Future Directions. In *2024 International Conference on Smart Technologies for Sustainable Development Goals (ICSTSDG)* (pp. 1-5). IEEE.

Su, Z., Wang, Y., Luan, T. H., Zhang, N., Li, F., Chen, T., & Cao, H. (2021). Secure and efficient federated learning for smart grid with edge-cloud collaboration. *IEEE Transactions on Industrial Informatics*, *18*(2), 1333–1344. DOI: 10.1109/TII.2021.3095506

Tan, X., Jiang, Y., Yang, Y., & Xu, H. (2024). Teola: Towards end-to-end optimization of llm-based applications. arXiv preprint arXiv:2407.00326. https://arxiv.org/pdf/2407.00326

Tanenbaum, M. L., Hanes, S. J., Miller, K. M., Naranjo, D., Bensen, R., & Hood, K. K. (2017). Diabetes device use in adults with type 1 diabetes: Barriers to uptake and potential intervention targets. *Diabetes Care*, *40*(2), 181–187. DOI: 10.2337/dc16-1536 PMID: 27899489

Tangari, G., Ikram, M., Sentana, I. W. B., Ijaz, K., Kaafar, M. A., & Berkovsky, S. (2021). Analyzing security issues of android mobile health and medical applications. *Journal of the American Medical Informatics Association : JAMIA*, *28*(Issue 10), 2074–2084. https://doi.org/. DOI: 10.1093/jamia/ocab131 PMID: 34338763

Teo, Z. L., Jin, L., Liu, N., Li, S., Miao, D., Zhang, X., Ng, W. Y., Tan, T. F., Lee, D. M., Chua, K. J., Heng, J., Liu, Y., Goh, R. S. M., & Ting, D. S. W. (2024). Federated machine learning in healthcare: A systematic review on clinical applications and technical architecture. *Cell Reports Medicine*, *5*(2), 101419. DOI: 10.1016/j.xcrm.2024.101419 PMID: 38340728

Thakur, D. (2021). Federated learning and privacy-preserving AI: Challenges and solutions in distributed machine learning. [IJARESM]. *International Journal of All Research Education and Scientific Methods*, *9*(6), 3763–3764.

Thilakarathne, N. N., Muneeswari, G., Parthasarathy, V., Alassery, F., Hamam, H., Mahendran, R. K., & Shafiq, M. (2022). Federated learning for privacy-preserved medical internet of things. *Intelligent Automation & Soft Computing*, *33*(1), 157–172. DOI: 10.32604/iasc.2022.023763

Thomas, M. G., Avari, P., Godsland, I. F., Lett, A. M., Reddy, M., & Oliver, N. (2021). Optimizing type 1 diabetes after multiple daily injections and capillary blood monitoring: Pump or sensor first? A meta-analysis using pooled differences in outcome measures. *Diabetes, Obesity & Metabolism*, *23*(11), 2521–2528. DOI: 10.1111/dom.14498 PMID: 34286892

Tonekaboni, S., Joshi, S., McCradden, M. D., & Goldenberg, A. (2019). What clinicians want: Contextualizing explainable machine learning for clinical end use. In Proceedings of the Machine Learning for Healthcare Conference (pp. 359–380). PMLR. http://proceedings.mlr.press/v106/tonekaboni19a/tonekaboni19a.pdf

Topol, E. J. (2019). High-performance medicine: The convergence of human and artificial intelligence. *Nature Medicine*, *25*(1), 44–56. DOI: 10.1038/s41591-018-0300-7 PMID: 30617339

Treloar, A. (2014). The Research Data Alliance: Globally co-ordinated action against barriers to data publishing and sharing. *Learned Publishing*, *27*(5), 9–13. DOI: 10.1087/20140503

Ullah, F., Srivastava, G., Xiao, H., Ullah, S., Lin, J. C. W., & Zhao, Y. (2024). A Scalable Federated Learning Approach for Collaborative Smart Healthcare Systems with Intermittent Clients Using Medical Imaging. *IEEE Journal of Biomedical and Health Informatics*, *28*(6), 3293–3304. DOI: 10.1109/JBHI.2023.3282955 PMID: 37279135

Upadhyay, D., Garg, P., Aldossary, S. M., Shafi, J., & Kumar, S. (2023). A linear quadratic regression-based synchronised health monitoring system (SHMS) for IoT applications. *Electronics (Basel)*, *12*(2), 309. DOI: 10.3390/electronics12020309

Upreti, D., Yang, E., Kim, H., & Seo, C. (2024). A Comprehensive Survey on Federated Learning in the Healthcare Area: Concept and Applications. *CMES-Computer Modeling in Engineering \& Sciences, 140*(3).

Vajpayee, A. (2019). Critical Issues of Early Intervention for the Amelioration of Social Isolation of Kharwar Children. In (Eds) Nagendra Kumar Singh, Tribal Communication Myth Metaphor and Reality. Iesha Gyandeep Publication, ISBN: 9788193790694. New Delhi (pp 169-181).

Vajpayee, A. (2021). Environmental challenges and critical issues of early intervention for the children of Kharwar tribe. In Pratap, A., Paranjape, B., Shyam, G. 2021 (Eds.). Tribal and Environmental History of India: New Perspectives. Research India Press. New Delhi, Pp-312-328.

Vajpayee, A. (2023). Intervention Studies for Mental Health: A Comprehensive Exploration of Historical Evolution, Theoretical Foundations, and Contemporary Applications. Journal of Humanities, Music and Dance, Vol-3, Issue-5, Pp-21-33. ISSN:2799-1180. https://doi.org/10.55529/jmhib.35.21.33

Vajpayee, A. (2024). Pixels, Perspectives, and Psychological Strain: Unravelling the Link Between Negative Body Image, Internet of Things (IOT), and Mental Health Challenges in Student Population. In: Gupta, S.K., Karras, D.A., Natarajan, R. (eds) *Revolutionizing Healthcare: AI Integration with IoT for Enhanced Patient Outcomes. Information Systems Engineering and Management*, (Pp-). vol 7. ISBN: 978-3-031-65021. Springer Nature, Switzerland, Cham. https://doi.org/ DOI: 10.1007/978-3-031-65022-2_17

Vajpayee, A. (2024). Traditional pedagogy to Technetronic Education. *Aspects of Quality Management in Value Creating in the Industry 5.0 Way*, 179. ISBN: 9781032677019 https://doi.org/DOI: 10.1201/9781032677040

Vajpayee, A., & Ramachandran, K. K. (2019) Reconnoitring Artificial Intelligence in Knowledge Management. International Journal of Innovative Technology and Exploring Engineering (IJITEE) ISSN: 2278-3075, Volume-8 Issue-7C May 2019. Pp; 114-117.

Vajpayee, A., Gupta, S. K., & Sanghani, P. (2025). Immersive Learning for Environmental Stewardship: Behavioural Effectiveness, Engagement, and Motivation to Act Through XR Technology. In: Gupta, S.K., Maurya, N., Le, DN., Mzili, T. (eds) Exploring the Impact of Extended Reality (XR) Technologies on Promoting Environmental Sustainability. Information Systems Engineering and Management, vol 38. Pp-383-480 Springer Nature, Switzerland Cham. ISBN: 978-3-031-88013-1. https://doi.org/DOI: 10.1007/978-3-031-88013-1_21

Vajpayee, A. (2017). Effect of Early Intervention on Pictorial Perception of Deprived and Non-Deprived Children. *Indian Journal of Psychological Science. Vol*, *9*(1).

Vajpayee, A. (2017). Impact of Visual Literacy Skill Program on Visual Literacy of Deprived Children and Non-Deprived Children. *Likars'ka Sprava*, (7), 75–80. https://liksprava.com/index.php/journal/article/view/314. DOI: 10.31640/LS-2017(7)15

Vajpayee, A. (2024). IoT in Daily Life: Investigating the Impact of IoT on Procrastination, Well-Being, Mental Health, and Healthcare Wizards. In Gupta, S. K., Karras, D. A., & Natarajan, R. (Eds.), *Revolutionizing Healthcare: AI Integration with IoT for Enhanced Patient Outcomes. Information Systems Engineering and Management, ISBN: 978-3-031-65021* (Vol. 7). Springer., DOI: 10.1007/978-3-031-65022-2_11

Vajpayee, A. (2025). AG-IoT and robotics solutions for early intervention in developmental delays among mentally retarded children. In Malik, M. M., Maryam, H., Khan, I. U., & Gupta, S. K. (Eds.), *Artificial General-Internet of Things (AG-IoT) for Robotics: Advanced computer vision applications and future trends* (Vol. 58, pp. 1–16). Springer., DOI: 10.1007/978-3-031-95302-6_1

Vajpayee, A., & Mishra, R. C. (2003). The Short and Long-Term Effect of Training on Cognitive Task Performance of Children. *Indian Journal of Psychology*, *10*, 6–12.

van Genderen, M. E., Cecconi, M., & Jung, C. (2024). Federated data access and Federated learning: Improved data sharing, AI model development, and learning in intensive care. *Intensive Care Medicine*, *50*(6), 974–977. DOI: 10.1007/s00134-024-07408-5 PMID: 38635044

Vasilev, Y., Rumyantsev, D., Vladzymyrskyy, A., Omelyanskaya, O., Pestrenin, L., Shulkin, I., Nikitin, E., Kapninskiy, A., & Arzamasov, K. (2025). Evolution of an Artificial Intelligence-Powered Application for Mammography. *Diagnostics (Basel)*, *15*(7), 822. DOI: 10.3390/diagnostics15070822 PMID: 40218172

Vepakomma, P., Gupta, O., Swedish, T., & Raskar, R. (2018). Split learning for health: Distributed deep learning without sharing raw patient data. *arXiv preprint arXiv:1812.00564*.

Verdejo Espinosa, Á., Lopez, J. L., Mata Mata, F., & Estevez, M. E. (2021). Application of IoT in healthcare: Keys to implementation of the sustainable development goals. *Sensors (Basel)*, *21*(7), 2330. DOI: 10.3390/s21072330 PMID: 33810606

Verma, A., & Khari, M. (2024). Vision-Based Accident Anticipation and Detection Using Deep Learning. *IEEE Instrumentation & Measurement Magazine*, *27*(3), 22–29. DOI: 10.1109/MIM.2024.10505198

Verma, S., & Kumar, M. (2024). Automatic classification of melanoma using Grab-Cut segmentation and convolutional neural network. *SN Computer Science*, *5*(5), 591. DOI: 10.1007/s42979-024-02949-4

Verma, S., & Kumar, M. (2025). A hybrid machine learning model for skin disease classification using discrete wavelet transform and gray level co-occurrence matrix (GLCM). *Multimedia Tools and Applications*, *84*(12), 12835–12853. DOI: 10.1007/s11042-024-19449-5

Vora, L. K., Gholap, A. D., Jetha, K., Thakur, R. R. S., Solanki, H. K., & Chavda, V. P. (2023). Artificial intelligence in pharmaceutical technology and drug delivery design. *Pharmaceutics*, *15*(7), 1916. DOI: 10.3390/pharmaceutics15071916 PMID: 37514102

Wåger, J., & Bagger, A. (2025). Didactic dimensions of teaching content for and with students with intellectual disabilities (ID): A scoping review. *European Journal of Special Needs Education, 40*(1), 53–68. DOI: 10.1080/08856257.2024.2323250

Wang, R., Gao, Z., Zhang, L., Yue, S., & Gao, Z. (2025). Empowering large language models to edge intelligence: A survey of edge efficient LLMs and techniques. *Computer Science Review, 57*, 100755. https://chinaxiv.org/abs/202411.00258V1. DOI: 10.1016/j.cosrev.2025.100755

Wang, S., Zhang, Y., & Zhang, Y. (2018). A blockchain-based framework for data sharing with fine-grained access control in decentralized storage systems. *IEEE Access : Practical Innovations, Open Solutions, 6*, 38437–38450. DOI: 10.1109/ACCESS.2018.2851611

Wang, T., Du, Y., Gong, Y., Choo, K.-K. R., & Guo, Y. (2023). Applications of federated learning in mobile health: Scoping review. *Journal of Medical Internet Research, 25*, e43006. Advance online publication. DOI: 10.2196/43006 PMID: 37126398

Wen, J., Li, X., Ye, X., Li, X., & Mao, H. (2025). A highly generalized federated learning algorithm for brain tumor segmentation. *Scientific Reports, 15*(1), 21053--. DOI: 10.1038/s41598-025-05297-2

Wen, Y., & Wen, Y. (2022, September 2). Federated learning powered by NVIDIA Clara. *NVIDIA Technical Blog*. https://developer.nvidia.com/blog/federated-learning-clara/

Wen, J., Zhang, Z., Lan, Y., Cui, Z., Cai, J., & Zhang, W. (2023). A survey on federated learning: Challenges and applications. *International Journal of Machine Learning and Cybernetics, 14*(2), 513–535. DOI: 10.1007/s13042-022-01647-y PMID: 36407495

Wiafe, E., & Azubuike, C. M. (2024). Juggling family commitments and responsibilities in North America: Narratives from female African graduate students. *Cuadernos del Centro de Estudios de Diseño y Comunicación*, 27(238).

Wibawa, F., Catak, F. O., Sarp, S., & Kuzlu, M. (2022). BFV-based homomorphic encryption for privacy-preserving CNN models. *Cryptography, 6*(3), 34. DOI: 10.3390/cryptography6030034

Wilson, L. M., & Castle, J. R. (2020). Recent advances in insulin therapy. *Diabetes Technology & Therapeutics, 22*(12), 929–936. DOI: 10.1089/dia.2020.0065 PMID: 32310681

Xia, Y., Yang, D., Li, W., Myronenko, A., Xu, D., Obinata, H., Mori, H., An, P., & Harmon, S. Turkbey Evrim and Turkbey, B., Wood, B., Patella Francesca and Stellato, E., Carrafiello, G., Ierardi, A., Yuille, A., & Roth, H. (2021). Auto-FedAvg: Learnable federated averaging for multi-institutional medical image segmentation. https://doi.org//arXiv.2104.10195DOI: 10.48550

Xing, H., Sun, R., Ren, J., Wei, J., Feng, C. M., Ding, X., Guo, Z., Wang, Y., Hu, Y., Wei, W., Ban, X., Xie, C., Tan, Y., Liu, X., Cui, S., Duan, X., & Li, Z. (2025). Achieving flexible fairness metrics in federated medical imaging. *Nature Communications, 16*(1), 3342--. DOI: 10.1038/s41467-025-58549-0

Xu, J., Glicksberg, B. S., Su, C., Walker, P., Bian, J., & Wang, F. (2021). Federated learning for healthcare informatics. *Journal of Healthcare Informatics Research, 5*(1), 1–19. DOI: 10.1007/s41666-020-00082-4 PMID: 33204939

Yala, A., Lehman, C., Schuster, T., Portnoi, T., & Barzilay, R. (2019). A deep learning mammography-based model for improved breast cancer risk prediction. *Radiology, 292*(1), 60–66. DOI: 10.1148/radiol.2019182716 PMID: 31063083

Yale, A., Dash, S., Dutta, R., Guyon, I., Pavao, A., & Bennett, K. P. (2019, April). Privacy preserving synthetic health data. In *ESANN 2019-European Symposium on Artificial Neural Networks, Computational Intelligence and Machine Learning*.

Yamini, B., Dinesh, M. G., Gracious, L. A., & Subramanian, R. S. (2025). Exploring Blockchain Technology: Concepts, Features, and Industry Transformations. In *Blockchain Applications for the Energy and Utilities Industry* (pp. 305-322). IGI Global Scientific Publishing.

Yang, B., Yuen, P. C., Zhang, Y., & Zeng, A. (2023). Allosteric feature collaboration for model-heterogeneous federated learning. *IEEE Transactions on Neural Networks and Learning Systems*. Advance online publication. DOI: 10.1109/TNNLS.2023.3335168 PMID: 38145509

Yang, Q., Liu, Y., Chen, T., & Tong, Y. (2019). Federated machine learning. *ACM Transactions on Intelligent Systems and Technology, 10*(2), 12. Advance online publication. DOI: 10.1145/3298981

Yang, X., & Xing, C. (2024). Federated medical learning framework based on blockchain and homomorphic encryption. *Wireless Communications and Mobile Computing, 2024*, 1–15. DOI: 10.1155/2024/8138644

Yang, X., Yu, H., Gao, X., Wang, H., Zhang, J., & Li, T. (2024). Federated continual learning via knowledge fusion: A survey. *IEEE Transactions on Knowledge and Data Engineering, 36*(8), 3832–3850. DOI: 10.1109/TKDE.2024.3363240

Yaqoob, M. M., Alsulami, M., Khan, M. A., Alsadie, D., Saudagar, A. K. J., AlKhathami, M., & Khattak, U. F. (2023). Symmetry in Privacy-Based Healthcare: A Review of Skin Cancer Detection and Classification Using Federated Learning. *Symmetry, 15*(7), 1369. DOI: 10.3390/sym15071369

Yin, L., Feng, J., Xun, H., Sun, Z., & Cheng, X. (2021). A privacy-preserving federated learning for multiparty data sharing in social IoTs. *IEEE Transactions on Network Science and Engineering*, *8*(3), 2706–2718. DOI: 10.1109/TNSE.2021.3074185

Yonemori, Y., Takahashi, E., Ren, H., Hayashi, T., & Endo, H. (2009). Biosensor system for continuous glucose monitoring in fish. *Analytica Chimica Acta*, *633*(1), 90–96. DOI: 10.1016/j.aca.2008.11.023 PMID: 19110121

Yu, C., Shen, S., Wang, S., Zhang, K., & Zhao, H. (2025). Communication-Efficient Hybrid Federated Learning for E-Health with Horizontal and Vertical Data Partitioning. *IEEE Transactions on Neural Networks and Learning Systems*, *36*(3), 5614–5628. DOI: 10.1109/TNNLS.2024.3383748 PMID: 38598400

Yurdem, B., Kuzlu, M., Gullu, M. K., Catak, F. O., & Tabassum, M. (2024). Federated learning: Overview, strategies, applications, tools and future directions. *Heliyon*, *10*(19), e38137. Advance online publication. DOI: 10.1016/j.heliyon.2024.e38137 PMID: 39391509

Zaeem, R. N., & Barber, K. S. (2020). The effect of the GDPR on privacy policies: Recent progress and future promise. [TMIS]. *ACM Transactions on Management Information Systems*, *12*(1), 1–20. DOI: 10.1145/3389685

Zhang, P., Li, Y., Zhou, Z., & Wang, J. (2024). TinyLLaMA: Compact and efficient language models for edge NLP applications. Proceedings of the 2024 International Conference on Computational Linguistics (COLING). https://arxiv.org/html/2401.02385v1

Zhang, T., Zhang, S., Chen, Z., & Liu, D. (2021). PMFL: Partial Meta-Federated Learning for heterogeneous tasks and its applications on real-world medical records.

Zhang, F., Kreuter, D., Chen, Y., Dittmer, S., Tull, S., Shadbahr, T., Schut, M., Asselbergs, F., Kar, S., Sivapalaratnam, S., Williams, S., Koh, M., Henskens, Y., de Wit, B., D'Alessandro, U., Bah, B., Secka, O., Nachev, P., Gupta, R., & Roberts, M. (2024). Recent methodological advances in Federated learning for healthcare. *Patterns (New York, N.Y.)*, *5*(6), 101006. DOI: 10.1016/j.patter.2024.101006 PMID: 39005485

Zhang, F., Shuai, Z., Kuang, K., Wu, F., Zhuang, Y., & Xiao, J. (2023). Unified fair federated learning for digital healthcare. *Patterns (New York, N.Y.)*, *5*(1), 100907. Advance online publication. DOI: 10.1016/j.patter.2023.100907 PMID: 38264718

Zhang, L., Fang, G., & Tan, Z. (2025). FedCCW: A privacy-preserving Byzantine-robust federated learning with local differential privacy for healthcare. *Cluster Computing*, *28*(3), 182. Advance online publication. DOI: 10.1007/s10586-024-04894-6

Zhang, X., Pan, S. L., Tim, Y., & Jiang, Z. (2025). Designing an immersive virtual reality artefact for disability inclusion: An action design research. *European Journal of Information Systems*, 1–30. DOI: 10.1080/0960085X.2025.2567670

Zhao, Y., Chen, J., Zhang, J., Yang, Z., Tu, H., Han, H., Zhu, K., & Chen, B. (2021). User-Level Membership Inference for Federated Learning in Wireless Network Environment. *Wireless Communications and Mobile Computing*, *2021*(1), 5534270. DOI: 10.1155/2021/5534270

Zhou, H., Tang, J., & Zheng, H. (2015). Machine learning for medical applications. *TheScientificWorldJournal*, *825267*(1), 825267. Advance online publication. DOI: 10.1155/2015/825267 PMID: 25692180

Zhou, L., Jain, A., Dubey, A. K., Singh, S. K., Gupta, N., Panwar, A., Kumar, S., Althaqafi, T. A., Arya, V., Alhalabi, W., & Gupta, B. B. (2025). FPA-based weighted average ensemble of deep learning models for classification of lung cancer using CT scan images. *Scientific Reports*, *15*(1), 19369. DOI: 10.1038/s41598-025-02015-w PMID: 40461493

Zhou, T., Lin, Z., Zhang, J., & Tsang, D. H. (2024). Understanding and improving model averaging in federated learning on heterogeneous data. *IEEE Transactions on Mobile Computing*, *23*(12), 12131–12145. DOI: 10.1109/TMC.2024.3406554

Zhou, Y., Wu, Y., Su, Y., Li, J., Cai, J., You, Y., Zhou, J., Guo, D., & Qu, X. (2025). Cloud-magnetic resonance imaging system: In the era of 6G and artificial intelligence. *Magnetic Resonance Letters*, *5*(1), 200138. DOI: 10.1016/j.mrl.2024.200138 PMID: 40918039

Ziller, A., Usynin, D., Braren, R., Makowski, M., Rueckert, D., & Kaissis, G. (2021). Medical imaging deep learning with differential privacy. *Scientific Reports*, *11*(1), 13524. DOI: 10.1038/s41598-021-93030-0 PMID: 34188157

About the Contributors

Ng Khai Mun currently serves as the Acting Deputy Vice Chancellor (Academic & Research) at Infrastructure University Kuala Lumpur, Malaysia. Before becoming Acting Deputy Vice Chancellor, he was the Dean of the Faculty of Engineering, Science & Technology. With over 15 years in academia, Dr. Ng has significantly contributed to engineering education and research. A Chartered Engineer with the Engineering Council UK, and a Professional Technologist with the Malaysia Board of Technologies, he actively engages in academic and industry collaborations. His scholarly work includes multiple journal publications, conference proceedings, and a registered copyright for a solar absorber system. He has been involved in various funded research projects. His research expertise spans renewable energy systems, thermo fluids, and sustainable engineering solutions. He has served as a reviewer for high-impact journals such as Solar Energy and the Journal of Building Engineering, as well as a panel evaluator for research funding proposals. Beyond his academic and research commitments, Dr. Ng is dedicated to fostering innovation and industry-driven research collaborations.

Chin-Shiuh Shieh received the M.S. degree in electrical engineering from National Taiwan University, Taipei, Taiwan, in 1991, and the Ph.D. degree from the Department of Computer Science and Engineering, National Sun Yat-Sen University, Kaohsiung, Taiwan, in 2009. In 1991, he joined the Department of Electronic Engineering, National Kaohsiung University of Science and Technology, Kaohsiung, as a Faculty Member, where he is currently an Associate Professor. His research interests include wireless networks and handover techniques.

Danish Ather is an accomplished book editor with a robust academic and professional background. Currently as Professor at Amity University in Tashkent, Uzbekistan, Dr. Ather brings over 18 years of experience in teaching, research, and administration. He holds dual Ph.D. degrees in Computer Science and Computer Science & Engineering. His editorial expertise is highlighted through his role as

Editor of the proceedings submitted yearly to IEEE USA for the SMART Series conferences. Dr. Ather has authored a book titled "Level up Your Programming with Core Dragon" and published 54 research papers in international journals and conferences, with 15 indexed in Scopus. He is a Senior Member of the IEEE Society and has received numerous awards, including a Certificate of Appreciation from the Ministry of Digital Technologies, Republic of Uzbekistan. His technical proficiency and dedication to advancing knowledge in fields such as IoT, AI, and programming make him a valuable asset in the realm of academic publishing.

Arvind Panwar is a distinguished researcher and academician with over 15 years of experience in Computer Science and Engineering. He holds a Ph.D. from Guru Gobind Singh Indraprastha University, where his thesis focused on designing a secure cloud-based blockchain framework for health record management. His expertise spans blockchain technology, information security, cybersecurity, and data analytics.Dr. Panwar is actively involved in academic publishing, having authored 9 SCI/SCOPUS-indexed journal articles, 15 conference papers, and 18 book chapters. He is currently editing three significant books for esteemed publishers: Data Analytics and Artificial Intelligence for Predictive Maintenance in Industry 4.0 for Bentham, Qubits Unveiled: Quantum Computing Solutions for Efficient Supply Logistics for Nova Publications, and Energy Efficient Internet of Things-Based Wireless Sensor Network for Wiley-Scrivener Publishing LLC. These works highlight his expertise in cutting-edge technologies and their applications in modern industry and logistics.A prolific innovator, Dr. Panwar holds 8 granted patents and 11 published patents in the domains of blockchain, AI, and IoT applications. His academic contributions include mentoring graduate students, spearheading interdisciplinary research, and engaging in global collaborations, such as his visiting professorship at South Kazakhstan Pedagogical University.Dr. Panwar's dedication to advancing technological innovation and his extensive academic achievements make him a leading figure in bridging research and industry.

Vishal Jain is pursuing Postdoc from Kuala Lumpur University of Science & Technology (KLUST) (formerly known as Infrastructure University Kuala Lumpur (IUKL)), Malaysia. He is presently working as a Professor (CSE) at the Department of Computer Science & Engineering, School of Engineering & Technology, Vivekananda Institute of Professional Studies - Technical Campus, New Delhi. Before that, he worked as Professor at Sharda University, Greater Noida and Associate Professor at Bharati Vidyapeeth's Institute of Computer Applications and Management (BVICAM), New Delhi. He has been associated as a member of the Faculty Board, Board of Planning and Management, Executive Council, Academic Council, Curriculum Development and Review Committee and Academic Audit of various higher education Institutions. His research areas include machine learning, information retrieval, semantic web, ontology engineering, data mining, ad hoc networks, sensor networks and network security.

Zamira Atamuratova is working at the Department of Pedagogy and Psychology, Urgench State University, Urgench, Uzbekistan.

Yamini B is an faculty member in the Department of Networking and Communications at SRM Institute of Science and Technology, Kattankulathur. She has expertise in networking technologies, communication systems, and related research domains. Her academic contributions focus on blending technical knowledge with practical applications for students. She is actively involved in research and scholarly activities within the institution. Through her dedication, she continues to motivate and guide students in the field of Networking and Communications.

Hina Bansal is an inspirational teacher and researcher with 16+ years of experience specializing in Bioinformatics/Computational Biology, working as an Assistant Professor in the centre for Bioinformatics and Computational Biology, Amity Institute of Biotechnology, Amity University, Noida since January 2008. Her research interest includes Network pharmacology, functional Genomics and Genome informatics, NGS, functional Proteomics, Molecular docking and simulation, Python, Artificial intelligence, and Machine learning. She has more than forty research publications in reputable peer reviewed journals, book, and book chapters. She has presented numerous papers in various national and international conferences. She has been an active member in organising several workshops and conferences. She is a dynamic reviewer for various peer reviewed journals including BMC Computational Biology and Scientific Reports. She is very proficient in programming languages like C, C++, Java and Python. With her perseverance, academic excellence, research capabilities, and leadership abilities, Dr. Hina a very potential candidate.

Vibha Bora is a Professor from Electronics Engineering, G H Raisoni College of Engineering, Nagpur, Maharashtra, India. She received her PhD in Electronics & Communication Engineering from Visvesvaraya National Institute of Technology, Nagpur, India in 2016. Master of Technology in Electronics from Yeshwantrao Chavan College of Engineering, Nagpur in 2006 and Bachelor of Engineering in Electronic & Communication Engineering from Government College of Engineering, Amravati in 1996. She is Incharge of Biomedical Engineering & Technology incubation Center (BETiC-GHRCE) in association with BETiC-IIT Bombay. Her research of interest includes Image Processing, Pattern Recognition, Machine Learning, Electromagnetic Theory and Electronics Devices. Currently she of chairman of Interdisciplinary Board of Studies. She is member of IEEE, IETE, ISTE.

Sanskruti Chandankar is a student at G H Raisoni College of Engineering, pursuing her studies in the Electronics Department. She recently completed a 6-month internship at BETiC - GHRCE, where she worked on an innovative project titled "Low-Cost Insulin Pump for Diabetes Management." She is eager to contribute to advancements in healthcare technology.

Asomi Chowdhury is currently pursuing a specialization in Biotechnology at Amity University, Noida, India.Their academic and research interests revolve around the integration of biotechnology with machine learning, and artificial intelligence. They are especially intrigued by how these cutting-edge technologies can revolutionize the healthcare industry and contribute to sustainable global development.

Manthan Ghosh is an Assistant Professor in Electronics Engineering at G H Raisoni College of Engineering, Nagpur, India. His research interests lie at the intersection of artificial intelligence, biomedical signal and image processing, and embedded systems. He has worked extensively on the development of intelligent diagnostic frameworks for healthcare, including deep learning-based systems for ocular disease detection, real-time biosignal analysis, and non-invasive health monitoring solutions. His contributions also extend to optical communication systems and smart sensing technologies. Manthan is an active contributor to journals, book chapters, and conferences, and he collaborates on interdisciplinary projects aimed at advancing cost-effective and scalable health technologies.

Lipika Goel is the Professor and Head of the Artificial Intelligence and Machine Learning (AIML) department at Sridevi Women's Engineering College, Hyderabad. With over 14 years of combined experience in both academia and industry, she is recognized for her expertise in the fields of Machine Learning, Software Reliability, and Software Engineering. Dr. Goel holds a Ph.D. and M.Tech from Amity University, Noida, and a B.Tech from Uttar Pradesh Technical University, Uttar Pradesh. Throughout her career, she has made significant contributions to research, publishing numerous articles in reputed journals, and presenting papers at various national and international conferences. In addition to her academic achievements, she has also been involved in government-funded projects, notably under the Technical Education Quality Improvement Programme (TEQIP) scheme, further solidifying her commitment to advancing technology and education in her field.

Dipta Gomes has completed their Higher Secondary Certificate from Notre Dame College, and then started their undergraduate in Computer Science at American International University-Bangladesh (AIUB). Since then, they fell in love with algorithms, programming languages and lastly Artificial Intelligence at all its diversities. Having taken part in various national and international events organized all around the country, one of the achievements they include is 2nd Runner's Up position in National Hackathon 2016 organized by ICT Ministry of Bangladesh. After finishing their undergraduate, they joined their College as a Lecturer of ICT department. Beside their job, they finished a Masters in Computer Science at AIUB once again specializing in Intelligent Systems. During their masters, they have carried out researches on Scheduling Algorithms, Graceful Labeling, Machine learning algorithms for prediction, Image Processing optimizations, Data Mining algorithms, Underwater Image Processing and Natural Language Processing algorithms. After their Masters, they joined American International University-Bangladesh (AIUB) as a Lecturer in Department of Computer Science.

Pradeep Gupta received his B.E. (CSE) in 2006, MTech (CSE) in 2011. He has 15 years of experience in teaching. He is currently employed as an Assistant Professor at Ghaziabad's Ajay Kumar Garg Engineering College. Artificial Intelligence, Machine Learning, Deep Learning, and Cyber Security are some of his research interests.

Noor Mohamed I is an Assistant Professor in the Department of Artificial Intelligence and Data Science at Panimalar Engineering College, Chennai. He specializes in artificial intelligence, data analytics, and emerging computational technologies. His teaching approach emphasizes practical problem-solving combined with strong theoretical foundations. He actively contributes to research initiatives, academic development, and student mentoring. With his expertise and dedication, he continues to inspire students to excel in the fields of AI and Data Science.

J. Balachandar is an Assistant Professor in the Department of Computer Science and Engineering at Chennai Institute of Technology. He is dedicated to teaching and guiding students in core areas of computer science. His academic interests include research, innovation, and fostering technical excellence among learners.

J. Bibija is an Assistant Professor in the Department of Computer Science and Business Systems at S.A. Engineering College. She is actively involved in teaching and mentoring students to build strong technical and analytical skills. Her academic interests focus on modern computing technologies and their applications in business and society.

Jaishree Jain, Associate Professor in Computer Science & Engineering Department, Ajay Kumar Garg Engineering College, Ghaziabad, affiliated to AKTU, Lucknow, Uttar Pradesh, INDIA. She have 14 years teaching experience in CSE & IT Departments that include Chandigarh University, Punjab and college of AKTU, University, Lucknow since July 2010. She had done her B.Tech. in Information Technology from Uttar Pradesh Technical University, Lucknow. She had done her M.Tech. in Software Engineering from MNNIT, Allahabad. She had qualified GATE two times in 2007 & 2008 with 94.86 percentile. She had done her Ph.D. from TMU, Moradabad in 2023. She had Published more than 50 research papers in SCI/SCOPUS/ UGC-Care/ UGC/National and International Journals, Conferences and 5 Book chapters published in International Book. She has received several best paper awards for her research papers at various international conferences.

Sachin Jain is an Associate Professor in the Department of Computer Science and Engineering at Ajay Kumar Garg Engineering College, Ghaziabad. He completed his B.Tech in Computer Science and Engineering in 2007 from UPTU, Lucknow and M.Tech in Computer Science and Engineering in 2010 from GGSIPU, Delhi. He has completed his Ph.D in Computer Science and Engineering from Sharda University Greater Noida in 2025. He is a UGC-NET qualified teacher and has total 15 years of teaching experience. His research interests lie in Artificial Intelligence, Deep Learning and Machine Learning. He has published several research papers in Peer-Reviewed Journals and Conference proceedings. Dr. Jain has filed several patents for his work.

Updesh Kumar Jaiswal is currently working as an Assistant Professor in the Computer Science and Engineering Department at AKGEC, Ghaziabad, UP, India. He received his Bachelor's degree in Information Technology in 2006 and his Master's in Computer Science and Engineering in 2008. He has 17 years of academic and research experience. His research interests include Software Engineering, Artificial Intelligence, Machine Learning, Cyber Security, Wireless Sensor Networks, and Algorithm Design. He has published many research papers in various reputed international Journals and Conferences so far.

Norbek Kholboyev is a faculty member in the Department of Medicine at Termez University of Economics and Service, Termez, Uzbekistan. His academic and professional interests focus on advancing medical education, healthcare practices, and fostering research-driven approaches to improve patient care and community health.

Nivas Kumar is an academic professional associated with Jawahar Engineering College, Chennai. He holds expertise in the field of Mechanical Engineering and is dedicated to nurturing student growth. With a strong passion for teaching, he emphasizes both technical skills and practical applications. He actively contributes to academic development and engages in knowledge-sharing initiatives. Residing in Chennai, he continues to inspire students through his commitment to education and research.

Arun Kumar is an interdisciplinary researcher in Clinical Psychology, currently serving as an Assistant Professor at Amity University, Noida and research Scholar at P P Savani University, Surat Gujarat. His scholarly work includes several peer reviewed publications and presentations at national and international seminars with clinical research.

Saroj Kushwah currently working as an Assistant Professor in the Computer Science and Engineering Department at AKGEC, Ghaziabad, UP, India. She received her Ph.D degree in "Machine Learning" in 2023. She received her Bachelor's degree in Information Technology in 2010-11, and her Master's in Computer Science and Engineering in 2013-14. He has 4.5 years of academic and research experience. Her research interests include Data Science, Big Data Analytics, Artificial Intelligence, Machine Learning, Cyber Security, Wireless Sensor Network, and Algorithm Design. She has attended several International and National conference and workshop as well as published many research papers and book Chapters in various reputed international Journals and Conferences till now.

Anto Gracious L. A. is a faculty member in the Department of Computer Science and Engineering at R.M.K. College of Engineering and Technology, Tiruvallur District, Tamil Nadu. He is committed to imparting quality education and guiding students in their academic and research pursuits. His professional interests include emerging trends in computer science and engineering applications

Sri Ram Macharla, Experienced Technical Manager-Architect with a demonstrated history of working in IT industry. Skilled in Machine Learning, Robotic Process Automation, Apache Spark, Big Data, Data Science, Linux, Python, and Firmware. Strong engineering professional with a Master of Technology - MTech focused in Data Analytics from Birla Institute of Technology & Science, Pilani.

Nishant Kumar Pathak, an Associate Professor at Ajay Kumar Garg Engineering College (AKGEC), Ghaziabad, Uttar Pradesh, is a distinguished educator, researcher, and author who has dedicated over 15 years to shaping the minds of future engineers and technologists. His profound commitment to academic excellence and student mentorship has left an indelible mark on countless learners and colleagues, inspiring them to pursue knowledge with passion and rigor. As a prolific author, Dr. Pathak has penned four acclaimed books that have contributed significantly to the body of knowledge in computer science and programming. His scholarly work includes more than 30 research papers published in prestigious national and international journals, highlighting his deep expertise and active engagement in advancing research. His remarkable contributions have been recognized by the Ministry of Human Resource Development (MHRD), a testament to his dedication to fostering academic growth and innovation. Additionally, Dr. Pathak was honored with an award from the Gyan Uday Foundation for his impactful work in writing motivational books that inspire and uplift readers. Beyond his academic pursuits, Dr. Pathak is passionately involved in social initiatives focused on community upliftment and empowerment. He believes strongly in the transformative power of education and the importance of empathy in creating a more just and compassionate society. His efforts reflect a holistic approach to education—one that integrates knowledge dissemination with societal responsibility. Dr. Nishant Kumar Pathak embodies the ideal of a modern educator—combining scholarly achievement with a heartfelt commitment to social betterment. Through his teaching, writing, research, and community engagement, he continues to inspire generations of students and professionals, championing the idea that education, when paired with empathy and action, is a powerful catalyst for a brighter and more equitable future.

Siva Subramanian R is a faculty member at SRM Institute of Science and Technology, Irungalur Campus, Tamil Nadu. He is actively engaged in teaching and guiding students in the field of computer science and related disciplines. His academic interests include research, innovation, and fostering technical skills among learners.

Ravikumar R. Natarajan is an experienced academician with over 12+ years of teaching and research expertise across institutions in India, the UAE, and the Maldives. He currently serves as an Assistant Professor at Marwadi University, Rajkot, specializing in Machine Learning, Recommender Systems, and AI-driven applications in healthcare and security. He holds a Ph.D. in Machine Learning and Recommender Systems from Amity University, Jaipur, a Master of Engineering in CSE from VMRF University, Salem, and a Bachelor of Engineering in CSE from Anna University. He also has a MiniMBA from the Swiss eLearning Institute. Dr. Ravikumar has authored more than 8+ multiple SCIE/Scopus-indexed journal articles, 25+ IEEE/Springer conference papers, and co-authored a book on Artificial Intelligence. He has also published 9 patents and contributed 10+ book chapters in emerging domains such as Federated Learning, Blockchain, and Digital Twins for IGI Global, Wiley and Springer publisher. He actively mentors students through initiatives like the Research Activities Club (RAC) and Student Research Internship Training (SRIT), promoting innovation and research culture.

Aarthi S is a dedicated Assistant Professor in Computer Science with over six years of teaching experience. She is currently pursuing her Ph.D. at Marwadi University, Gujarat, and holds an M.Phil. and MCA from Bharathiar University, Tamil Nadu. Throughout her academic career, Aarthi has specialized in programming languages such as C++, Java, and C, and contributed to research in recommender systems and AI-related data privacy. She has published journal articles, contributed to book chapters, and actively participated in technical workshops. Known for her student mentorship and engagement in academic events, Aarthi remains committed to fostering innovation and excellence in computer science education.

Anusha S, received her B.E degree in Computer Science Engineering from Coimbatore Institute of Engineering and Information Technology, affiliated to Anna University, Chennai in the year 2009. She completed her M.E degree in Computer Science Engineering from Rajalakshmi Engineering College, affiliated to Anna University, Chennai in the year of 2011. She pursuing her Ph.D in Anna university, Chennai under the department of Electronics and Communication Engineering at Dr.Sivanthi Aditanar College Of Engineering. She is working as an assistant professor in the Information Technology, Easwari Engineering College, Chennai. Her research interests include Image processing, Medical Image Processing, Neural Network, Machine learning, Computer Networks.

S. Sindhuja is an Assistant Professor in the Department of Computer Technology at Kongu Engineering College, Erode. She is dedicated to teaching and guiding students in the field of computer technology, with a focus on fostering innovation, technical skills, and academic excellence.

Tafhimul Haque Sadi is a researcher and professional in the field of Computer Science, specializing in machine learning, artificial intelligence, and data science. He is currently affiliated with the Machine Intelligence Research Lab (AMIR) and has contributed to advancements in intelligent systems and computational methodologies. His work emphasizes innovation and collaboration within academic and industry settings.

Parag Sanghani is an Endeavour Fellow from QUT, Australia and has a global exposure of education systems in Europe, Australia and UK. He has worked with a leading university in UAE as the Head of Academics. He has in the past handled 250 Million USD PPP mode projects in education and infrastructure sector in India. He has trained several executives in different parts of world. For several years he has taught subjects like Innovation & Creativity, Information Systems and Operation Management to students globally. He has published more than twenty research papers and articles in journals of great repute. He has worked with agencies like NAAC, India and QS, Singapore to enhance the quality of Higher education. Currently Dr. Parag Sanghani is ProVost of P P Savani University.

Valisher Sapayev is an Assistant Professor working in the Department of General Professional Sciences, Uzbekistan.

Dip Sarker is currently pursuing a Bachelor's degree in Computer Science and Engineering and has accumulated over a year of experience working in a dynamic startup environment. During this time, they have developed strong skills in algorithm design and optimization, with a focus on large-scale data analysis and high-performance computing. Their practical experience, combined with their academic research, has allowed them to explore cutting-edge solutions for efficient data processing.

Narinderjit Singh Sawaran Singh is an Associate Professor at INTI International University, Malaysia. He graduated from Universiti Teknologi PETRONAS (UTP) in 2016 with Ph.D in Electrical & Electronic Engineering specialized in Probabilistic Methods for Fault Tolerant Computing. Currently, he is appointed as the research cluster head for Computational Mathematics and Technology focuses on the areas like Expert Systems and Artificial Intelligence, Exploratory Data Analysis, Optimization Algorithms, Data Modelling and Computational Intelligence - Swarm Intelligence. He is one of the appointed Editorial Board Members for Journal of Data Science (JoDS) - an international journal indexed by Google Scholar and MyJurnal. He is a very dedicated and committed academician with 20+ years of experience in teaching and more than 10 years of research experience. He is a very resourceful researcher with wide-ranging research interests - Computational, Modeling & Simulation, Mathematical & Statistical Modeling, Fault-tolerant Computing (reliability - VLSI circuit design), Data Modelling & Computational Intelligence and Healthcare Data Analysis are on the top of the list.

Mandeep Singh is an accomplished academician and Assistant Professor in the School of Computer Science, Engineering, and Technology (SCSET) at Bennett University, Greater Noida, India. He holds a Master's degree with Distinction in Information Security from Ambedkar Institute of Advanced Communication Technologies and Research (AIACTR) (now NSUT East Campus). With over nine years of teaching experience, he is currently pursuing a Ph.D. in Computer Science & Engineering from Dr. B.R. Ambedkar National Institute of Technology (NIT) Jalandhar, where he completed his coursework with Distinction (8.00 CGPA). Mr.

Singh's expertise spans Computer Networks, Mobile Ad Hoc Networks (MANETs), Machine Learning, and Deep Learning. His research contributions include book chapters, international journals, and conference proceedings, alongside a notable track record of patent publications. His dedication to excellence has earned him awards and recognition from the Institute of Industrial Development (IID) and MSME, Government of India for contributions to research and entrepreneurship.

Sanket Somkuwar is a student at G H Raisoni College of Engineering, pursuing his studies in the Electronics Department. He recently completed a 6-month internship at BETiC - GHRCE, where he worked on an innovative project titled "Low-Cost Insulin Pump for Diabetes Management." He is eager to contribute to advancements in healthcare technology.

Nancy Soni is a student at Amity University, Noida, India, specializing in Biotechnology. Their academic and research interests lie in the convergence of biotechnology, information technology, machine learning, and artificial intelligence. They are particularly focused on the transformative potential of these emerging technologies in the healthcare sector and their broader impact on sustainable global development. They are dedicated to advancing interdisciplinary research and continuously seek opportunities to explore innovative solutions at the intersection of science and technology.

Thilagam T is an faculty member in the Department of Computer Science and Engineering at Vel Tech Rangarajan Dr. Sagunthala R&D Institute of Science and Technology, Chennai. She specializes in core areas of computer science with a strong interest in emerging research domains. Her teaching emphasizes blending theoretical knowledge with practical applications to enhance learning outcomes. She actively contributes to academic development, research initiatives, and student mentoring. Through her dedication and expertise, she continues to inspire students to pursue excellence in computer science and engineering.

Thilagam T is a faculty member in the Department of Computer Science and Engineering at Vel Tech Rangarajan Dr. Sagunthala R&D Institute of Science and Technology, Avadi, Chennai. She is dedicated to teaching, research, and mentoring students in the field of computer science. Her academic interests include advanced computing technologies and innovative research in engineering education.

Anish T. P. is a faculty member in the Department of Computer Science and Engineering at R.M.K. College of Engineering and Technology, Tiruvallur District, Tamil Nadu. He is dedicated to teaching, research, and mentoring students in the field of computer science. His academic interests include emerging technologies, innovative computing solutions, and advancing engineering education

Aparna Vajpayee is a distinguished academician and researcher at the School of Liberal Arts and Management Studies, PP Savani University. Her research spans spatial cognition, language schematization, educational psychology, and cognitive processes in learning, extending to industrial relations, organizational culture, Buddhist studies, and Artificial Intelligence. Recipient of multiple national and international awards, she has authored over 90 publications and nine patents and published in reputed publishers like Sage, Routledge, Springer, Cambridge Publishing, and Emerald, etc., and has established herself as a leading voice in interdisciplinary cognitive and behavioural research.

Index

A

B

C

D

E

F

G

H

S

W

www.ingramcontent.com/pod-product-compliance
Lightning Source LLC
LaVergne TN
LVHW062337300926
849161LV00007B/1732